Improve International

NURSING ANAESTHESIA

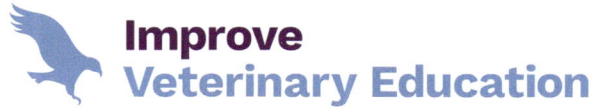

First published 2023

Copyright © Improve International 2023

All rights reserved. No part of this publication may be reproduced, stored in a retrieval system, or transmitted, in anyform or by any means, electronic, mechanical, photocopying, recording or otherwise, without prior permission of the copyright holder.

Published by
Improve International Ltd.
Alexandra House, Whittingham Drive
Wroughton, Swindon,
Wiltshire SN4 0QJ
United Kingdom

Tel: +44 (0) 1 793 759 159
https://improveinternational.com/uk/

Important note
Medicine is an ever-changing science, so the contents of this publication, especially recommendations concerning diagnostic and therapeutic procedures, can only give an account of the knowledge at the time of publication. While utmost care has been taken to ensure that all specifications regarding drug selection and dosage and treatment options are accurate, readers are urged to review the product information sheet and any relevant material supplied by the manufacturer, and, in case of doubt, to consult a specialist. From both an editorial and public interest perspective, the publisher welcomes notification of possible inconsistencies. The ultimate responsibility for any diagnostic or therapeutic application lies with the reader.

A Catalogue record for this book is available from the British Library

ISBN: 978-1-913352-19-6

Copywriter: Dr. Pippa Elliot
Illustrator: Elaine Leggett
Photos by the authors unless otherwise indicated.

Authors

Nicola Grint

BVSc PhD CertVA DVA DiplECVAA MRCVS

Nicki graduated from Bristol Vet School in 2000, and stayed on to undertake an internship and then residency in veterinary anaesthesia. In 2005, she moved to Liverpool Vet School to undertake a three year lectureship post, becoming head of division in 2007. After leaving Liverpool, Nicki locumed at the Animal Health Trust, the Royal Veterinary College, and Ross University School of Veterinary Medicine. She completed her PhD in analgesia at Bristol University and holds the RCVS Certificate and Diploma in Veterinary Anaesthesia, and is also a European Diplomate in Veterinary Anaesthesia and Analgesia. She ran the anaesthesia service at Cave Veterinary Specialists for 8 years and is now an independent anaesthesia consultant.

Emma Love

BVMS CertVA DipECVAA DVA PhD FHEA FRCVS

Emma graduated from the University of Glasgow Veterinary School in July 2000 and completed a residency in veterinary anaesthesia at the University of Bristol. She holds RCVS and European College of Veterinary Anaesthesia and Analgesia Diplomas and is an RCVS Specialist in Veterinary Anaesthesia. Emma completed a PhD in 2009 Advances in the Objective Evaluation of Pain and Analgesic Efficacy in Horses and her clinical and research interests include pain assessment and analgesia in animals. Emma is currently a Senior Teaching Fellow in Veterinary Anaesthesia at the University of Bristol.

Pamela Murison

BVMS PhD DipECVAA DVA PGCert(HE) FHEA MRCVS

Pamela Murison is Professor of Veterinary Anaesthesia at the University of Glasgow. She has over 25 years of experience working in a veterinary school environment teaching veterinary and veterinary nursing students. Her research interests include assessing efficacy of novel analgesics and factors which could have an effect on ventilation during anaesthesia.

Contents

The Anaesthetic Machine and Monitoring Equipment
Emma Love
- Anaesthetic Machines 2
- Preparing for Anaesthesia 10
- Breathing Systems 10
- Ancillary Anaesthetic Equipment 19
- Ventilation 20
- Monitoring Anaesthesia and the Cardiovascular System 22
- What To Do When the Alarm Sounds 30
- References and Further Reading 34
- Self-assessment 35

Preanaesthetic Assessment and Premedication. Intravenous and Inhalant Anaesthetics
Emma Love
- Anaesthetic Risk 38
- Core Pharmacology 41
- Principles of Premedication 43
- Induction of Anaesthesia 47
- Inhalational Anaesthetic Agents 52
- Maintenance of Anaesthesia 56
- References 57
- Self-assessment 58

CPR and Emergencies
Pamela Murison
- Introduction 62
- Accidents and Emergencies 64
- Cardiopulmonary Resuscitation 81
- References 90
- Self-assessment 91

Anaesthesia of Exotics and the Horse
Pamela Murison
- Outline and Principles 96
- Equine Anaesthesia 98
- Steps in Equine Anaesthesia 106
- Small Mammals Anaesthesia 114
- Anaesthesia in Birds 126
- Anaesthesia in Reptiles 131
- References 136
- Self-assessment 137

Fluid Therapy and Critical Care Nutrition
Nicki Grint
- The Principles of Fluid Therapy 144
- Blood Products 150
- Nutrition for the Critical Patient 155
- Suggested Reading 157
- Self-assessment 158

Analgesia
Nicki Grint
- Pain Assessment 162
- Difficulties in Pain Assessment 165
- Physiology of Pain 165
- Analgesic Drugs 167
- Pre-emptive Analgesia 169
- Constant Rate Infusions (CRIs) for Analgesia 173
- Chronic Pain 175
- References 182
- Self-assessment 183

Anaesthetic Considerations for Specific Conditions I
Nicki Grint
- Neuromuscular Blockade 188
- Effects of Neuromuscular Blockade on Muscles ... 190
- Anaesthesia for Thoracic Surgery 194
- Anaesthesia for Head and Neck Surgery 198
- Anaesthesia for Cardiac Patients 202
- Anaesthesia for Neurological Patients 206
- References 209
- Self-assessment 210

Anaesthetic Considerations for Specific Conditions II
Nicki Grint
- Pregnancy and Anaesthesia 214
- Anaesthesia of Paediatric and Neonatal Patients . 217
- Anaesthetising the Geriatric Patient 221
- Anaesthesia for Liver Dysfunction 223
- Renal Dysfunction and Anaesthesia 226
- Anaesthesia for Endocrinopathies 230
- References 237
- Self-assessment 238

The Anaesthetic Machine and Monitoring Equipment

Emma Love

Chapter Summary:

- The anaesthetic machine: components, medical gases.
- Preparing for anaesthesia: required equipment, record keeping.
- Breathing systems.
- Ancillary anaesthetic equipment.
- Ventilation: IPPV.
- Monitoring anaesthesia and the cardiovascular system.

ANAESTHETIC MACHINES

Components of the Modern Anaesthetic Machine

Anaesthetic machines (Figure 1) vary in complexity and appearance. **Modern machines have gas supplies, pressure gauges, pressure regulators (reducing valves), flowmeters, vaporisers, a pressure relief valve, oxygen flush, and a common gas outlet.** Some machines also include oxygen supply failure alarms, nitrous oxide cut out, and other safety mechanisms to prevent delivery of a hypoxic gas mixture. Anaesthetic machines marketed for veterinary practices may not have the safety features that are mandatory on those for human use.

Medical Gas

Types of Medical Gases

Delivering a reliable and adequate source of the correct compressed medical gas to the patient is a vital part of safe anaesthesia (e.g. oxygen, medical air, nitrous oxide).

Medical gases offer health and safety considerations from the veterinary team's perspective. Unfortunately, due to inadequate knowledge, accidents associated with medical gases have caused morbidity and mortality not only of patients but also operating personnel.

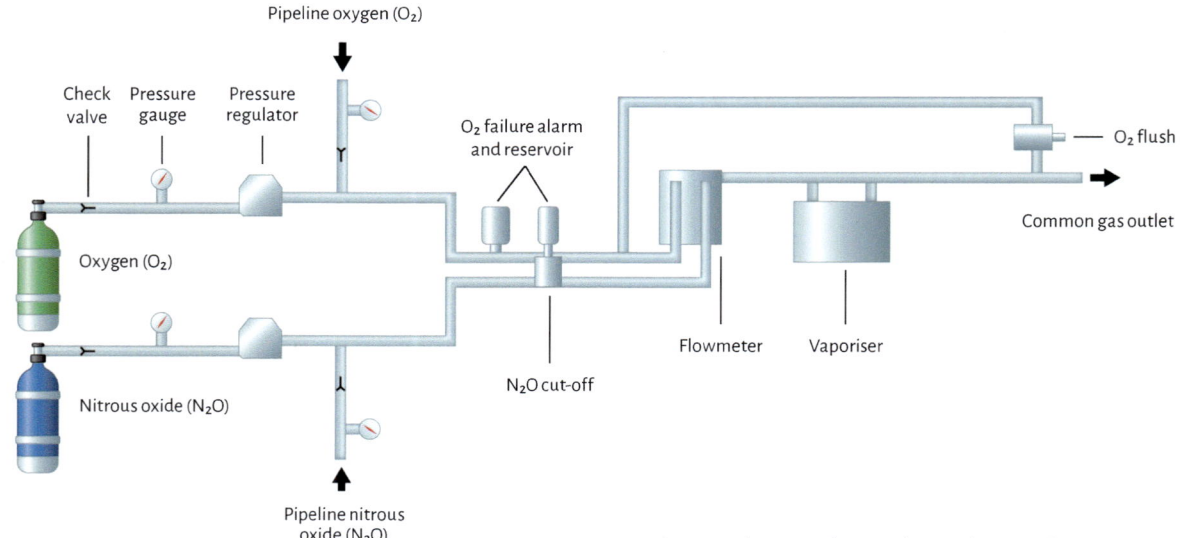

Figure 1. Schematic of a typical anaesthetic machine.

Anaesthetic machines have the capacity to use and administer a variety of medical gases including oxygen, medical air, and nitrous oxide. These gases may **be referred to as carrier gases** reflecting their role in the delivery of the volatile anaesthetic from the vaporiser to the patient.

OXYGEN

The primary gas used in anaesthesia is oxygen. Many factors (e.g. drugs, patient comorbidities) in anaesthesia can cause hypoventilation so it is recommended to supplement inspired oxygen during anaesthesia. Healthy small animals with no airway disease require a **minimum delivery of 33% inspired oxygen** to maintain adequate haemoglobin oxygen saturation during anaesthesia. However, a **higher percentage of inspired oxygen may be required in sick animals.**

Oxygen can be supplied as a compressed gas in cylinders (Table 1), as a liquid in a vacuum insulated evaporator (VIE) or generated by an oxygen concentrator.

Some anaesthetic machines have a medical air supply, in addition to oxygen, so that air oxygen mixtures can be administered. The advantage of air oxygen mixtures is they may **reduce the development of absorption atelectasis** which can develop when high inspired fractions of oxygen are administered during anaesthesia. **Some clinicians prefer to use air oxygen mixtures during anaesthesia for prolonged procedures.** The percentage of oxygen can be varied depending on the animals' individual requirements.

Prolonged administration of high inspired fractions of oxygen (more than 12 hours) can lead to **oxygen toxicity.** The duration of anaesthesia in veterinary practice is usually considerably less than this, so oxygen toxicity is not often a concern in surgical patients. However, the percentages of oxygen used for supplementation in the **intensive care unit (ICU) setting** should be carefully evaluated, particularly if the animal's lungs are ventilated for prolonged periods, and it may be appropriate to use air oxygen mixtures in that context.

Oxygen supports combustion so care is imperative when used near naked flames (e.g. during disbudding of goat kids) or diathermy (e.g. airway surgery).

NITROUS OXIDE

In the past, nitrous oxide was commonly included in anaesthetic machines due to its beneficial analgesic effects and subsequent reduction in inhalational anaesthetic requirements. In recent years this has changed with **nitrous oxide becoming less commonly used** due to growing concern over the environmental impact of nitrous oxide and its role in the destruction of the ozone layer. In addition, there is concern over exposure of nitrous oxide to staff (especially, although not exclusively, pregnant women) and the security aspects of storing a substance that is subject to abuse.

Table 1. The colour coding system used in the UK for cylinders, pipelines, and flowmeters. However, it is important to note that the colour coding of medical gases varies internationally so the definitive way to determine content is to read the labels.

Gas	Colour coding system (UK)
Oxygen	White
Medical air	Black and white
Nitrous oxide	Blue

Methods of Gas Supply

CYLINDERS

Cylinders are the main way that medical gases are stored for use in practice; these can either be attached to the anaesthetic machine or used to supply a larger scale pipeline system.

Cylinders are usually **made of molybdenum steel and stored carefully in a dry, well ventilated, and fireproof area.** They should not be exposed to extremes of heat or moisture, and kept away from oil/grease/flammable materials. Small, portable, lightweight cylinders made from aluminium wrapped in carbon or aramid (e.g. Kevlar®) fibre are also available and may be useful when transporting animals around the hospital.

E-sized cylinders are usually used on anaesthetic machines, and these can be stored horizontally on shelves, whereas bigger cylinders should be stored upright.

Oxygen cylinders made from molybdenum steel are ferromagnetic which has **significant implications in proximity to magnetic resonance imaging (MRI) equipment.** A standard operating procedure for changing oxygen cylinders should be developed and followed by all staff to ensure safe handling in this environment.

Oxygen is stored as a compressed gas at a pressure of 13 700 kPa whereas nitrous oxide is stored as a liquid with its vapour at the top of the cylinder at a pressure of 4 400 kPa. **Cylinder valves seal the contents** at these high pressures and are mounted on top of the cylinder. There is a noninterchangeable safety system (pin index system) on the cylinder valve which fits into the yoke of the anaesthetic machine or pipeline system. The yoke has corresponding pins which interdigitate with the holes in the cylinder valve (pin index system) and this geometric feature means that **only the correct gas cylinder can be fitted into the yoke,** preventing accidental connection of the incorrect cylinder. A compressible sealing washer (Bodok seal) must be placed between the anaesthetic machine yoke and the cylinder's valve outlet.

Cylinders should be turned on slowly (to prevent a rapid release of pressure which can generate heat) and the apparatus checked to ensure that the cylinder/anaesthetic machine seal is gas tight. Lubricant should never be used to open a cylinder and care should be taken not to over tighten when closing cylinders.

A one way valve or **backflow check valve** next to the inlet of the yoke prevents loss of gas from an empty yoke and prevents the transfer of contents between cylinders if there is the capacity to have more than one cylinder fitted to the system.

Cracking cylinders (opening briefly then closing them before connecting them to the yoke) **is no longer recommended.** Instead, it is important to check that the cylinder valve is clean, dry, and free from dust or other debris.

Liquid Oxygen

Storing oxygen in a liquid form is an effective and economical way to store and supply large amounts of oxygen when the requirements are very high (for example, a large veterinary hospital). The **vacuum insulated evaporator (VIE)** stores the liquid oxygen at very low temperatures (-150 to -170 °C) and at high pressures (500–1000 kPa).

The VIE is a fire hazard and therefore the unit should be situated in a site away from hospital buildings. There must be vehicle access so that a tanker has access for refilling. **Filling the VIE is a specialist procedure** as there is the risks of burns, frostbite, and hypothermia from the cryogenic liquid. Gaseous oxygen is transported to the hospital via a pipeline system.

Oxygen Concentrators

Oxygen concentrators come in a variety of sizes and may be used to supply oxygen to a single patient (e.g. ICU setting), supply a single anaesthetic machine, or supply a pipeline system. The former two uses are more likely to be used in veterinary practice.

Concentrators use zeolite (hydrated aluminium silicates of alkaline earth materials) molecular sieves which selectively retain nitrogen and other components of air to **produce a maximum oxygen concentration of 95%.** If using oxygen from an oxygen concentrator with a circle breathing system, **care should be taken when using very low flow techniques** due to the potential for accumulation of argon (not removed by the zeolite sieves). At the higher fresh gas flow rates often used in practice, this is not a concern. However, as the environmental awareness of the impact of anaesthesia becomes more widespread and people begin to adopt low flow anaesthesia, this should be considered when formulating new protocols.

Pipeline Supplies

Piped gas supplies for oxygen, medical air, and nitrous oxide are a convenient way of supplying medical gases to anaesthetic machines in practices where there **are multiple anaesthetic machines and throughput is high.** (Machines still require size E oxygen cylinders as back up.)

The piped gas has a central gas supply (cylinder banks or liquid oxygen), copper pipework, and outlets supplying gas at a pressure of 400 kPa which are identified by colour coding, gas name, and shape. Colour coded hoses run from the anaesthetic machine to the outlet.

These hoses have a Schraeder probe which is gas specific with a unique collar indexing system and a diameter that fits into the pipeline's terminal outlet for that specific gas only. This ensures only the correct hose can be plugged into the outlet (oxygen is white and nitrous oxide is blue). A noninterchangeable screw thread (NIST) attaches the hose to the anaesthetic machine.

Systems which use cylinders as the central gas supply (instead of liquid gas) have a cylinder manifold which should be **located in a separate, fire proof building to the hospital.** There are often two groups of cylinders called primary and secondary banks. The valves of all the cylinders (in both groups) are open and the supply changes automatically between banks when a pressure sensitive device which detects when the cylinders are nearly empty. An alarm (usually located in a busy area of the hospital) sounds to warn staff when one of the banks needs replenishing.

It is important any interruption to the power supply does not impact on oxygen delivery via the pipeline system. There should also be a means of isolating the gas supply to specific parts of the hospital in the event of fire or maintenance work being required.

Gas Delivery to the Patient

Pressure Regulators

A pressure regulator (reducing valve) is used to reduce the high and variable cylinder pressures (with a nominal full pressure of: O_2: 13 700 kPa and N_2O: 4400 kPa) to approximately 400 kPa. Pressure regulators are positioned between the cylinders and the rest of the anaesthetic machine and protect the anaesthetic machine while allowing fine control of gas flow (through the flow meter). In a pipeline system, pressure regulators are also used to ensure the supply to the terminal outlets is 400 kPa.

Flowmeters: Control and Measurement of Gas Flow

A conventional flowmeter has three main components:

- flow control valve
- tapered tube
- bobbin or ball.

The flow control valve **reduces the pressure of the gas** from 400 kPa to just above atmospheric pressure (1–8 kPa). A **flow control knob** controls the entry of gas into the tapered tube.

Conventional flowmeters have a needle valve, valve seat and a tapered and calibrated glass sight tube, which are individually calibrated for each gas and accurate (+/- 2.5%).

Flowmeters in series enable accurate delivery of oxygen in low flow systems. There may be a single flowmeter for each gas or two flow meters in series (the first calibrated 0.1–1 l and the second 1 l+). The gas entering the tapered tube lifts the bobbin or ball in proportion to the flow and it rotates without touching the sides of the glass tube. Readings should be taken from the top of a bobbin or the centre of a ball.

The oxygen flush button bypasses the flow meter and vaporiser, and oxygen is delivered out of the common gas outlet at a flow rate of 30–70 l/min as it comes directly from the oxygen source at 400 kPa. This can cause potentially fatal consequences (e.g. barotrauma, volutrauma) if the breathing system is connected to the anaesthesia machine and the patient.

When a machine is able to administer more than one gas, the **oxygen flow control knob is located to the far left of the bank,** (although in other countries it may be positioned to the far right). This latter configuration makes it technically easier to ensure that oxygen is the last gas added to the mixture; in the event of damage to the nitrous oxide or medical air flowmeter tubes this means that the oxygen does not escape. UK machines are configured so that the oxygen is fed into the mixture down stream of other gases (the last gas added to the fresh gas flow despite the knob being on the left of the machine) and is known as baffling the oxygen tube. In the USA the positions of the oxygen and nitrous oxide flowmeters are reversed to ensure that oxygen is the final gas to be added.

The oxygen flowmeter flow control knob is designed so that it can be located and differentiated from the others in the dark. It protrudes further than other knobs, is larger and has a coarsely fluted profile. The names of the gases are written on the knobs and the back of the tubes are fluorescent, so they glow in the event of a power cut.

There may be an on/off switch on the anaesthesia machine and minimum flow through the flowmeter. This is a safety feature to ensure that adequate oxygen for metabolic purposes is delivered to a patient should the anaesthetist forget to turn the flowmeter dial.

Electronically controlled flowmeters may be found on some anaesthetic machines. These have a pneumatic backup to ensure delivery of oxygen in the event of a power failure.

Prevention of Delivery of a Hypoxic Gas Mixture

There are three measures in the anaesthetic machine designed to **prevent delivery of a hypoxic gas mixture:**
- oxygen fail safe
- oxygen failure alarm
- hypoxic guard.

The oxygen fails safe cuts off delivery of nitrous oxide when the oxygen pressure (and flow) falls. An audible alarm sounds to alert the anaesthetist that the oxygen supply has failed, and some machines also have a visual cue. Some machines incorporate an air intake valve to enable room air to be entrained into the anaesthetic machine in the event of oxygen failure.

Hypoxic guard with interlocked oxygen and nitrous oxide flow controls prevent accidental delivery of a hypoxic gas mixture, as the **ratio of oxygen to nitrous oxide cannot be decreased below 1:4** (25% oxygen). Individual machines differ in how this is achieved; mechanical, pneumatic, and electronic mechanisms exist.

Older anaesthetic machines and machines designed for the veterinary market may not incorporate an oxygen fail safe, oxygen alarm or hypoxic guard. Even if a machine incorporates these features vigilance during anaesthesia to ensure delivery of an appropriate gas mixture is still required, particularly if using low flows.

Delivery of Anaesthetic Gases and Vapours

The Vaporiser

The vaporiser enables a controlled and predictable amount of anaesthetic vapour to be added to the carrier gases (usually oxygen) for administration to the animal. It sits on the back bar of the anaesthetic machine, down steam from the flowmeters.

Some anaesthetic machines have fixed vaporisers which are integral to the machine and cannot easily be removed from the back bar, whereas others can be moved between machines. Machines that can accommodate more than one vaporiser should ideally have an interlock system to prevent more than one vaporiser being turned on simultaneously.

When filling the vaporiser with the volatile agent, **key fill systems** (with grooves and shapes that only fit specific bottles to vaporisers), and systems designed to engage the bottle of the anaesthetic agent (like the Quik-Fil sevoflurane bottle) with the vaporiser help. Advantages include reduced spillage and ensuring the correct agent is used.

Some vaporisers are filled by pouring anaesthetic agent, via a funnel, directly into it; but this increases the potential for spillage, occupational exposure, and the risk of accidental filling with the wrong agent. There is the potential to overfill some types of vaporisers depending on the position of the dial; for example, the Tec 7 vaporiser should be filled with the dial in the off position to prevent this.

More modern vaporisers are classified by their Tec number, with the more recently designed (improved features and safety) vaporisers having a higher number. Currently, the most common Tec vaporisers used in practice are from 3 to 7.

There are two ways for gas to pass through a vaporiser: it can be pushed through under positive pressure from the fresh gas flow into a plenum (pressurised) vaporiser or pulled over the open jar type vaporisers (draw over vaporisers).

The Plenum Vaporiser
Most vaporisers are of **the plenum type with two chambers:**
- a **pressurised vaporising chamber** within which the carrier gas becomes fully saturated with anaesthetic vapour; and
- a **bypass chamber** which does not have any anaesthetic agent in it.

The proportions of the carrier gas entering each chamber are controlled by the dial on the vaporiser.

Factors Affecting Vaporisation
Several factors influence how much volatile agent is vaporised.

Surface Area for Vaporisation
Within the vaporisation chamber there is a system of wicks and baffles to increase the surface area and improve the efficiency of vaporisation (Figure 2).

Temperature
The saturated vapour pressure of the anaesthetic agent varies with temperature. For the liquid volatile anaesthetic agent to change into a vapour within the vaporiser, there must be a constant ambient temperature surrounding it (i.e. not too close to its boiling temperature, and not too cold). Vaporisers employ two mechanisms to ensure that their output is constant, despite fluctuations in temperature:

They are manufactured from copper and brass (which explains their heavyweight) and they act as a heat sink. Depending

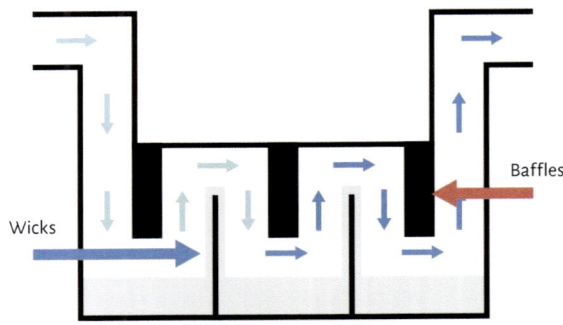

Figure 2. Diagrammatic representation of the interior of a plenum vaporizer showing wicks and baffles.

on temperature, a bimetallic strip and valve alter the proportion of gas entering the vaporisation chamber. This is referred to as the temperature compensation mechanism – TEC and explains the trade names of some vaporisers (e.g. Fluotec®).

Fresh Gas Flow
Changes in carrier gas flows may influence the vaporiser output by either altering the proportion of the total gas flow that passes through the vaporisation chamber or the efficiency of vaporisation (the gas flow is moving too quickly to contact vapour molecules to pick it up).

Although it is not a big concern with modern vaporisers when used at usual flows, it is worth consulting the vaporisers manual when using very low flow anaesthesia (e.g. less than 500 ml/min).

Tilting of the Vaporiser
Tilting a vaporiser can lead to the inhalant anaesthetic liquid entering the bypass chamber. This means gas which normally passes through the bypass chamber unchanged could be fully saturated with vapour, resulting in administration of a much higher percentage of the inhalant anaesthetic than intended. In the worst case scenario this could result in administration of almost 33% isoflurane. The amount of tolerance varies depending on the vaporiser brand and series.

Electronically Controlled Vaporisers
Traditionally plenum vaporisers have been used to administer inhalant anaesthetic agents like **isoflurane and sevoflurane.** Another inhalant agent, desflurane, may also be used in some specialist hospitals. However, since desflurane has a boiling point close to room temperature, administration of reliable and safe concentrations using conventional vaporisers is not possible. An electronically controlled, heated vaporiser is required.

Recently, electronically controlled anaesthetic machines with lightweight vaporiser cassettes have become available. These vaporisers look completely different to conventional ones, with the advantages of requiring virtually no servicing, can be tilted, and are very accurate. An example is the Aladin® cassette vaporiser for use with the GE Healthcare Anaesthesia Delivery Unit.

Nonreturn Pressure Relief Safety Valve

Downstream from the vaporiser, there is a **spring loaded nonreturn valve** which prevents damage to vaporisers and flow meters in the event of back pressure through the system, e.g. if the common gas outlet is occluded. There is also a pressure relief valve which opens when pressure in the back bar reaches 30–40 kPa. It is worth noting that **this is a safety mechanism for the anaesthetic machine only.** Pressures of this magnitude have the potential to cause considerable damage to the animal's lungs and cardiovascular compromise.

Common Gas Outlet

The anaesthesia machine only has one common gas outlet from which all anaesthesia gases are delivered to the patient; it connects the anaesthesia machine to the breathing system. The common gas outlet on the anaesthetic machine is a standard size; a 22 mm male and 15 mm female connection, allowing all sizes of breathing systems to be attached. An oxygen analyser can be placed between the common gas outlet and the breathing system to enable the anaesthetist to check the percentage of oxygen administered.

Oxygen Flush

The emergency oxygen flush supplies oxygen at a high flow (35–75 l/min) directly from the oxygen source (usually 400 kPa). It bypasses the flowmeter and the vaporiser.

As the source of the oxygen is upstream from the flowmeters, the high flow and high pressures have the potential to cause barotrauma to the animal's lungs if the flush button is pushed when the patient is attached to the breathing system. Therefore, it's use should be restricted to:
– testing breathing systems
– emergencies only.

When oxygen needs to be flushed through the breathing system quickly, the breathing system must be disconnected from the endotracheal tube and occluded at the patient end to prevent contamination of the environment with waste anaesthetic gases.

The emergency oxygen flush should not be used routinely during anaesthesia.

At the end of anaesthesia, before disconnecting the animal from the breathing system, flushing the system with oxygen should be done by increasing the fresh gas flow and manually emptying the reservoir bag of the breathing system into the scavenge, rather than by using the oxygen flush button.

Breathing Systems

The breathing system provides the connection from the common gas outlet of the anaesthetic machine to the animal to facilitate delivery of gases and anaesthetic vapours, and removal of waste gases, which are vented through the adjustable pressure limiting (APL) to the scavenging system.

Scavenging Systems

Excess and waste anaesthetic gases and vapour from the patient are usually vented from the breathing system through the **adjustable pressure limiting (APL) valve** (colloquially known as the pop off valve), and into the scavenging system.

It is important these gases are removed from the operating theatre environment **for health and safety reasons.** This is covered by regulations including the Control of Substances Hazardous to Human Health (COSHH). Excessive exposure to waste anaesthetic gases may have negative effects on many body systems including the reproductive, hepatic, and renal systems, it increases the risk of haematological cancers and decrease the mental performance of theatre staff.

In the UK, the maximum accepted standards for anaesthetic waste gas exposure over an eight hour time weighted average are:
– halothane 10 parts per million (ppm)
– isoflurane 50 ppm
– sevoflurane 60 ppm
– nitrous oxide 100 ppm.

Isoflurane and sevoflurane gas monitoring badges help measure the individual exposure level of staff. These badges are worn for one day near the collar of a top (e.g. scrub top) and then analysed and a report is provided by the monitoring company.

Scavenging tubing is a different colour to the other tubes in the breathing system (e.g. pink, green, or blue). The tubing is connected to the APL valve by a 30 mm male connector with 22 mm tubing.

There are two classifications for scavenging systems:
- passive scavenging which relies on the flow of gases
- active scavenging where suction removes the gases.

Passive Scavenging Systems

The most common form of passive scavenging is a **canister** which contains charcoal particles (e.g. F-air® canister and Cardiff Aldasorber®). The scavenge tubing from the breathing system connects directly to the top of the canister.

The **charcoal absorbs volatile agents only,** not nitrous oxide or expired carbon dioxide (CO_2). The canister should be placed on a flat surface to allow the expired CO_2 to flow from the bottom vents and should be placed below the level of the patient (or APL valve) and away from heat sources (as heat can cause the vapours to be released).

There is no indicator to tell the anaesthetist that the canister is full and no longer has any more absorption capacity. Therefore, **the canister should be weighed before every anaesthetic** to ensure it has not exceeded the absorption capacity, which is usually detailed on the canister, but is typically 1400 g.

Active Scavenging Systems

Active scavenging has a similar basic design to the passive version described above but **incorporates a fan or pump to draw the patient's expiratory breath from the breathing system.** It is important to incorporate features that prevent both negative pressure (i.e. suction) being applied to the animal's airway and also the build-up of pressure in the system in the event of inadequate suction or failure.

An air break is a device that draws in room air from below where the scavenge is attached; the top part of the air break has a valve which can be tightened or loosened to change suction pressure.

Active scavenging systems have **an on/off switch** which must be turned on to ensure the system works correctly. It is usually labelled AGS (anaesthetic gas scavenge system/disposal system).

Minimizing Risk

An anaesthetic safety checklist should be completed for every patient in between procedures. Checklists reduce the opportunity for human error and encourage a systematic approach to preparation for anaesthesia and surgery; checking the anaesthetic machine is an important component of this process and should be documented.

The Association of Veterinary Anaesthetists (AVA) has developed an anaesthesia safety checklist which incorporates all aspects of the anaesthesia process but also has a specific section on checking the anaesthesia machine.

Checking the Anaesthetic Machine: Oxygen Delivery Only

The anaesthetic machine and all equipment should be checked prior to use, including in between patients. The following checklist is a modified version of the Association of Anaesthetists of Great Britain and Ireland (AAGBI) document which has gained widespread acceptance in hospitals.
- The scavenging system should be turned on (if active scavenging system is used) or charcoal canisters should be weighed (if passive scavenging system is used):
    - correct scavenging tubing configuration should be confirmed, ensuring it is plugged into correct outlets;
    - the machine should be visually checked looking for signs of damage.
- The oxygen cylinders should be turned on or the oxygen pipeline hose from the anaesthesia machine should be inserted into the correct pipeline outlet, tugging to ensure it is correctly inserted and secure:
    - cylinder pressures should be confirmed as adequate (and therefore have enough oxygen for the planned procedure) and cylinders should be changed if required;
    - the pipeline pressure gauge should be checked (should be 400 kPa) if piped from a larger oxygen supply.
- A fresh gas flow of oxygen should be set (e.g. 2–4 l/min).
- The oxygen cylinder should be turned off or the oxygen unplugged from the wall outlet, leaving the flowmeter knob on at 2–4 l/min:
    - the oxygen flowmeter bobbin should fall to zero and an alarm should sound;
    - the oxygen supply and the oxygen failure alarm system has now been checked.
- The oxygen source should be turned back on or reconnected.
- The oxygen flush button function should be confirmed.
- A fresh gas flow of oxygen should be set (e.g. 2–4 l/min):
    - the common gas outlet should be occluded completely (with thumb). The oxygen flowmeter bobbin should fall slightly indicating a build-up of pressure and therefore no leaks in the pipework within the anaesthesia machine or backbar. This safety feature (fall in flow) in the machine ensures no damage is caused to the pipeline or vaporisers due to the high pressure;
    - leaks around the vaporiser should be listened for. The nonreturn pressure relief safety valve may open (a hissing sound should be listened for and

gas flow around the valve on back bar can be felt for). This usually opens at pressures of 30 kPa. The oxygen delivery system within the anaesthesia machine or back bar has now been checked.
- Oxygen flow should be turned off.
- The vaporiser should be visually checked for any signs of damage:
    - the vaporiser should be turned on and off (without oxygen flow), ensuring the dial turns smoothly.
- The desired breathing system and ancillary equipment should be checked.

Checking the Anaesthetic Machine: Oxygen and Nitrous Oxide Delivery

- **The previous oxygen safety checks should be completed** ensuring the oxygen source is connected and turned on. Charcoal passive scavenging systems must not be used when nitrous oxide is being delivered to the patient.
- The nitrous oxide cylinder should be turned on or the oxygen pipeline hose from the anaesthetic machine should be inserted into the correct pipeline outlet, tugging to ensure that it is correctly inserted and secure:
    - cylinder pressure should be confirmed as adequate and the cylinder changed if required;
    - it is important to note the pressure gauge on the nitrous oxide cylinder does not measure its contents. It measures the saturated vapor pressure of nitrous oxide in equilibrium with its liquid phase. This means the pressure remains constant until all the liquid has evaporated (at a pressure of 4 400 kPa).
- **A breathing system should be connected** to the common gas outlet and the patient end of the breathing system occluded so all waste gas goes out via the scavenging system. Fresh gas flows of oxygen and nitrous oxide should be set to 4 l/min.
- The oxygen cylinder should be turned off or the oxygen unplugged from the wall outlet, leaving both the flowmeter knobs on 2–4 l/min. The oxygen flowmeter bobbin should fall to zero and an alarm should sound while the nitrous oxide should simultaneously "cut out" and delivery should cease. This safety check ensures that nitrous oxide is not the only gas delivered to the patient if oxygen delivery were to fail.
- Nitrous oxide flow should be turned off via the flowmeter knob. The oxygen source should be turned back on or reconnected:
    - with the closed breathing system still connected to the common gas outlet and the patient end occluded, fresh gas flows of oxygen and nitrous oxide should be set to 4 l/min. Oxygen flow should be decreased, and it should be ensured that the flow of nitrous oxide also decreases. The nitrous oxide flow should be increased, and it should be ensured that

the oxygen flow also increases. The **hypoxic guard** within the flowmeter unit has now been checked.

Minimising Exposure to Anaesthetic Gases

Working Practices

Effective scavenging of waste anaesthetic gases is very important for minimising occupational exposure to anaesthetic gases. Checking the scavenging system works and is intact is an important part of the preanaesthetic machine check. However, scavenging is only part of a series of measures that should be taken in veterinary practice to minimise exposure to anaesthetic gases. As mentioned previously, it is vital the working environment is safe at all times and for all people, as excessive exposure to waste anaesthetic gases may cause significant problems for human health.

Isoflurane and sevoflurane gas **monitoring badges** are used to measure the individual exposure level of staff. These badges are worn for one day near the collar of a shirt and are then analysed and a report is provided by the monitoring company.

Other measures taken to minimise exposure to anaesthesia gases (in addition to machine checks and a functioning scavenging system) include:
- well ventilated theatres and recovery areas (15–20 air changes per hour). The recovery area is an area where people are exposed to high levels of anaesthetic gases;
- intravenous (IV) induction agents should be used wherever possible, with intramuscular drug administration options considered if IV access is not feasible. This may be challenging in exotic animal anaesthesia, though it should always be considered;
- cuffed endotracheal tubes should be used as appropriate, the animal should be connected to the breathing system, and the cuff of the endotracheal tube inflated, and leak checked with oxygen before turning inhalant anaesthetic agents are turned on;
- low oxygen flow rates should be used where possible;
- the breathing system should be filled with oxygen before disconnecting the animal (oxygen flow should be increased at the end of the procedure);
- Key-fill or Quik-fil attachments should be used on the volatile agent bottle to attach directly to the vaporiser instead of a funnel;
- vaporisers should be filled at the end of the day when fewer people are working in the area. Swapping vaporisers should be considered if the supply of inhalational agent becomes inadequate during anaesthesia rather than refilling them in theatre.

Preparing for Anaesthesia

Required Equipment

In addition to preparing and checking the anaesthetic machine and breathing system prior to use, it is advantageous to prepare other equipment required in advance.

Equipment to Place an IV Catheter

- clean, sharp clippers and blades to clip the fur
- skin preparation (usually chlorhexidine based and alcohol)
- hand sanitiser for the person placing the catheter
- two appropriately sized catheters
- tape to secure the catheter
- swab or cotton wool ball to clean any blood that may escape from the catheter hub
- preflushed T-port connector or extension set
- sterile saline flush to ensure catheter patency
- bandage material.

Equipment for Tracheal Intubation

- laryngoscope
- gauze swab to hold the tongue
- endotracheal tubes of suitable sizes (or other airway management device such as a supraglottic airway) and a tie to secure in place
- bougie if difficult intubation is anticipated
- cuff inflation syringe
- cuff pressure manometer
- suction if regurgitation or vomiting during induction of anaesthesia is a risk.

Other Equipment

- monitoring equipment should be prepared in advance
- a mask to supplement inspired oxygen before induction.

Record Keeping

An anaesthetic record should be completed for every animal that undergoes an anaesthesia. It helps identify immediate patient trends and provides data for future anaesthetics for that patient.

It is helpful to start the anaesthesia record during the preparation phase of anaesthesia. This is to capture all relevant information (the findings of any diagnostic testing, considerations of any patient comorbidities) and helps prompt thoughts to form an individual and tailored anaesthesia plan.

Relevant data includes:
- date
- surgeon and anaesthetist
- patient signalment and relevant history
- procedure performed
- drugs administered (dose, route, time) and their effects
- timing of critical events (e.g. start/end of surgery, checklists, extubation, and head lift).

The patient's physiological variables should be recorded every five minutes, of which a minimum heart rate and respiratory rate should be included. Other monitoring parameters include:
- eye position
- palpebral reflex
- pedal reflex
- jaw tone
- oxygen saturation (SpO_2)
- end tidal carbon dioxide ($ETCO_2$)
- blood pressure
- temperature
- ventilation information if measurable: tidal volume, inspiratory pressure.

Alongside patient parameters, **the oxygen and gas flow (l/min) and vaporiser setting (%) should also be recorded.** Recording IV fluid therapy rates and blood loss volumes (where appropriate) is also recommended.

Some monitors can produce electronic versions of anaesthetic records to print or download to the patient's file. Developing a database of easily searchable anaesthetic records facilitates clinical audit. Anaesthetic records, recommended by the RCVS Practice Standards Scheme, are available on the Association of Veterinary Anaesthetists website.

Breathing Systems

Key Terms in Respiratory Physiology

An understanding of respiratory physiology and its terminology is important during anaesthesia.

Dead Space

The volume of gas not involved in gas exchange. Gas exchange from the respiratory system into the vascular system only occurs within the alveoli.

Tidal Volume

The volume of gas entering the lungs with each inspiration. There are many ranges for the tidal volumes of dogs and cats in the literature. For the purposes of breathing system calculations (which are estimations) 10 ml/kg is adequate.

Minute Volume

The volume of gas entering the lungs in one minute. This is equivalent to the tidal volume multiplied by respiratory rate. If the respiratory rate is unknown or the animal is panting 200 ml/kg/minute can be used to estimate minute volume for breathing system calculations.

Metabolic Oxygen Requirements

The amount of oxygen required each minute for metabolic processes. For the purposes of breathing system estimations, 10 ml/kg/minute is adequate for small animals and 5 ml/kg/minute for large animals. Please note that these are likely to be overestimates in most cases.

Rebreathing

"Rebreathing occurs when the inspired gases reaching the alveoli contain more carbon dioxide than can be accounted for by mere reinhalation from the patient's dead space gas (should be negligible)" (West, 2012).

Breathing Systems

Function of Breathing Systems

An anaesthetic breathing system is used to connect the anaesthetic machine to the patient, either with a mask or connected to an endotracheal tube. The breathing system is used to deliver oxygen (+/- nitrous oxide) and volatile anaesthetic (if an inhalational technique is being used) to the animal, and to ensure exhaled carbon dioxide and volatile anaesthetic are removed safely.

Removing exhaled carbon dioxide from the expiratory breath is important to prevent hypercapnia, or a build-up of carbon dioxide in the blood. Hypercapnia causes respiratory acidosis, as well as sympathetic stimulation leading to tachycardia, increased blood pressure, sweating, tachypnoea, and cardiac arrhythmias. These signs can look similar to a light plane of anaesthesia. The mucous membranes may also turn a brick red colour.

The incorrect use of a breathing system or faulty equipment can lead to anaesthetic complications and contribute to morbidity and mortality associated with anaesthesia. Therefore, it is essential to check the breathing system thoroughly before each use.

Factors Influencing the Choice of Breathing System

Breathing systems are classified as non-rebreathing or rebreathing based on the method of removal of expired carbon dioxide.

The choice of breathing system is influenced by factors including:
- resistance
- mechanical dead space
- equipment drag: how heavy the breathing system is and the pull on the endotracheal tube
- type of ventilation: spontaneous or intermittent positive pressure ventilation (IPPV)
- fresh gas and inhalational anaesthetic requirements
- valve position and scavenging.

Soda Lime

Soda lime is a component of rebreathing systems such as the circle system. **Its function is to absorb exhaled carbon dioxide via a chemical reaction.** The reaction is exothermic, so it produces heat and water, which can be helpful in maintaining the animal's body temperature (though care should be taken on hot days) and humidifies inspired gases.

$$H_2O + CO_2 \rightarrow H_2CO_2$$

$$2H_2CO_3 + 2NaOH + Ca(OH)_2 \rightarrow CaCO_3 + Na_2CO_3 + 4H_2O$$

Soda lime contains calcium hydroxide, sodium hydroxide, water and an indicator dye. **The granules change colour (indicator dye) when exhausted,** which lets the anaesthetist know that the soda lime should be changed as it can no longer absorb any more carbon dioxide.

Modern inhalant anaesthetics produce carbon monoxide when in contact with desiccated soda lime, so it is important to change the soda lime regularly even if the breathing system is used infrequently and the soda lime dye colour has not changed.

The frequency of this change is indicated in the manufacturers recommendations and varies between brands, but the soda lime should be changed when rebreathing is seen on the capnograph, or **when 50% of the granules have changed colour.**

Soda lime is caustic. Appropriate PPE including gloves and a face mask should be worn when changing the soda lime and care should be taken to prevent inhalation of dust (by staff or patients).

There are also carbon dioxide absorbents without sodium, potassium, or barium hydroxides that have been produced more recently (e.g. Amsorb Plus®). These have the advantage of not generating carbon monoxide, compound A, or formaldehyde. The colour change is preserved.

Components of Breathing Systems

Reservoir Bag

The reservoir bag is made of antistatic rubber and plastic. **Observing movement of the reservoir bag** during anaesthesia is useful to monitor ventilatory pattern, detect disconnection from the breathing system, and detect overinflation of the bag (e.g. adjustable pressure limiting valve closed, twisted bag on T-piece with Jackson-Rees modification). The volumes of bags available commercially range from 0.5 to 6 l.

A guide for selection of an **appropriately sized bag, is that it should be three to six times the animal's tidal volume,** based on an approximation of 10 ml/kg for tidal volume. For a 20 kg dog tidal volume would be 200 ml, so the bag required would be at least 600 ml. Since bags come in a limited range of sizes, the most appropriate reservoir bag for this patient would be 1 to 2 l bag (2 l most likely used in practice).

Adjustable Pressure Limiting (APL) Valve

Adjustable pressure limiting (APL) valves are one way, adjustable, spring loaded valves, which **allow exhaled gases and excess fresh gas flow to leave the breathing system,** but do not allow room air to enter the breathing system. These are often connected to the scavenging system. **The APL valve should be left open during spontaneous ventilation,** and between breaths during intermittent positive pressure ventilation (IPPV). When the APL valve is closed, gas cannot pass into the scavenging tubing and pressure builds up within the system.

The APL valve can be adjusted (or "closed") up to a certain pressure before it pops open as a safety feature to prevent barotrauma or volutrauma to the patient if accidently left closed.

Breathing System Tubing
The radius and length of breathing system tubing impacts the resistance to breathing, and therefore influences the selection of tubing. Poiseuille's law describes the relationship between the resistance of the tubing and the diameter and length of the tubing during laminar flow.

This equation **shows the resistance to airflow is inversely proportional to the radius of the tubing,** so halving the radius of the tubing increases the resistance 16 fold. Doubling the length of the tubing has a less profound effect and doubles the resistance.

$$R = 8\eta l / \pi r^4$$

- where R is resistance
- η is the viscosity of the substance
- l and r are the length and radius of the tubing

Coaxial Configuration
In these breathing systems, **one tube runs within the other.** In the Bain system, the inner tube is the inspiratory limb, which has the theoretical advantage of expired air warming inspired air. However, in practice, movement of gases is so quick there is insufficient time for heat transfer. There is a risk of disconnection, fracture, or kinking of the inner tube.

Parallel Configuration
The two tubes run parallel to one another. No warming of inspired air occurs but damage to the tubes is more easily detected compared to a coaxial configuration. Parallel systems may exert more equipment drag than coaxial ones.

Types of Breathing Systems

Non-rebreathing Systems

Carbon Dioxide Removal
It is important carbon dioxide is removed during ventilation to **prevent the adverse effects of hypercapnia.** Hypercapnia may cause respiratory acidosis, tachycardia, increased blood pressure, tachypnoea, and cardiac arrhythmias.

Non-rebreathing systems remove expired carbon dioxide (and other gases and vapours) from the breathing system by the use of relatively high fresh gas flows (flushing the carbon dioxide into the scavenging system). This means each inhalation consists of fresh gas from the anaesthetic machine, plus or minus a small amount of expired dead space gas (in which the concentration of carbon dioxide should be negligible).

Advantages and Disadvantages
Advantages
- Rapid changes in the depth of anaesthesia can be achieved as the inspired vapour concentration is similar to settings on the vaporiser on the anaesthetic machine.
- It enables the of use nitrous oxide, a useful analgesic, though its use is declining due to environmental impact (depletion of the ozone layer).
- It is relatively cheap to purchase and maintain with no soda lime to change, and the circuits can be discarded after use in an animal with infectious respiratory disease or if contaminated with body fluids.
- It has a lower resistance, which is useful for smaller animals.

Disadvantages
- It has high fresh gas flows and volatile agent requirements, which contributes to environmental pollution and has cost implications.
- Heat and moisture loss and the cold dry gases may contribute to hypothermia and impair the function of the mucociliary escalator in the respiratory tract.
- Not all breathing systems can be used for prolonged ventilation.
- Flow rates may become impractically high for larger animals.

Calculating Fresh Gas Flow Rates
Fresh gas flow (FGF) requirements are calculated using the animal's weight, minute volume and the circuit factor for the breathing system.

> Minute volume = tidal volume × respiratory rate

A value of 10 ml/kg estimates the tidal volume in dogs and cats, for the purposes of breathing system calculations the respiratory rate can be counted (however this is not accurate if animal panting). Various figures for tidal and minute volumes for different sized dogs and cats appear in textbooks; oxygen fresh gas flow calculations typically overestimate volumes to be on the safe side. A reasonable approximation for minute volume in dogs and cats is 200 ml/kg/min. which is preferred in calculations to tidal volume x respiratory rate.

> For example, for a 15 kg dog:
> Minute volume = 200 ml/kg/minute
> = 200 × 15/minute = 3 l/minute

To calculate the fresh gas glow (FGF), the patient's minute volume should be multiplied by the circuit factor to ensure the breathing system supplies the patient with fresh gas and a high enough flow to remove carbon dioxide. This calculation guides the anaesthetist as to the flow rate of oxygen (or other gases) that should be delivered via the flowmeter.

> Fresh gas flow (ml/min) = minute volume x circuit factor
>
> Circuit factors:
> - Bain and the Ayre T-piece are approximately 2–3.
> - Magill and Lack are approximately 0.8–1.
>
> Note: Only non-rebreathing systems have a circuit factor.

Mixtures of medical air and oxygen may be used during anaesthesia and have the advantages of **reducing absorption atelectasis** and the negative effects that high inspired fractions of oxygen have on the respiratory tract structure and function when administered over prolonged periods (oxygen toxicity).

When using nitrous oxide, this is delivered using a ratio of 1:2 of oxygen:nitrous oxide. To prevent diffusion hypoxia **the nitrous oxide is turned off five minutes before the end of anaesthesia** and the oxygen flow is increased to 3 litres/minute.

Fresh gas flow calculations are estimates of the fresh gas flows required. The calculations are often generous, and it is possible to use lower fresh gas flows than the calculations suggest when **monitoring the capnograph carefully.** The fresh gas flow can be reduced in a stepwise way from the value calculated while carefully monitoring for any evidence of rebreathing of expired carbon dioxide. It is important this is monitored throughout anaesthesia as increases in the animal's minute volume (e.g. in response to a light plane of anaesthesia or nociception) increase fresh gas flow requirement and, if this is not met, lead to rebreathing and potentially hypercapnia.

Without capnography, it is not advisable to reduce fresh gas flows below the estimate. In addition, it is important to be aware that changes in the respiratory pattern, particularly if the duration of the end expiratory pause is reduced, (e.g. by tachypnoea), may increase fresh gas flow requirements.

Reducing fresh gas flows where feasible and in conjunction with capnography enables oxygen and anaesthetic agent conservation and has the advantage of reducing atmospheric pollution and cost.

Types of Non-rebreathing Systems
Bain (Mapleson D) (Figure 3)
Features
- weight range: 8+ kg
- IPPV can be used, and also makes the system more efficient so lower fresh gas flows can be used
- circuit factor: two to three

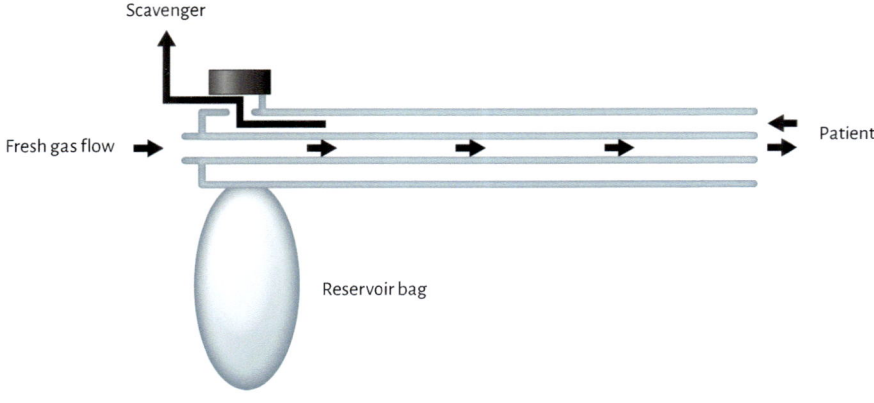

Figure 3. Diagram of a Bain breathing system showing the direction of gas flow.

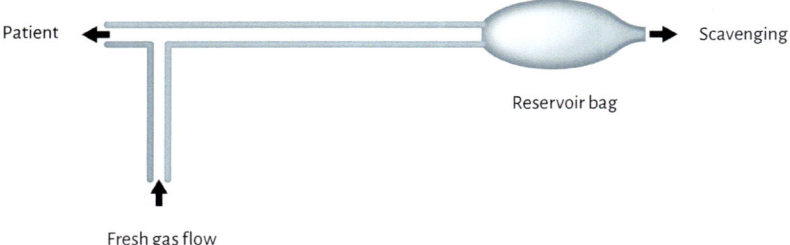

Figure 4. Diagram of a T-piece.

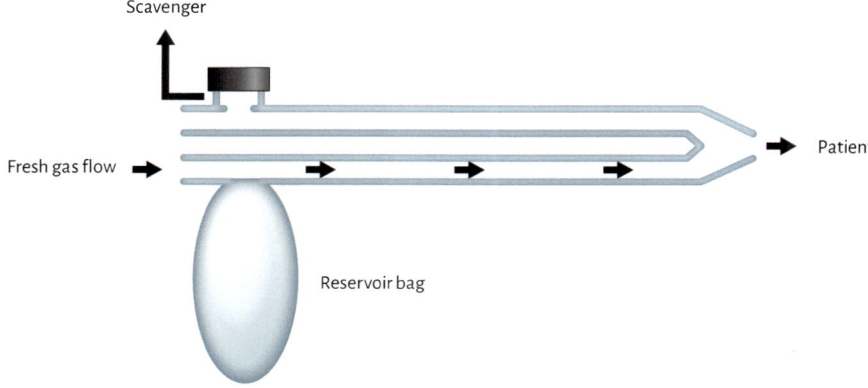

Figure 5. Diagram showing fresh gas flow in a parallel Lack breathing system.

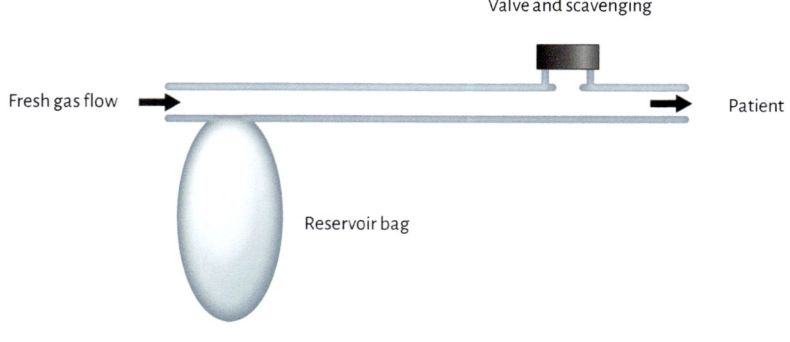

Figure 6. Diagram of a Magill breathing system.

- resistance: moderate
- drag: low
- dead space: low/moderate
- valves and scavenging positioned at anaesthetic machine end
- the reservoir bag is positioned on the **expiratory limb** of the breathing system.

Due to the configuration of the coaxial tubing, it is possible for the **inner tubing to become damaged, altering gas flow within the system.** It is therefore essential that the integrity of the inner tube is confirmed before use. This can be achieved by connecting the system to the anaesthetic machine and setting the oxygen flow to 4 l/min, then transiently occluding the patient end of the inner tube with either the tool provided or a fingertip (the plunger of a 5 ml syringe can also be used though there is the potential that the rubber tip may become dislodged, blocking the breathing system). During occlusion the oxygen flowmeter bobbin should dip and the pressure relief valve hiss. Immediately after the occlusion is released, the bobbin on the oxygen flowmeter jumps briefly to a value above 4 l/min before returning to 4 l/min.

Ayres T-piece with Jackson-Rees modification (Mapleson F) (Figure 4)

The original form of the T-piece consisted of tubing, which was open ended on the expiratory limb (no bag; connected directly to scavenging tubing). Figure 4 shows the Ayres T-piece with Jackson-Rees modification (Mapleson F) where the reservoir bag is open ended and scavenging is connected directly to this. A version with an APL valve is available; the paediatric T-piece with an APL valve (Mapleson D), and the addition of the valve facilitates scavenging and a safe location of the reservoir bag for IPPV.

Features
- weight range: up to 7.5–10 kg
- IPPV can be used
- circuit factor: two to three
- dead space: low
- resistance: low
- drag: low/moderate (two tubes present)
- difficult to scavenge in original format with open ended bag.

LACK (MAPLESON A) (FIGURE 5)
Features
- weight range: 10+ kg
- IPPV: no
- circuit factor: one
- resistance: high if coaxial, lower if parallel
- drag: moderate
- dead space: moderate
- position of valves and scavenging: anaesthetic machine end

- the reservoir bag is positioned on the **inspiratory limb** of the breathing system
- lower flows utilise dead space gases that have not undergone gas exchange.

The Lack should not be used for prolonged IPPV though it is possible to use it for manual ventilation for short periods, e.g. management of postinduction apnoea, or if the fresh gas flow is increased.

A miniature version (Mini Lack) is available and can be used in animals weighing less than 10 kg, including cats.

Magill (Mapleson A) (Figure 6)
Features
- weight range: 5+ kg
- IPPV: no
- circuit factor: one
- resistance: moderate
- drag: high
- dead space: moderate
- position of valves and scavenging: next to patient's head (inconvenient).

The Magill is rarely used in veterinary practice nowadays.

Rebreathing Systems

CARBON DIOXIDE REMOVAL
Expired carbon dioxide is removed from the patient's exhaled breath by an absorber, such as soda lime. The remaining gases and anaesthetic vapour are recirculated in the breathing system, mixed with fresh gas and vapour from the anaesthetic machine, and form a mixture of fresh gas and previously expired gas (minus carbon dioxide) which is reinhaled by the animal.

ADVANTAGES AND DISADVANTAGES
Advantages
- low fresh gas flow and volatile agent consumption: the lower the fresh gas flow the less waste gases and vapours contaminate the environment
- heat and moisture conserved
- easy to change between spontaneous ventilation and IPPV.

Disadvantages
- slower changes in depth of anaesthesia
- nitrous oxide should not be used at low fresh gas flow rates
- higher resistance may be problematic in smaller animals
- may contribute to patient hyperthermia.

CALCULATING FRESH GAS FLOW RATES
Fresh gas flows for rebreathing systems are calculated using an estimate of the animal's metabolic oxygen consumption

(not minute volume). Approximations of 5–10 ml/kg/min are used in the estimations.

Metabolic oxygen consumption is what is used at a cellular level and is what is taken from the alveoli. It is important to remember that the circle system removes carbon dioxide and reuses gases from the patient's dead space, and between breaths.

Vaporiser performance should also be considered as some do not function as expected at very low flows (usually 0.5 l/min minimum).

Features
- high fresh gas flow for the first 15 minutes of anaesthesia, traditionally called denitrogenation, to eliminate nitrogen (air) from the system. Nowadays this is still used to enable adequate concentrations of anaesthetic vapour to be achieved during the uptake phase of anaesthesia
- nitrous oxide cannot be used in closed systems (the FGF = oxygen requirement)
- volatile agent concentration does not equal the vaporiser setting, as it is diluted
- depth of anaesthesia is slow to change.

Low Flow
The valve is open and oxygen, in excess of the animal's metabolic oxygen requirement, is added. This is less economic than a closed system and less heat and moisture is preserved. However, **running a circle with a low flow** (rather than closed), is more realistic and achievable in practice. Accurate flow meters are required.

High fresh gas flows are administered for the first 15 minutes of anaesthesia to achieve adequate concentrations of anaesthetic vapour during the uptake phase of anaesthesia.

> - **Nitrous oxide can only be used if the inspired oxygen concentration is measured at a ratio of 1:1 oxygen:nitrous oxide.**
> - **Volatile agent concentration does not equal the vaporiser setting.**
> - **Depth of anaesthesia is slow to change.**

As oxygen is constantly used by the patient and replaced at a low flow with both oxygen and nitrous oxide, eventually the ratio of nitrous oxide within the breathing system is disrupted (it is not consumed by the patient; it is inhaled and exhaled) and the system is filled with less oxygen.

Initially, a higher flow should be used for the first 10–15 minutes of anaesthesia and then the oxygen turned down to 500–1000 ml/min. Traditionally the use of higher flows at the start of anaesthesia have been used for denitrogenation though more recently air/oxygen mixtures have been used in anaesthesia and the value of denitrogenation is questionable. However, the higher fresh gas flow establishes the inhalant agent concentration more quickly during the uptake phase of anaesthesia. **Higher flows are also used to change the depth of anaesthesia quickly** after changing the vaporiser setting. For example, if the animal is light and the vaporiser setting increased, it is worthwhile simultaneously increasing the oxygen flow.

In most small animals, weighing 50 kg or less an oxygen flow of 500–1000 ml/min is adequate for a circle system.

Types of Rebreathing Systems
Circle Circuit (Figure 7)
The weight ranges for circle circuits is variable and depends on the size of the circle system components.

Traditionally circle circuits designed for adult humans were used and were **suitable for animals above 15–20 kg.** However, there are now some on the market that can be used in smaller animals, even cats when paediatric tubing is used. This has the advantage of significantly decreasing the amount of inhalant agent required and has environmental benefits.

Features
- suitable for prolonged intermittent positive pressure ventilation (IPPV)
- resistance is higher than non-rebreathing systems as there are two unidirectional valves. It is important to be aware that during anaesthesia, heat and moisture accumulates and this can make the valves sticky
- drag: moderate/high
- valve and scavenge position: modern machines, away from patient.

To and Fro (Figure 8)
The to and fro is almost obsolete in veterinary practice but included in this chapter for completeness.

Features
- IPPV is possible but valve position inconvenient
- resistance: moderate
- drag: high
- older versions difficult to scavenge
- risk of chemical bronchiolitis
- mechanical dead space increases over time as soda lime becomes exhausted
- risk of gas channelling over the top of the soda lime (carbon dioxide not removed by passage through soda lime) if the canister is in a horizontal position.

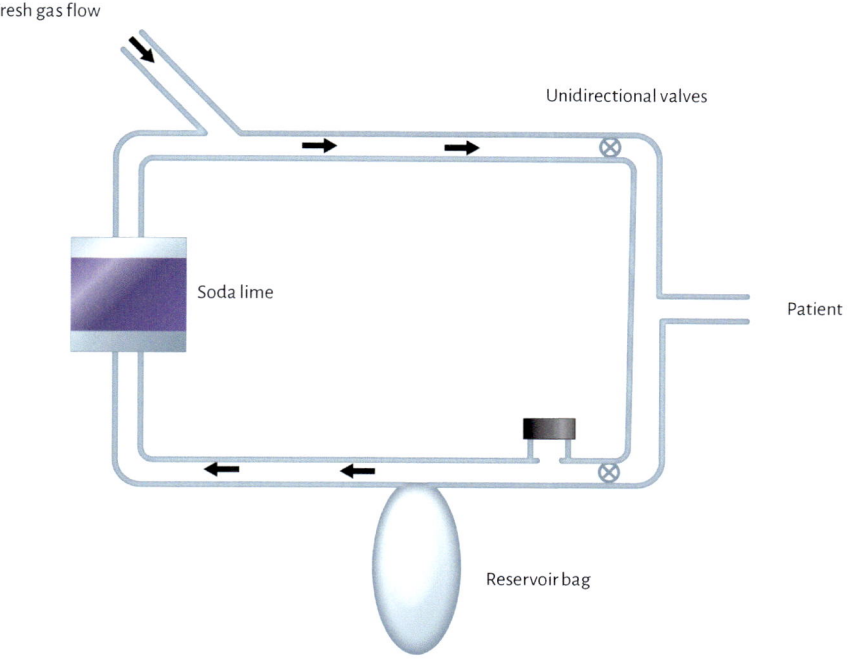

Figure 7. Diagram of a circle breathing system.

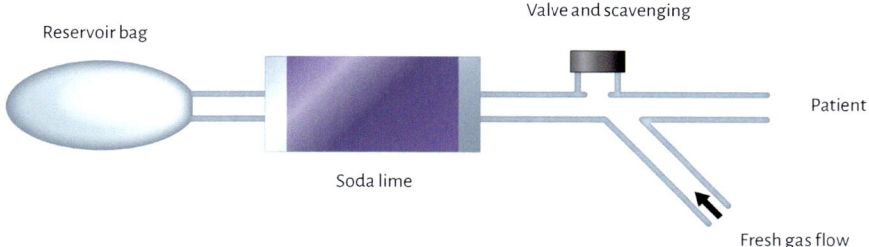

Figure 8. Diagram of a to and fro breathing system.

Hybrid Breathing System
Humphrey ADE Circle

The Humphrey ADE breathing system incorporates Mapleson A, D and E configurations and can be used for a wide range of patient weights. The fresh gas flows required are lower than those needed for the Lack, T-piece or Bain circuits so it is an economical system to run. It is also possible to attach a removable soda lime canister so that it functions as a circle system.

Ventilation Issues

Leaks Within the System

Breathing systems should always be checked before use. An initial visual check should be undertaken before attaching the system to the common gas outlet, looking for splits, cracks, or tubing disconnection. A physical check should then be performed, including the following:
- the APL valve should be closed and the patient connector occluded (e.g. with a thumb) before filling the system with oxygen until either a pressure of 30–40 cmH$_2$O is reached or the bag is turgid (if no pressure gauge);
- the oxygen flow should be turned off and the pressure should be maintained within the system for 10 seconds;
- to release the pressure, the APL valve should be opened before removing the occlusion from the patient connector.

During use, APL valves have been reported to malfunction when gas sampling lines and other tubing became caught within them.

The Circle and Bain systems require additional checks:

CIRCLE
- the unidirectional valves should be visually inspected and then the system partially filled with oxygen by closing the APL valve and occluding the patient connector;
- the reservoir bag should be squeezed a couple of times while watching that the unidirectional valves open and close;
- the APL valve should be left open after this check.

BAIN
The integrity of the inspiratory inner tube of the Bain system should be checked using the procedure described in the section describing this breathing system (occluding the tube and observing the flowmeter bobbin dipping).

APL Left Closed

One of the most common anaesthetic related accidents is leaving the APL valve closed. This results in **pressure building up in the system** and in the patient, causing barotrauma and volutrauma.

Signs the APL valve is closed include:
- distended reservoir bag as pressure increases
- reduced thoracic movements and low end tidal CO_2 as the animal's ability to ventilate is compromised
- leaking round endotracheal (ET) tube if uncuffed tubes are used or the cuff has not yet been inflated
- tachycardia if cardiac output is affected and a drop in oxygen saturation (SpO_2).

At this point, in a previously healthy animal, opening the APL valve is likely to resolve the situation. In an animal with pre-existing disease, it is possible that compromised ventilation will contribute to a significant anaesthetic emergency.

If the closed APL valve is not noticed relatively quickly, the increased pressure within the system can lead to rupture within the respiratory tract leading to pneumothorax or pneumomediastinum. This is potentially fatal unless recognised and treated very quickly.

Preventing Accidents

When checking breathing systems, the pressure within the filled system should always be released by opening the APL valve before removing the occlusion at the patient connector end to ensure that the system is ready for use.

A preinduction checklist that requires the anaesthetist to confirm the breathing system has been checked and the APL valve is open should be implemented.

There are commercially available spring loaded devices that attach to the scavenger side of the APL valve. These enable temporary occlusion of the breathing system to facilitate manual ventilation without the operator having to close the APL valve.

Excessive Resistance within the Breathing System

Features of breathing systems such as tubing diameter and length, valves, and soda lime canisters contribute to resistance to breathing. It is important that anaesthetists are aware of the **signs indicating excessive resistance for an individual animal.**

Signs associated with excessive resistance within the breathing system include:
- altered respiratory rate: low or occasionally fast
- decreased tidal volume
- hypoventilation and hypercapnia: increased end tidal CO_2
- hypoxia
- a light plane of anaesthesia due to reduced alveolar ventilation
- altered respiratory pattern: paradoxical ventilation or increased effort.

The signs of excessive resistance are unpredictable. Therefore, it is important to remember that **weight ranges for breathing systems are only guidelines** and an animal may not be able to cope with the resistance in a system despite being within the correct weight range.

Excessive Apparatus Dead Space

Apparatus dead space is described as **space beyond the patient's anatomical dead space,** and the equipment dead space beyond where fresh and expiratory gases are separated in the breathing system; this may be an integral part of the breathing system (e.g. in the Y connector of the tubing) or an excessively long endotracheal tube protruding from the animal's mouth.

In small animals, increasing the **apparatus dead space to tidal volume ratio** may increase the work of breathing as the minute volume needs to increase to maintain $PaCO_2$ at normal levels (because rebreathing of expired gases is likely to occur). In animals that cannot cope with the increased workload, the $PaCO_2$ will rise.

The volume of dead space in the breathing system should be considered when selecting the breathing system and tubing for an individual animal. It is important to remember that additional connectors (e.g. for airway gas sampling) and heat and moisture exchangers also contribute to dead space.

Endotracheal tubes may need to be shortened. These can be premeasured and cut before anaesthesia, using **the point of the shoulder and incisor arcade as external landmarks** to indicate approximate length.

Cutting the tube after insertion according to the markings on the tube (that should sit just above the larynx) is not commonly recommended due to the potential for trauma to the airway when trying to refit the connector and the inevitable delay in achieving a secure airway (protected from regurgitation) and administering oxygen.

Premeasuring and cutting endotracheal tubes should be done for brachycephalic dogs. These brachy tubes (which are shorter than for other breeds) can be put aside especially for anaesthetising these patients.

Ancillary Anaesthetic Equipment

Endotracheal Tubes

Endotracheal intubation protects the airway and facilitates ventilation. In most cats and dogs, the technique for tracheal intubation is relatively straightforward, although it can be challenging in some species (e.g. rabbits), and not feasible in others (e.g. mice).

Tubes are now mainly **made from PVC or silicone,** though red rubber tubes may occasionally be used in practice. **Armoured tubes** are useful to prevent occlusion of the tube when animals are positioned with their necks flexed (e.g. CSF sampling or certain ophthalmic surgeries); these are reinforced with wire embedded in the wall of the tube.

Correct endotracheal tube placement can be verified by:
- presence of a trace on the capnograph (optimal and recommended method)
- direct visualisation of the tube passing through the larynx
- condensation on the inside of the tube during breathing
- simultaneous movement of the thorax and reservoir bag.

Most tubes have a cuff which, when correctly inflated, protects the patient's airway against potential aspiration and reduces the exposure of staff to inhalant anaesthetic agents.

The use of cuffed tubes in cats is controversial; if used incorrectly they can contribute to anaesthetic related morbidity (e.g. if the tube twists within the trachea when the cat is turned, tracheal rupture is possible). In addition, when red rubber tubes were commonly used, the cuff restricted the diameter of tube; this is less of a concern with modern materials and tube design. On a positive note, a correctly inflated cuff produces an effective seal to reduce waste anaesthetic gas exposure.

The pilot balloon of the cuff may be used to determine only if the cuff is inflated or not and should not be used to assess the adequacy of cuff inflation after intubation.

To inflate the cuff of the endotracheal tube (after verification of correct placement and before the inhalational anaesthetic agent is turned on), the oxygen flow should be turned on and the breathing system connected to the endotracheal tube. An assistant should close the APL valve and squeeze the reservoir bag while, simultaneously, the anaesthetist listens for leaks and carefully inflates the cuff until no gas can be heard escaping.

Manometers may be used to measure cuff pressure (usually 20–30 cmH$_2$O) and guide cuff inflation but should be used in conjunction with the method described above.

Supraglottic Airway Devices

Supraglottic airway devices, including laryngeal mask airways and the veterinary specific V-Gel airways, sit above the larynx and may be **easier to insert** compared to an endotracheal tube, in species such as rabbits.

These have the advantage of reducing trauma to the airway which can be a problem with repeated attempts to intubate. The use of a supraglottic airway device is difficult to justify in dogs in which intubation of the trachea is relatively easy, and they **are most likely to be of value in cats and rabbits.**

They do not fully protect the airway against aspiration, and it can be difficult to achieve an effective seal during IPPV. Capnography helps verify correct positioning of the device.

Laryngoscopes

Laryngoscopes facilitate intubation by **enabling the anaesthetist to clearly visualise the larynx.** This is achieved by using the blade of the laryngoscope to depress the base of the tongue (without depressing the epiglottis).

Although it is possible to perform endotracheal intubation without a laryngoscope, their **routine use is recommended.** This enables the operator to develop the manual dexterity required in animals with difficult airways (e.g. brachycephalic animals), or those with pathology in the laryngeal or pharyngeal region. It also familiarises clinicians with normal upper airway anatomy.

Two main designs of blade are available (straight or curved) in different lengths. Laryngoscopes should always be cleaned and disinfected after use.

Heat and Moisture Exchanger

Heat and moisture exchangers (HMEs) are used to **reduce the incidence of hypothermia during anaesthesia and to minimise drying of the respiratory tract epithelium.**

They are placed between the breathing system and endotracheal tube. When the animal exhales, moisture condenses on the cooler HME surface. This condensed moisture evaporates with the next breath of cold, dry gas. Some HMEs incorporate a bacterial filter and a sampling port that the respiratory gas module (capnography) of a monitor can be connected to.

They do contribute to apparatus dead space and this factor should be considered when deciding whether to use one or not.

Masks and Anaesthetic Chambers

Facemasks are useful to facilitate oxygen supplementation. It is desirable to be able to visualise the animal's mouth and mucous membrane colour, and care should be taken not to obstruct the nares with the mask or rub against the eyes in brachycephalic breeds.

Although facemasks may be used to deliver inhalant anaesthetic agents, they have significant **disadvantages including atmospheric pollution and lack of airway protection.** They should only be used for delivery of inhalant anaesthetics if intubation or the use of a supraglottic airway device is not possible.

Anaesthetic induction chambers may be used for induction of anaesthesia or for oxygen supplementation. The transparent plastic should enable the anaesthetist to watch the animal carefully.

It is worth noting that induction of anaesthesia with an inhalational agent increased the risk of anaesthetic related death in the CEPSAF study. Use of both masks and chambers for this purpose both incur significant environmental pollution and exposure of personnel to anaesthetic gases. Therefore, induction of anaesthesia with an inhalant agent should be **reserved only for those few circumstances where no other anaesthetic technique is feasible.**

Ventilation

Indications for Intermittent Positive Pressure Ventilation (IPPV)

Mechanical ventilators are often used to deliver intermittent positive pressure ventilation (IPPV) to anaesthetised animals.

They are also used in the intensive care unit (ICU) setting, though there are additional considerations for long term ventilation which are beyond the scope of this chapter, which focuses on the short term provision of IPPV in the anaesthetic setting.

Indications for the use of IPPV include:
- **Management of hypoventilation (hypercapnia).** In conscious animals, $PaCO_2$ ranges between 35–45 mmHg, though many anaesthetised animals have a degree of respiratory depression and may hypoventilate. The point at which to initiate IPPV is controversial, and it is important to take into account any preexisting conditions and evaluate the physiological status of the animal when deciding whether or not to initiate ventilation.
- **Inclusion of infusions of opioids** such as fentanyl or alfentanil in the anaesthetic technique. Both opioids can produce significant respiratory depression so IPPV may be required to manage this.
- **Open thorax** surgical procedures that enter the thorax abolish the animal's ability to generate the negative pressure which drives the inflow of gas during inspiration. Therefore, IPPV is required during procedures such as thoracotomy, laparotomy for diaphragmatic rupture repair, and thoracoscopy.
- **Respiratory compromise:** IPPV may be considered in animals with conditions affecting the respiratory system, on an individual case basis.
- **Animal with head injuries** and increased intracranial pressure (ICP) or intraocular pressure (IOP). Careful implementation of mechanical ventilation may be appropriate in some animals with head injuries and those with increased intracranial or intraocular pressure as hypercapnia increases intracranial pressure.
- **Neuromuscular blocking drugs:** if neuromuscular blocking drugs are administered as part of the anaesthetic technique, IPPV is essential as spontaneous ventilation

either ceases completely or is significantly compromised due to paralysis of the respiratory muscles.
- **Compliance** is an important term when considering ventilation. It can be defined as the volume change per unit pressure change and classified into thoracic wall, lung, or total lung compliance. The inspiratory curve is different to the expiratory curve on a graph of lung compliance; this is known as **hysteresis**. Neonatal animals often have good pulmonary compliance whereas compliance can be reduced by conditions such as pulmonary fibrosis ("Westie lung") and pneumothorax.

Physiological Effects of Intermittent Positive Pressure Ventilation (IPPV)

Intermittent positive pressure produces significant physiological effects; during inspiration, IPPV results in a **reverse in interpleural pressures** (inspiration occurs when interpleural pressure is increased) compared to during spontaneous ventilation (inspiration occurs when interpleural pressure is decreased).

Effects on Circulation

It is thought that venous return to the heart is facilitated by the negative interpleural pressures that are generated during inspiration during spontaneous ventilation. During IPPV, the intrathoracic pressure increases, and this reduces venous return and consequently cardiac output (due to compression of the vena cava). These effects are most pronounced if IPPV is performed with long expiratory times, high airway pressures, and the addition of **positive end expiratory pressure (PEEP)**.

The effects of IPPV on reducing cardiac output are relatively well tolerated in healthy, normovolaemic animals, but are **more significant in hypovolaemic animals or those with cardiovascular disease.**

Renal plasma flow is reduced during IPPV and with increased production of antidiuretic hormone (reduces urine production). There may be hepatic venous congestion as a consequence of increased intrathoracic pressure and this, in combination with the decrease in cardiac output and subsequently blood pressure, may result in **reduced arterial blood flow to the liver.**

There is a direct relationship between PaCO$_2$ and cerebral blood flow. IPPV enables anaesthetists to manipulate PaCO$_2$ and this can be beneficial when dealing with animals with raised intracranial pressure (as the PaCO$_2$ increases, cerebral vasodilation occurs, potentially increasing the volume within the rigid cranium). However, care should be taken since inadvertent hypocapnia can reduce cerebral blood flow; **monitoring ETCO$_2$** (and possibly blood gases in selected animals) is important during ventilation.

Volutrauma and Barotrauma

Mechanical ventilation has the potential to result in **iatrogenic lung injury:**
- **barotrauma is caused by high airway pressures** and characterised by air outside the alveoli as a consequence of alveolar rupture (e.g. pneumothorax);
- **volutrauma,** which causes alterations in gaseous exchange, is caused by **repeated stretch and overinflation of the alveoli.**

Inflation of Stomach

Normally, IPPV is performed with the trachea intubated, but this may not be possible in very small animals such as mice. **When IPPV is performed with a facemask, oxygen is forced into the stomach (as well as the trachea)** and the distended viscus can press on the diaphragm, and compromise ventilation.

Types of Ventilators

A wide variety of ventilators are found in veterinary practice; classified according to how gas is delivered to the animal:
- **volume controlled:** time cycled, volume cycled, pressure cycled
- **pressure controlled:** time cycled.

The most common ventilator in small animal practice is **volume controlled and time cycled.**

A volume controlled ventilator delivers a constant flow of gas to the animal, whereas a pressure controlled ventilator delivers a constant pressure of gas. Cycling refers to the process which signals the end of inspiration and the start of expiration.

Volume Controlled and Time Cycled Ventilation

These ventilators deliver a constant flow of gas to the animals' lungs over a defined time. After the time has elapsed, expiration begins. Increasing either the inspiratory flow or the inspiratory time will increase the tidal volume delivered. Any increases in airway resistance or reduction in compliance result in an increased airway pressure.

These ventilators often have a **high pressure alarm** which warns the anaesthetist of increased airway pressure. This warning alarm requires the anaesthetist to take appropriate action as the ventilator continues to deliver gas flow over the predetermined time and it is possible for volutrauma to occur at high pressures.

Volume Controlled and Volume Cycled Ventilation

These ventilators **deliver a constant flow of gas until the predetermined tidal volume** (approximately 10 ml/kg) is delivered. Increases in resistance or decreases in compliance result in an increased airway pressure like those found with volume controlled, time cycled ventilators. Increasing the flow increases the respiratory rate, as the preset tidal volume is achieved more quickly.

Volume Controlled and Pressure Cycled Ventilation

A constant flow of gas is delivered until a preset peak airway pressure (usually 10–15 cmH$_2$O in small animals) is reached at which point inspiration is terminated.

The tidal volume delivered may be variable and depends on the compliance of the lungs and airway resistance.

Pressure Controlled and Time Cycled Ventilation

During inspiration, gas pressure delivery is maintained at a consistent level.

Lung compliance means the flow of gas decreases during inspiration.

Once the set pressure is achieved the gas flow reduces to effectively hold the lungs at the preset pressure, until the set time has elapsed, at which point expiration begins.

These types of ventilators are unusual in veterinary practice.

PEEP and CPAP

PEEP is the application of positive end expiratory pressure during IPPV, whereas CPAP is continuous positive airway pressure during spontaneous ventilation.

Both involve the application of expiratory resistance with the aim of improving functional residual capacity by holding the alveoli open at the end of a breath. However, they can have deleterious effects on cardiovascular function so judicious use is essential.

Monitoring Anaesthesia and the Cardiovascular System

Record Keeping

Nurses play a major role in monitoring anaesthesia in practice, which is vitally important as all anaesthetics carry a risk. The aim of monitoring anaesthesia is to **detect changes in physiological variables and recognise trends before the animal's condition deteriorates** so appropriate corrective action can be taken.

Anaesthetising animals for surgery and diagnostic procedures requires a team approach. Nurses play a key role in co-ordinating the team and communicating with stakeholders while advocating for the animal by their input into planning effective analgesic and other care.

The depth of anaesthesia should be assessed regularly with the aim being for a patient to be in **stage III (light or medium)** depending on how stimulating the procedure is. At this plane the patient has **minimal jaw tone, a ventromedially rotated eye, and a sluggish to absent palpebral reflex.** There should be no laryngeal or pharyngeal reflexes, and an absence of lacrimation. The respiratory pattern should be regular. (See Table 2).

It is important to regularly observe movements of the thoracic wall and reservoir bag and palpate the peripheral pulses.

When palpating the pulse the following factors should be considered:
- what is the rate?
- is the pulse regular?
- does the pulse match the heart rate?
- is the pulse easy to palpate?
- is it easy or difficult to occlude the pulse?

Situational awareness is an important skill to develop. In addition to monitoring the animal the nurse should monitor the anaesthetic machine function, the animal's fluid balance, the stage of surgery, and watch for factors that may impact on the animal or people working within the room.

Anticipating potential problems, planning appropriately, plus effective planning ahead helps smooth the course of anaesthesia and reduce stress.

Table 2. Table showing some features of ventilation, ocular signs, and response to surgical stimulation at the different stages and planes of anaesthesia as described by Guedel.

Stages		Ventilation			Pupil	Eyeball position	Eye reflexes	Lacrimation	Response to surgical stim.
		Intercostal	Diaphragm	Pattern					
Awake				Irregular panting					
Stage II				Irregular breath-holding			Palpebral		
Stage III	Light plane 1			Regular					
	Medium plane 2			Regular shallow					
	Deep plane 3			Jerky				Corneal	
Stage IV						↓			

Monitoring and Checklists

Observation of the animal should start prior to preanaesthetic medication administration.

Continuous, hands on monitoring is appropriate after administration of preanaesthetic medication (e.g. in sick animals or those with brachycephalic airways) and for all other animals must be **continuous throughout the period of anaesthesia until the animal has recovered from anaesthesia.**

Guidelines released in 2020 by the American Animal Hospital Association (AAHA) **recommend that sedated patients are monitored as thoroughly as patients under general anaesthesia.** The AAHA also recommends **diligent monitoring during recovery from anaesthesia.**

The anaesthesia record is a legal document. It helps identify trends, provides a database for future anaesthetics, and a medicolegal record for any investigations that may arise. Some monitors produce electronic versions of anaesthetic records which can be printed or downloaded to the patient's file.

> A complete anaesthetic record should be kept, which includes:
> - **General details:** date, animal details, personnel details, procedure performed, drugs administered (dosage, route, and time), drug effects, timing of critical events (e.g. start/end of surgery, checklists, extubation and head lift).
> - **Physiological variables:** heart and respiratory rates, and temperature recorded as a minimum, and if data from monitors is available this should be added.

Nurses often take the lead with anaesthetic checklists; these play an important role in improving the safety of anaesthesia and are proven to reduce patient morbidity and mortality from human error. Anaesthetic records and checklists can be downloaded from the Association of Veterinary Anaesthetists.

Implementation of clinical audits can help improve standards in practice and there are many opportunities to audit anaesthetic related topics. Good record keeping is essential to facilitate this process.

Monitoring equipment is a useful adjunct to the monitoring of anaesthesia. Knowledge of the equipment is essential to allow interpretation of the information it provides. The use of equipment in healthy cases is useful to build familiarity with use and how to interpret the data prior to use in a high risk patient. Monitoring devices do provide useful additional information and are essential in some cases but are never a substitute for careful hands on monitoring of anaesthesia.

The Association of Veterinary Anaesthetists Guidelines for Safer Anaesthesia (https://ava.eu.com/resources/anaesthesia-guidelines/) state that when monitoring anaesthesia there should be:
- a dedicated anaesthetist monitoring each case
- additional monitoring equipment such as pulse oximetry, capnography, and blood pressure monitor available and utilised.

These emphasise the importance of the hands on nurse's role in addition to the use of equipment.

Patient Support

Thermoregulation

Anaesthesia may interfere with the normal homeostatic processes that regulate body temperature. **Hypothermia is common,** particularly in smaller patients, and is a risk factor in the increase of patient morbidity and mortality. It can have profound effects on drug pharmacokinetics (particularly metabolism), reduce anaesthetic requirements, prolong recovery from anaesthesia, cause bradycardia and arrhythmias, negatively impact wound healing, and increase infection rates.

Hypothermia reduces the MAC of inhalational anaesthetic agents and therefore the percentage provided of inhalational agent should be reduced.

Hyperthermia is less common, but can occur in animals with infections, rare disorders (malignant hyperthermia), or iatrogenically (e.g. low flow anaesthesia using a circle system on a large breed dog with a dense coat or overzealous use of warming aids).

A rectal thermometer is usually adequate to check body temperature before and after anaesthesia. Body temperature should always be checked regularly during anaesthesia; when access for repeated measurements could compromise the sterility of the surgical field, **a thermistor or thermocouple incorporated into an oesophageal probe** is often used. In addition, skin temperature can be measured.

Blood Glucose

It is appropriate to measure blood glucose in animals with certain clinical conditions, such as:
- diabetes mellitus
- sepsis
- hepatic dysfunction
- neonatal animals.

When sampling blood from an intravenous catheter for glucose measurement, it is important to ensure that it has not been used to infuse fluids containing glucose.

Urine Output

Urine output is not routinely measured during anaesthesia, but it **is a useful indicator of renal perfusion.** If a urinary catheter and collection system is in situ as part of patient care (unrelated to anaesthesia) it is sensible to monitor urine output, particularly in sicker animals or those having prolonged procedures.

Urine output should be at least 1–2 ml/kg/hr but may be more for patients on intravenous fluid therapy.

Monitoring the Cardiovascular System

Oesophageal Stethoscope

Heart rate can be measured by auscultation with a standard stethoscope, but this is often inconvenient in the anaesthetised animal. **Instead, an oesophageal stethoscope is useful, inserted to the level of the heart base** (the 5/6th rib or point of the elbow when flexed into the patient's thorax).

Monitoring benefits include:
- heart and respiratory sounds heard without disturbing draping
- gives an indication of the mechanical activity of the heart, though use in conjunction with pulse palpation is recommended.

Electrocardiogram (ECG)

The ECG can give information on the electrical activity of the heart and is **useful to detect arrhythmias** (Figures 9 and 10).

The P wave is generated from the atria, when the electrical impulse moves from the sinoatrial node (SA node, the pacemaker) to the atrioventricular node (AV node). The QRS complex occurs when the electrical impulse moves through

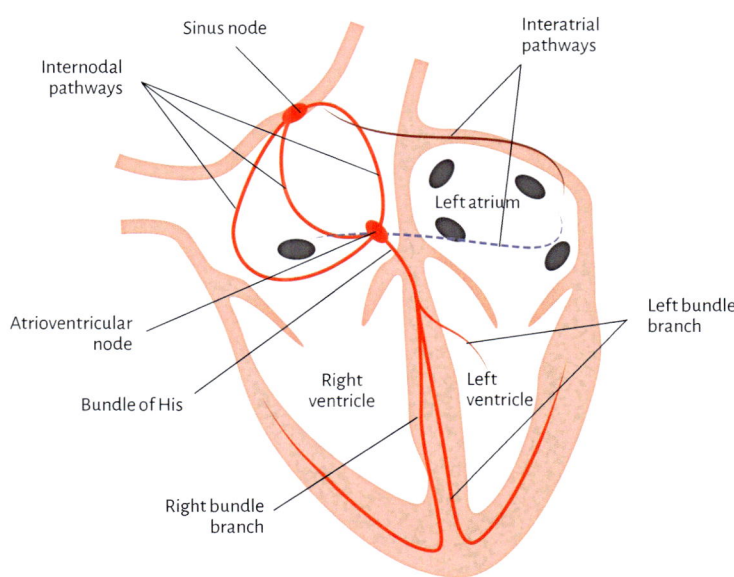

Figure 9. Diagram of the electrical conduction pathways within the heart.

the ventricles, down the bundle of His and up the Purkinje fibres. Understanding how the P and the QRS are formed, helps troubleshoot any abnormal complexes or arrhythmias.

It is worth recognising that an ECG can double count the T and QRS waves giving an inaccurate heart rate value, **therefore heart rate should be counted from pulse palpation or auscultation** rather than relying on the ECG.

The ECG is easy to connect. Three electrodes are attached to the patients:

In **small animals:**
 — red: right forelimb
 — yellow: left forelimb
 — black/green: left hindlimb.

In **horses** a base apex configuration is used:
 — red: jugular furrow
 — yellow: sternum
 — black: ribcage.

> The direction of how the electrical impulse is read is based on what lead the ECG is reading. **Lead II is the most commonly read lead** in veterinary anaesthesia.
> - Lead I: right forelimb to left forelimb.
> - Lead II: right forelimb to left hindlimb.
> - Lead III: left forelimb to left hindlimb.

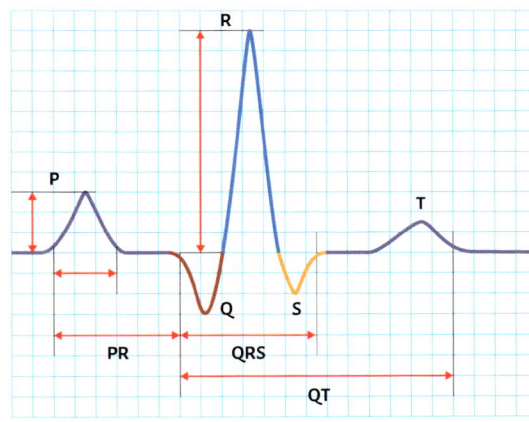

Figure 10. Diagram of a labelled electrocardiogram (ECG) trace.

Other considerations for ECG use include:
 — good contact with the electrodes is important, adhesive pads on the paws are more comfortable in the conscious animal than crocodile clips;
 — electrical activity in the heart does not mean there is a cardiac output;
 — dead animals may have relatively normal ECG for several minutes;
 — Oesophageal ECG probes may be useful though care should be taken with diathermy (a faulty diathermy unit has been reported to cause oesophageal burns).

Arterial Blood Pressure

Arterial blood pressure is the pressure of blood in an artery which is determined by blood volume, vascular tone, and cardiac output.

> Blood pressure =
> cardiac output × systemic vascular resistance

Systemic vascular resistance (SVR) refers to the resistance to blood flow offered by all of the systemic vasculature, excluding the pulmonary vasculature. Mechanisms that cause vasoconstriction increase SVR and those mechanisms that cause vasodilation decrease SVR. Although SVR is primarily determined by changes in blood vessel diameters, changes in blood viscosity also affect SVR.

> Cardiac output = heart rate × stroke volume

Stroke volume is the volume of blood ejected from the heart with every beat, which is influenced by the preload, afterload, and contractility of the heart.

Blood pressure measurement has limitations since it is the product of two factors. For example, blood pressure may appear normal in an animal with low cardiac output and high systemic vascular resistance, but in this case tissue perfusion is likely to be poor. It is important to understand the blood pressure calculation when troubleshooting hypo/hypertension, as there may be different factors including the heart rate, fluid volume, drugs affecting cardiac contractility strength etc.

Mean arterial blood pressure (MAP) should remain above 60 mmHg to preserve tissue perfusion.

> Approximate MAP = diastolic pressure +
> 1/3 (systolic pressure - diastolic pressure)

There are several methods of assessing MAP:
- invasively
- using oscillometric devices
- using Doppler methods.

INVASIVE ARTERIAL BLOOD PRESSURE MEASUREMENT

This is optimal in terms of the accuracy of measurement and providing continuous information. However, it carries risks associated with potential complications (including haemorrhage, haematoma formation, infection, thrombosis) and is usually reserved for high risk patients.

Key points to consider:
- requires cannulation of an artery, which may be technically challenging, e.g. in cats;
- transducer should be positioned at level of right atrium, using the point of the shoulder in dorsal recumbency and sternum in lateral recumbency;
- the transducer should be set to zero before use;
- monitoring is expensive and there are ongoing costs with transducer purchase.

NON-INVASIVE BLOOD PRESSURE MONITORING

There are two main methods of noninvasive blood pressure measurement: oscillometry and Doppler.

These are relatively straightforward to use though are less accurate than invasive blood pressure monitoring and provide intermittent measurements rather than continuous ones.

Both use cuffs applied to the distal limb or tail. The cuff width should be approximately 40% of the limb circumference, otherwise there may be errors in the readings:
- cuff too small: erroneously high readings
- cuff too large: erroneously low readings.

Oscillometric Devices
Key points:
- detects changes in cuff pressure as the cuff deflates (caused by pulses in the artery);
- provides systolic, diastolic, and mean blood pressure values, and heart rate;
- HR should be compared to measured pulse rate to assess if reading is believable;
- more accurate if normal sinus rhythm;
- movement artefacts restrict use during recovery or in conscious animals;
- may be difficult to obtain snug fit for cuff in hairy or chondrodystrophoid breeds (a ring bark clip of the leg should be considered to get more accurate readings in hairy breeds, like Newfoundlands);
- data at three to five minute intervals.

High definition oscillometry has recently become available with a veterinary specific algorithm. One of the advantages is its ability to recognise artefacts.

Doppler Technique
Key points:
- ultrasound probe placed over artery in distal limb or tail and position confirmed by listening to pulsatile blood flow;
- cuff placed proximal to probe and inflated with a sphygmomanometer until no sounds are heard;

- sounds reappear when the pressure in the cuff falls below systolic blood pressure.

Considerations with the use of Doppler include:
- can be difficult to keep probe in position;
- useful in cats as oscillometric methods can be harder to obtain readings;
- systolic blood pressure only. In cats the reading underestimates systolic pressure and is in between the mean and systolic arterial pressures;
- expensive;
- detects blood flow: may be useful for monitoring pulses if challenging to reach under drapes or difficult to palpate (e.g. in reptiles).

CENTRAL VENOUS PRESSURE

Central venous pressure is a pressure measurement of the blood in the cranial vena cava. It is affected by venous return, blood volume, and cardiac output.

Procedure:
- catheter placed in jugular vein and advanced until its tip lies in cranial vena cava;
- alternatively, a catheter may be inserted into the femoral vein and advanced until the tip lies in the thoracic portion of the caudal vena cava;
- saline manometer connected and zero reference point established at level of right atrium (sternal manubrium), or electronic transducer may be used;
- may be used to guide fluid therapy by monitoring the trend in a hypovolaemic patient and to assess the heart's ability to pump the blood being returned to it.

Monitoring the Respiratory System

Pulse Oximetry

Oxygen is essential for life and metabolic processes. The partial pressure of oxygen within the alveoli (PaO_2) is related to the fraction of inspired oxygen (FiO_2), atmospheric pressure (PATM), water vapour pressure (PH_2O), the partial pressure of carbon dioxide ($PaCO_2$), and the respiratory quotient (RQ) as shown in the following alveolar gas equation.

$$PaO_2 = FiO_2(PATM - PH_2O) - PaCO_2/RQ$$

Fortunately, at sea level the following abbreviation can be used:

$$PaO_2 = 5 \times FiO_2$$

This means when an animal is breathing room air (21% oxygen) the PaO_2 is approximately 100 mmHg and when an animal is breathing 100% oxygen during anaesthesia the PaO_2 is approximately 500 mmHg.

Inspired oxygen crosses the alveolar capillary membrane and after equilibration the partial pressure of oxygen in the alveoli (PaO_2) should be the same as the partial pressure of oxygen dissolved in blood (PaO_2). This assumes relatively normal lung function.

When measuring blood gases from an arterial blood sample, it is this dissolved fraction of oxygen, the PaO_2 that is measured.

Most oxygen within the blood is carried bound to haemoglobin, the rest is dissolved in plasma. The oxyhaemoglobin dissociation curve (Figure 11) relates the PaO_2 to the haemoglobin saturation of oxygen. The curve is sigmoid shaped; the affinity of haemoglobin for oxygen changes with the binding of the four sites on the haemoglobin molecule.

Haemoglobin must have all four sites bound with oxygen to be saturated; there is no such thing as a partially saturated red blood cell.

The oxygen content of blood (CaO_2) depends primarily on haemoglobin concentration and saturation, as seen from this equation:

$$CaO_2 = (1.31 \times Hb \times SaO_2) + 0.003 \times PaO_2$$

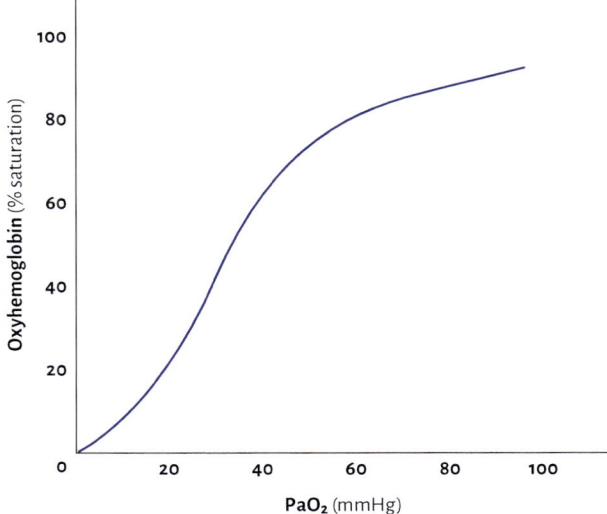

Figure 11. The oxyhaemoglobin dissociation curve.

Therefore, **anaemia has a big impact on blood oxygen content** and consequently oxygen delivery to the tissues; there may not be as many red blood cells circulating, and although they are fully saturated with oxygen, it is still not enough to oxygenate the tissue.

The pulse oximeter measures the haemoglobin oxygen saturation in arterial blood of the available red blood cells. The relationship between SpO_2 and PO_2 is summarised in table 3 and highlights why **an SpO_2 of 90% or less is cause for concern.**

Table 3. Relationship between SpO_2 and PO_2.

SpO_2	PO_2 (mmHg)
98%	100
95%	80
90%	60 (Hypoxaemia <60)
75% (cyanosis observable)	40

An SpO_2 of 90% is the value at which the curve declines precipitously down the steep slope and this point is known as the shoulder.

Underlying Physiology
Pulse oximeters use the differential absorbance of red and infrared light by oxyhaemoglobin and deoxyhaemoglobin to estimate the SpO_2. The probe is usually **placed on a relatively thin tissue** (e.g. the tongue or unpigmented tissue such as a toe) and the monitoring unit displays the pulse rate and SpO_2. Some monitors may also display a plethysmograph.

A variety of pulse oximeter probes are available including **rectal and skin probes.** Considerations when using a pulse oximeter include:
- be aware of the sigmoid shape of the oxyhaemoglobin dissociation curve;
- SpO_2 should be **above 90%, and above 95% when breathing 100% oxygen;**
- readings are affected by movement, ambient light, pigmentation, hair, and carboxyhaemoglobin/methoxyhaemoglobin;
- the probe may not be able to take readings when perfusion is poor (e.g. if vasoconstriction due to hypothermia or after (dex)medetomidine);
- easy to attach and noninvasive;
- a good SpO_2 in an anaemic animal may give a false sense of security.

Indications for Pulse Oximetry
Pulse oximetry is often used during anaesthesia although, as can be appreciated from the oxyhaemoglobin dissociation curve, when an animal is receiving 100% inspired oxygen a drop in **SpO_2 is a late warning sign of problems with oxygenation.**

Pulse oximetry is a useful tool to determine if oxygen supplementation is necessary:
- during sedation
- during recovery from anaesthesia.

Capnography

Underlying Physiology
During anaesthesia, some respiratory information can be gained from observing movement of the animal's thoracic cage and the reservoir bag on the breathing system as the animal breathes.

More information on the efficiency of ventilation can be gathered from evaluating the capnograph. **A capnograph is the trace of end tidal carbon dioxide during the respiratory cycle;** the graphs obtained over several breaths are referred to as the capnogram.

Carbon dioxide is produced in the tissues because of cellular metabolism. The circulation then transports it to the lungs where it is eliminated by ventilation. Capnography therefore **assesses both the circulatory system** (ability and strength of circulation to transport the CO_2 to the lungs), **respiratory system** (ventilation), and **metabolism** within the tissues.

Normal end tidal CO_2 tensions ($ETCO_2$) in conscious animals are approximately 35–45 mmHg. Figure 12 shows a capnograph trace with the end tidal carbon dioxide plotted against time.

Evaluation of the capnogram includes an assessment of **whether the trace returns to baseline between breaths;** if it does not, rebreathing of carbon dioxide is occurring (i.e. the patient is breathing in carbon dioxide in the fresh gas. The shape of the trace should also be evaluated).

Hypoventilation frequently occurs during anaesthesia and in an otherwise healthy animal $ETCO_2$ values in the mid 50's may be tolerated if everything else is normal. In animals with increased intracranial pressure (ICP), careful management of ventilation is required to maintain $ETCO_2$ levels around 30–35 mmHg and prevent further increases in ICP.

Types of Capnography
There are two methods used to measure end tidal carbon dioxide:
- mainstream capnography
- sidestream capnography.

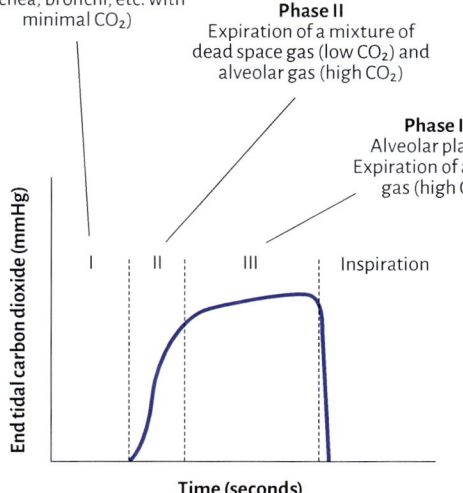

Figure 12. Capnograph trace with the end tidal carbon dioxide plotted against time.

Most capnographs work by **shining infrared light through a sample of expired gas and evaluating how much has been absorbed by carbon dioxide molecules.**

Mainstream Capnography

Mainstream capnography performs the measurement within **a sensor placed between the endotracheal tube and breathing system.**

Key points:
- provides rapid, real time results
- the monitors are compact and portable
- the sensor adds dead space, which can be problematic in small animals
- the sensor is vulnerable to damage
- capnography cannot be used in an MRI.

Sidestream Capnography

Sidestream capnography continuously withdraws gas from an attachment between the endotracheal tube and the breathing system, where sampling tubing connects to the monitor where the measurement is performed.

Key points:
- slower response than mainstream capnography; delay relates to length of sampling line;
- the water trap removes water vapour from sample and needs emptying/replacing when saturated;
- low dead space connectors are available;
- sidestream capnography can be used in an MRI;
- exhaust gases should be scavenged from the monitor to prevent environmental contamination.

Interpretation
Cardiogenic Oscillations

These are considered normal and occur at relatively low respiratory rates when cardiac output is good. Changes in pressure within the thorax due to the beating heart cause small changes in lung volume which is seen on the capnogram.

Rebreathing

The **capnogram does not return to baseline** between breaths. "Rebreathing occurs when gas/es reaching the alveoli contain more CO_2 than can be accounted for by mere reinhalation from the patients dead space gas (should be negligible)". (West, 2012).

Leaks

Leaks often result in **a lack of alveolar plateau.**

Bronchoconstriction/Shark Fin

This occurs when there is resistance within the airway or endotracheal tube, due to asthma, bronchoconstriction, or a mucous plug in the endotracheal tube.

Inspired Oxygen Monitoring

Inspired oxygen monitoring informs the anaesthetist about **the inspired (and often expired) oxygen percentage.** This allows the anaesthetist to ensure the patient is not breathing a hypoxic gas mixture. It is particularly useful if using nitrous oxide or air in addition to oxygen in a circle breathing system; and also recommended if using oxygen concentrators as a gas supply. These modules are not available on all monitoring devices.

Anaesthetic Agent Monitoring

Anaesthetic agent monitoring informs the anaesthetist about **the inspired and expired concentrations of the anaesthetic agent.** This is useful if using a circle breathing system where the volatile agent is diluted due to the lower fresh gas flow.

It is useful to know end tidal agent values as this is what MAC (minimum alveolar concentration) is measured with and best reflects the concentration of the volatile agent in the brain (which is where the volatile agents have their main effects).

SPIROMETRY

Gas flow and volume can be measured during breathing with spirometers. Simple mechanical devices can be used to measure tidal volume though more complex ones are also available.

Sidestream spirometry can be used during anaesthesia. This enables measurement of flow, volume and pressure and generates pressure volume and flow volume loops that can be used to assess the function of the respiratory tract, which is useful when using mechanical ventilation techniques. During inspiration the airway pressure is negative, and the trace starts at zero, however, this is reversed during mechanical ventilation. The measured tidal volume is displayed. The work of breathing is related to the area inside the loop.

Blood Gas Analysis

Blood gas analysis is used to **evaluate acid-base balance, ventilatory efficiency, and blood oxygenation.** Some blood gas analysers also measure parameters such as electrolytes or lactate.
- Arterial or central venous samples are used to assess acid-base balance and ventilation.
- An arterial sample is required to assess oxygenation.
- Arterial blood gas analysis is the gold standard to assess adequacy of ventilation.

What To Do When the Alarm Sounds

General Principles

As a rough guide, normal heart rates under anaesthesia for adult animals are approximately **100–200 beats per minute (bpm) in cats, and 60–120 bpm in dogs** (although when interpreting heart rates breed and anaesthetic protocols should be taken into account, e.g. heart rates may be lower in protocols that include α-2 adrenoreceptor agonists).

Blood pressure should be above 60 mmHg (mean), 40 mmHg (diastolic) and 90–100 mmHg (systolic) and SpO$_2$ should be 98–99% (95% may be a first warning that something is amiss and should be investigated; whilst values of 90% or lower require immediate attention).

In the conscious animal, end tidal CO$_2$ is approximately 35–45 mmHg. During anaesthesia higher values may be encountered due to anaesthetic induced hypoventilation and other causes.

The point at which to intervene depends on the animal and the effects that hypercapnia is having on other body systems. A fall in end tidal CO$_2$ may be something simple e.g. disconnection, or it may indicate something more sinister e.g. cardiac arrest. This is because blood flow is required to bring CO$_2$ produced by cells back to the lungs for elimination. If the alarms on the monitor sound, the following steps should be followed:
- **confirmation whether the heart is beating** by auscultation or an oesophageal stethoscope (if one is in place);
- **pulse assessment:** assess rate, regularity, and pulse pressure (whether it can be felt easily). Ideally a peripheral pulse (metatarsal or metacarpal sites) should be assessed first, moving up to femoral pulses, and then the apex beat;
- **mucous membrane colour should be checked:** assessing whether they are pink, pale, congested or cyanotic;
- **depth of anaesthesia should be assessed** and the stage of the procedure considered: for example, if the surgeon has just started to exteriorise the ovary during a spay, or if the animal has just been moved;
- **respiratory function should be assessed:** is the animal still connected to the anaesthetic machine and is oxygen being administered? If a capnograph is available, end tidal CO$_2$ should be checked. Pulse oximeters may not work well at high heart rates or if perfusion is poor but if it is working, the probe should be moved to a new location and SpO$_2$ checked;
- **body temperature should be measured;**
- **blood loss should be quantified;**
- **drugs** which have been administered should be taken into consideration;
- if possible, **blood pressure should be measured:** oscillometric devices may not work well at very low or high heart rates. Doppler ultrasound can be useful in these situations to monitor trends but only give information on systolic blood pressure.

When an alarm sounds it is important to have a logical approach that focusses on the patient. Alarms should not be dismissed as an equipment problem until the animal has been evaluated.

The best case scenario is that something straightforward has happened e.g. compression of tissue under the pulse oximeter probe or saturated water trap on a capnograph. However, if not, prompt action and identification of the problem facilitates management.

Commonly Encountered Problems

Tachycardia and Bradycardia

Tachycardia and bradycardia may occur during anaesthesia and influence cardiac output as illustrated below:

> **Cardiac output = heart rate × stroke volume**
>
> Stroke volume is the volume of blood ejected from the heart with every beat.

It is important to evaluate the effect on the animal if the tachycardia or bradycardia is affecting the animal.

Measurement of blood pressure and SpO_2, palpation of pulses, checking mucous membrane colour, assessment of the ECG to check for any abnormalities and interpretation of the capnograph give additional information, as well as assessing depth of anaesthesia in the context of what is happening during surgery.

Tachycardia

Although a slight increase in heart rate may improve cardiac output, severe tachycardia reduces diastolic filling time, with a subsequent reduction in stroke volume and therefore a fall in cardiac output.

Common causes of tachycardia are:
- inadequate anaesthesia or analgesia
- hypotension/hypovolaemia
- hypercapnia.

Drug administration can produce a direct effect on heart rate (e.g. antimuscarinics such as atropine) or indirect effect (e.g. hypotension as part of an anaphylactoid reaction, or bleeding). **Hypoxia and hyperthermia can increase heart rate, as can anaemia.**

Less commonly electrolyte abnormalities such as hypokalaemia may be responsible. Rarely, previously undiagnosed conditions such as hyperthyroidism, DCM (dilated cardiomyopathy), or phaeochromocytoma may result in an unexplained tachycardia during anaesthesia (although ideally most preexisting conditions are identified before anaesthesia).

The treatment of tachycardia is directed at addressing the primary cause. Administration of additional analgesia, fluid therapy, and IPPV may be appropriate in straightforward cases. Other animals may require more complex intervention to address the primary cause.

Bradycardia

Bradycardia can result in a decrease in cardiac output; maximum stroke volume is limited. The most common causes of bradycardia are deep anaesthesia, hypothermia, and drug administration (e.g. dexmedetomidine or fentanyl).

Hyperkalaemia should be considered as a cause in animals with a history of trauma or those with urinary tract obstruction. Hypertension can result in a reflex **bradycardia.**

Occasionally, **vagal stimulation** can lower the heart rate. Although traditionally associated with ocular surgery it can also occur during other procedures (e.g. during traction on viscera).

Severe hypoxia can result in bradycardia; this is often a near terminal event. Rarely, severe metabolic abnormalities such as hypoglycaemia or acidaemia may cause bradycardia.

Treatment should be informed by the cause and efforts should be directed to addressing this. In selected cases, administration of an antimuscarinic is appropriate though this can result in an initial bradycardia before the heart rate increases and then a subsequent tachycardia. It is important to be aware that increasing the heart rate in the face of hypertension, increases myocardial oxygen demand. In addition, the heart rates of hypothermic animals often fail to respond to antimuscarinic administration.

Abnormal ECG Traces

If an abnormal ECG trace is detected, first **a pulse or heartbeat should be checked for** while simultaneously informing the veterinary surgeon.

Occasionally ECG clips/pads become disconnected but it is important not to assume that this is the case if the ECG trace goes flat and the alarm sounds. Conversely, a relatively normal ECG may be observed in an animal with no cardiac output. This is called pulseless electrical activity.

> In the event of an arrhythmia, additional useful information is:
> - Pulse assessment:
>   — **Is there a pulse for every ECG complex?**
>   — **What is the pulse rate?**
>   — **How often are the abnormal complexes occurring?**
> - **When were the abnormal complexes first noticed and are they becoming more or less frequent?**
> - **Are the abnormal complexes associated with particular events (e.g. surgical manipulations)?**
> - **What is the arterial blood pressure?**
>   — **Has it changed since the abnormality was noticed?**
>   — **Can the monitor still get a reading?**

Hypotension

Blood flow to major organs (kidney, brain) is autoregulated **over a range of mean blood pressure from 60–120 mmHg**. Noninvasive methods of measuring blood pressure, including oscillometric and Doppler, are increasingly used during anaesthesia with the advantages of being relatively easy to use and safe for the animal. The Association of Veterinary Anaesthetists recommends blood pressure measurement during anaesthesia.

Monitoring trends is important when evaluating blood pressure readings.

It is important to remember that blood pressure does not directly indicate tissue perfusion so should be interpreted in light of all of the other clinical variables. It may be difficult to obtain readings from oscillometric devices if the blood pressure or heart rates are very low/high or there is an arrythmia. It is essential to remember that cuff width should be 40% of limb circumference.

If hypotension is detected (MAP less than 60 mmHg):
- **pulses should be checked** manually;
- **reading should be verified as repeatable** (cuff size should be checked, heart rate reading on monitor vs true HR, another location should be used) while evaluating the animal;
- assessment if the **depth of anaesthesia** is too deep;
- **additional analgesia should be checked** (so volatile agent percentage can be reduced);
- **heart rate should be checked** and consider management of bradycardia or tachycardia as appropriate;
- **blood loss should be checked:** if haemorrhage has occurred then the hypovolaemia should be managed with appropriate fluid therapy.

There are different approaches to the use of fluid therapy and the use of inotropes and vasopressors to treat hypotension, and clinical judgement based on the presence or absence of existing diseases should always be used. Regardless of the fluids and drugs chosen, it is important to evaluate how the animal responds. The following treatments can be considered:
- **10 ml/kg IV crystalloid fluid bolus**
- **10 ml/kg colloid bolus**
- **inotropes/vasopressors**.

Low Pulse Oximeter Reading

The alarm on a pulse oximeter sounds if haemoglobin oxygen saturation is low. A low SpO_2 indicates hypoxaemia (a decrease in partial pressure of oxygen in the blood) which means that the animal is at risk of hypoxia (reduced tissue oxygenation). Pulses should be palpated and the mucous membrane colour checked.

It is important to remember that cyanosis is not usually detectable by the human eye until SpO_2 <75%, so if the mucous membranes are blue, it is a real emergency.

A low SpO_2 may result from:
- failure of oxygen delivery to the animal
- disturbances of gas exchange within the lung
- circulatory failure.

> A stepwise approach to evaluating these three potential causes helps determine the cause of the low SpO_2.
> - **Oxygen delivery to animal should be ensured:**
>   — The oxygen supply on the anaesthetic machine should be checked and adequate flow of oxygen via rotameter ensured.
>   — Administration of nitrous oxide should be discontinued if being used.
>   — The breathing system should be checked. Looking in particular for sticky valves, damaged tubes and confirming it is attached to the endotracheal tube.
>   — Correct placement of the endotracheal tube should be confirmed.
> - **Disturbances of gas exchange within the lung:**
>   — Manual IPPV should be performed while watching movement of thoracic wall/feeling compliance/ensuring no leak around tube/checking the $ETCO_2$ value and capnogram.
>   — The veterinary surgeon may choose to do further diagnostic tests e.g. radiography, thoracocentesis etc. as appropriate depending on findings.
> - **Circulatory failure:**
>   — The presence or absence of a pulse should be confirmed, which in addition to poor perfusion may influence the pulse oximeter reading.
>   — Blood pressure should be measured.

Other factors that may influence pulse oximeter readings are:
- bradycardia and tachycardia
- patient movement: this is less of a problem with modern pulse oximeters
- ambient light
- skin pigmentation, presence of hair or excessively thick tissue
- compression of tissue by the probe: the probe should be moved to a new site.

The person monitoring the anaesthetic may be lulled **into a false sense of security by a normal pulse oximetry reading** since this does not equate to adequate oxygen delivery to the tissues. It may also be misleading in animals with anaemia and only indicates that the haemoglobin is saturated, not that there is enough of it.

Capnography

INCREASED END TIDAL CARBON DIOXIDE
The most common cause of an increase in end tidal CO_2 during anaesthesia is anaesthetic induced hypoventilation. The depth of anaesthesia should be checked and recently administered drugs considered (e.g. methadone or other opioids).

Assuming there is no rebreathing, and the level of hypercapnia is a concern for the anaesthetist, it can be managed by increasing minute volume, e.g. by IPPV. The decision as to when to initiate IPPV should be guided by the history of the animal and clinical evaluation. The heart rate, temperature, and blood pressure should be assessed; and the ECG checked for the presence of abnormal complexes. Rarely, an increase in metabolic rate may cause hypercapnia.

REBREATHING
If rebreathing is evident on the capnogram, the following should be checked:
- adequate fresh gas flow to a non-rebreathing breathing system should be ensured: the fresh gas flow can be increased as part of the troubleshooting process;
- it should be ensured the inner tubing of a coaxial Bain is patent and not disconnected: in practice, it is worth changing to another breathing system or other Bain circuit while this is checked;
- on a circle breathing system, the valves should be checked to ensure they are functioning correctly and not stuck and it should be ensured that the soda lime is not exhausted (the colour should be observed and the canister felt, which should be warm if the absorbent is working);
- a breath should be given by squeezing the reservoir bag while checking chest wall movement, whilst concurrently feeling for abnormal resistance to the process and listening for any abnormal sounds (e.g. mucus in ET tube);
- the dead space of the breathing system and any connectors should be evaluated and the ratio of dead space to tidal volume considered.

DECREASED END TIDAL CARBON DIOXIDE
A decrease in end tidal CO_2 may be due to an increase in minute volume in response to nociception, circulatory compromise, or a reduction in metabolism (e.g. due to severe hypothermia).

The end tidal CO_2 may be low compared to $PaCO_2$ if the animal is panting as this increases the ventilation of anatomical dead space and decreases alveolar ventilation.

Gas flow from the inspiratory limb of a T-piece is close to the sampling port for the capnograph and this gas may mix with expired alveolar gas, reducing the measured end tidal CO_2.

A manual supramaximal breath will reveal the true end tidal CO_2. This may also be seen if there is significant ventilation perfusion mismatch or leaks around the endotracheal tube or capnograph connector.

ABSENCE OF END TIDAL CARBON DIOXIDE
Absence of end tidal CO_2 may be due to cardiac arrest, respiratory arrest, disconnection of the endotracheal tube from the sampling connector, an incorrectly placed endotracheal tube, or an obstructed endotracheal tube or sampling line. Occasionally there may be loss of the capnograph trace due to a saturated water trap although an error message indicating this usually appears on the screen of the monitor.

> If the alarm sounds due to low or absent $ETCO_2$:
> - Pulse/HR etc. should be checked as potentially due to cardiac arrest.
> - The breathing system should be checked to ensure it has not become disconnected.
> - The endotracheal tube position should be confirmed as in the trachea.
> - The sampling line should be checked for breakage or occlusion.
> - Manual IPPV should be performed while watching movement of the thoracic wall/feeling compliance/ensuring there is no leak around the tube/checking the $ETCO_2$ value.

Understanding the information that anaesthetic monitoring equipment provides and being able to integrate it with clinical assessment of the animal should enable early detection of problems associated with anaesthesia. Early intervention and management of anaesthetic related complications is essential to ensuring a good outcome for the animal.

References and Further Reading

- *Anaesthetic records* (2022) Association of Veterinary Anaesthetists. (https://ava.eu.com/resources/checklists/) [accessed 02/09/2022]
- *Anaesthesia safety checklist* (2022) Association of Veterinary Anaesthetists (AVA). (https://ava.eu.com/wp-content/uploads/2015/11/AVA-Anaesthetic-Safety-Checklist-FINAL-UK-WEB-copy-2.pdf) [accessed 02/09/2022]
- *Technical information sheet 6 gas cylinder identification. Label and colour coding requirements. Revision 3.* (2018). British Compressed Gases Association. (https://bcga.co.uk/publications/tis6-gas-cylinder-identification-label-and-colour-coding-requirements-revision-3-2018/) [accessed 02/09/2022]
- Grubb, T., Sager, J., Gaynor, J.S., Montgomery, E., Parker, J., Shafford, H., Tearney, C. (2020) 2020 AAHA Anaesthesia and Monitoring Guidelines for Dogs and Cats. *JAAHA*. 56(2).
- West (2012) *Respiratory Physiology, The Essentials.* 9th Edition. Baltimore, Lippincott Williams & Wilkins.

Test

Answers on page 36

1. What is the primary reason that nitrous oxide use has decreased or been phased out in many veterinary practices?
    a. Difficulty delivering accurate concentrations.
    b. Environmental impact.
    c. Expense.
    d. Incompatible with sevoflurane.

2. What is the function of the non-return pressure relief safety valve on an anaesthetic machine?
    a. Prevent barotrauma in the event of the APL valve being left closed and excessive pressure in the breathing system.
    b. Prevent damage to the vaporizers and flow meters in the event of excessive back pressure through the system.
    c. Prevent the oxygen cylinder being over filled from the pipeline supply and developing excessive pressures.
    d. Prevent the delivery of a hypoxic gas mixture when air-oxygen or nitrous oxide- oxygen gas mixes are being used.

3. Which inhalational anaesthetic agent requires an electronically controlled, heated vaporizer for safe administration?
    a. Desflurane.
    b. Halothane.
    c. Isoflurane.
    d. Sevoflurane.

4. What is the definition of tidal volume?
    a. The volume of gas not involved in gas exchange.
    b. The volume of gas entering the lungs with each inspiration.
    c. The volume of gas entering the lungs each minute.
    d. The volume of gas required for metabolic purposes each minute.

5. What would be the most efficient breathing system to use for a 30 kg dog during anaesthesia?
    a. Bain.
    b. Circle.
    c. Lack.
    d. Magill.

6. When checking a Bain breathing system what should happen to confirm the integrity of the inner tube when it is occluded?
    a. Oxygen flow should cut out and the alarm should sound.
    b. Oxygen flow should "dip" and the pressure relief safety valve should open.
    c. The reservoir bag should fill to capacity and appear turgid.
    d. The APL valve on the breathing system should open.

7. What is the optimal method for confirming correct endotracheal intubation in a rabbit?
    a. Direct visualisation of the tube passing through the larynx.
    b. Exhalation audible through the tube when thorax compressed.
    c. Presence of a trace on the capnograph.
    d. Movement of hair placed in front of the tube in response to breathing.

8. In which species is the use of supraglottic airway devices most appropriate during routine anaesthesia?
    a. Dog.
    b. Goat.
    c. Horse.
    d. Rabbit.

9. What does a pulse oximeter measure?
    a. Haemoglobin oxygen saturation.
    b. Fraction of oxygen dissolved in plasma.
    c. Oxygen content of blood.
    d. Venous oxygen concentration.

10. You are monitoring anaesthesia in a cat. The cat weighs 5 kg, a T-piece is being used and the oxygen flow is set at 0.5 l/min. The following trace on the capnograph is observed:

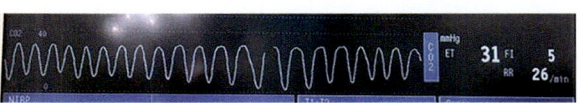

What is the most appropriate course of action?
    a. Change the soda lime.
    b. Ensure the APL valve is fully open.
    c. Start intermittent positive pressure ventilation.
    d. Increase the oxygen flow.

Self-assessment

CORRECT ANSWERS:

1. b
2. b
3. a
4. b
5. b
6. b
7. c
8. d
9. a
10. d

Notes

Preanaesthetic Assessment and Premedication. Intravenous and Inhalant Anaesthetics

Emma Love

Chapter Summary:

- The role of preanaesthetic assessment.
- Core pharmacology.
- Principles of premedication.
- Induction of anaesthesia: injectable and inhalation anaesthetics.
- Maintenance of anaesthesia.

Table 1. Table summarising the study by Brodbelt et al. (2008). The risk of death: the confidential enquiry into perioperative small animal fatalities.

Species	Subset	Risk of anaesthetic and sedation related death	
Dog	Overall	0.17%	1 in 601
	Healthy	0.05%	1 in 1849
	Sick	1.33%	1 in 75
Cat	Overall	0.24%	1 in 419
	Healthy	0.11%	1 in 895
	Sick	1.4%	1 in 71
Rabbit	Overall	1.39%	1 in 72
	Healthy	0.73%	1 in 137
	Sick	7.37%	1 in 14

ANAESTHETIC RISK

The **Confidential Enquiry into Perioperative Small Animal Fatalities (CEPSAF)** was a large scale prospective study designed to investigate the rate and risk factors for sedation and anaesthetic related mortality in small animal practice within 48 hours of the procedure. Although the data was collected almost 20 years ago the lessons learnt are still relevant to the conduct of anaesthesia in practice today.

Table 1 summarises the data taken from Brodbelt et al. (2008) in relation to anaesthetic and sedation related risk of death in cats, dogs, and rabbits. An important result from the study was that **more than half of anaesthetic related deaths occurred in the recovery period.** Therefore, there is significant scope for nurses to implement and evaluate nursing protocols designed to **improve monitoring during this critical period** with a positive impact on anaesthetic related safety.

The American Society of Anaesthesiologists' Classification system (see later in chapter) sorts patients into categories; **healthy patients or those with mild systemic disease are awarded an ASA grade of between I–II and sick patients an ASA grade of III or greater.**

For comparison, the confidential enquiry into perioperative equine fatalities (CEPEF) reported an overall death rate of 1.9% within seven days of anaesthesia. When horses undergoing emergency exploratory laparotomy were excluded the risk was 0.9% (Johnston et al., 2002).

Factors that Increase and Decrease Anaesthetic Risk

Factors reported to **increase** the risk of anaesthetic related death include:
- illness and comorbidities
- age: older animals at increased risk
- over or underweight
- emergency procedures
- complex procedures
- increased duration of procedures
- endotracheal intubation in cats: cats can be more difficult to intubate and rotation of the endotracheal tube (ETT) within the trachea can cause tracheal tears if the ETT is not disconnected from the breathing tube while the patient is repositioned
- fluid therapy in cats: cats are more at risk of volume overload if a precise means of fluid delivery (such as a syringe pump) is not available
- inhalation induction of anaesthesia
- controlled ventilation.

Factors reported to **decrease** the risk of anaesthetic related death include:

- preanaesthetic physical examinations
- premedication with medetomidine or acepromazine (compared to no premedication)
- an intravenous catheter for easy administration of medications if required
- monitoring cardiovascular function via pulse rate, heart rate, and blood pressure
- recording the cardiac rhythm (ECG)
- using a pulse oximeter
- monitoring body temperature and actively supporting the maintenance of body temperature
- keeping an anaesthetic record: recording parameters during the anaesthetic and recovery period
- close observation and patient support during the recovery period.

Most anaesthetic related deaths are multifactorial. A comprehensive and thorough approach to **preanaesthetic assessment** of the animal helps identify potential problems which may occur during anaesthesia. **Careful preparation of the animal and equipment** may also help reduce anaesthetic related accidents.

Patient Assessment

Clinical Assessment, Signalment, and History

A **thorough history should be taken and a full physical examination performed** before anaesthesia. This facilitates detection of potential problems which require further investigation prior to anaesthesia and/or influence the anaesthetic management and **enables tailoring the anaesthetic plan to the individual.** The early identification of potential problems, however small, is important.

Nurses play a key role in liaising with the pet owner before and after anaesthesia. In addition to discussing what is involved in the anaesthetic, confirming the procedure, arranging arrival/collection times, and arrangements for contacting the owner postoperatively (including the correct phone numbers), the nurse should **check with the owner that the history is still valid.** In particular, factors which should be double checked include **changes in exercise tolerance or demeanour** which may give clues as to the animal's health status. Sometimes vital information about the animal is gleamed from an owner's throw away comment.

Informed consent for the anaesthetic and procedure should be obtained, along with consent for the administration of unlicensed drugs (if appropriate). The following information contributes to the optimal nursing and anaesthetic plan for the individual animal:

- animal details: name, species, breed, age, gender, weight, temperament
- brief history: including coughing, polyurea/polydipsia (PU/PD), vomiting/diarrhoea, previous anaesthetics
- time of last feed and any specific nutritional requirements
- current medication: including dose and time of last administration
- vaccination status.

It is important to check if a patient is on any **long term medication,** particularly in their preoperative assessment. Patients on certain long term medications may require weaning prior to surgery (e.g. anticoagulant medications, steroids) or in the case of diabetic patients, the owners should be informed in advance of the required adjustments to the dosage regime for the day of surgery (diabetic patients should not be given a full dose of insulin if they have been fasted as this can cause dangerous hypoglycaemia).

There are **many breed predispositions** to diseases which may influence the course of anaesthesia and the amount of time dedicated to their management before and after anaesthesia. For example:
- Persian cats: polycystic kidney disease
- giant breed dogs: dilated cardiac myopathy (DCM), atrial fibrillation
- Bulldog: brachycephalic airway syndrome
- Sighthounds: altered metabolism of barbiturates.

The **animal's morphology should be considered:**
- IV catheterisation in chondrodystrophic breeds, such as Bassett Hounds, may be challenging (marginal ear veins can be used);
- thin animals are prone to hypothermia and low weight may be an indicator of another disease process;
- obesity or abdominal distension may impair ventilation during anaesthesia due to compression of the diaphragm.

The age of the animal is also significant:
- **neonatal and young animals** have poorly developed renal/hepatic function, an immature cardiovascular system, are prone to hypothermia and hypoglycaemia and drug distribution and drug effects may vary;
- **geriatric animals** may have reduced cardiorespiratory reserve and an increased risk of concurrent disease.

Physical Examination

The main areas of interest when performing a physical examination are the cardiovascular and respiratory system. **Baseline data should be recorded on the anaesthetic record** including pulse rate/quality; mucous membrane colour; respiratory rate; presence of ocular/nasal discharge and temperature.

During the examination, the following should be checked:
- mucous membranes: colour, capillary refill time, whether they are moist or dry
- airway patency: any abnormal respiratory sounds, problems opening the mouth
- thoracic auscultation: heart and pulse rates, pulse deficits, murmurs, arrythmias, and the lung sounds
- venous access: potential problems, previous IV catheter placement (note any evidence of thrombosis/infection/bruising
- peripheral lymph nodes: swellings or enlargement
- abdominal palpation: pain, distension, kidneys, or bladder palpable
- pain score: preexisting painful conditions.

Every animal that is anaesthetised or sedated should be examined, even if it has been examined before. Ideally, **a full physical examination should be performed 12–24 hours prior to anaesthesia** (or at the preoperative appointment) to give sufficient time for any additional tests to be performed. Then the physical examination should be repeated just prior to anaesthesia.

Physiological status can change rapidly, particularly in sick animals, and people are not infallible; one person may pick up something significant that another person has missed or has just become apparent. Fostering a team spirit where people's opinions are listened to and valued, regardless of job title or status, is important. It not only promotes a positive working environment but improves the safety and care of the animal.

Supplementary Tests

The physical examination and patient history may raise issues which require further investigation under veterinary direction, including radiography, ultrasound, ECG evaluation, haematology, biochemistry, and or blood gas analysis. **It is important to differentiate running additional tests to investigate findings of the clinical examination, versus running tests to screen for conditions.** Many of these tests have limited value as screening tests and the physical examination is important. For example, an ECG is not necessary to screen for arrhythmias as these should be detectable on auscultation and pulse palpation. However, if an abnormal rate or rhythm is detected during the examination then an ECG is indicated.

Preanaesthetic blood testing in apparently healthy young animals is a contentious issue. There is no evidence that this improves the safety of anaesthesia in this subset of animals; safety is better addressed by using checklists and training personnel to diligently monitor anaesthesia and interpret their findings, rather than running blood tests. Preanaesthetic blood **testing may be indicated in geriatric animals** (>80% of anticipated lifespan), to look for breed related conditions (e.g. polycystic kidney disease in Persian cats), and in sick animals. The results should be used to guide the preanaesthetic management of the animal, optimise their condition before anaesthesia, and choose the appropriate anaesthetic protocol and management.

ASA Classification

The American Society of Anaesthesiologists Classification may be used to describe patient physical status. The numeral may have the letter E as a suffix for emergency cases.
- **ASA I:** normal healthy animal.
- **ASA II:** an animal with mild systemic disease which is compensating well.
- **ASA III:** an animal with severe systemic disease which is not compensating fully.
- **ASA IV:** an animal that has severe uncompensated systemic disease which is a constant threat to their life.
- **ASA V:** a moribund patient which is not going to survive 24 hours without surgery.

(Note the further classification relating to organ donation is not applicable to veterinary medicine).

This classification system is a useful guide to focus the anaesthetist on the health status of the animal and question whether interventions are required before anaesthesia which could improve the ASA classification. Over the course of the day a patient's health status may change, therefore **an assessment and ASA classification should be performed immediately prior to anaesthesia** and after stabilisation (if necessary). It is worth noting this classification system does not take into account the procedure or the experience of the surgeon/anaesthetist, both of which influence anaesthetic risk.

Preparation for Anaesthesia

Withholding Food and Water

Healthy animals should have free access to water until the time of premedication administration. In certain circumstances, such as prior to endoscopy of the gastrointestinal tract, or conditions that alter mentation, water may need to be withheld and, in these cases, careful attention paid to fluid balance. Administration of intravenous fluids may be appropriate in these cases.

Food is often withheld before anaesthesia to reduce the risk of vomiting or regurgitation and aspiration. There is some debate about the optimal timing of food withdrawal before anaesthesia, though **fasting for 4–6 hours is usually appropriate for healthy adult dogs and cats.** Fasting for longer periods may be associated with an increased risk of regurgitation during anaesthesia. Younger animals require shorter fasting times due to the risk of hypoglycaemia, (no longer than 1–2 hours in paediatric patients less than eight weeks of age or those less than 2 kg in body weight).

Food is not withheld from rabbits due to the risk of hypoglycaemia and in order to maintain gastrointestinal function. It may not be possible to fast animals that require emergency procedures; the owner should be consulted as to when these animals last ate. It is important to be aware that factors such as stress and pain (as well as some gastrointestinal diseases) can delay gastric emptying and some individuals may have a full stomach despite being fasted. Profound sedation should be avoided when the airway is unprotected. In these animals a swift anaesthetic induction, ensuring endotracheal intubation (including inflation of the endotracheal cuff) with the patient's head lifted until the airway is secured, and preparing suction equipment before induction is recommended.

Effective communication of the instructions for food and water intake before anaesthesia to the owner is important, as is **ascertaining when the animal last ate/drank on admission. It is best to tell owners the time at which they should give the last meal to their pet,** rather than the time to starve the animal from; these specific instructions prevent long starvation times.

Protocol Planning

Successful anaesthesia is much more than an exercise in applied pharmacology. Drug selection is part of anaesthetic planning and should be guided by the results of the preanaesthetic assessment, although a more holistic approach is recommended, taking all aspects of anaesthesia into consideration.

After performing the preanaesthetic assessment of the animal and confirming the planned procedure, it is important to reflect on the following:
- anaesthetic considerations for the individual animal
- considerations for the proposed procedure
- how the above will be addressed.

Recognising potential complications and identifying how to manage them is easier at this stage than during an emergency in theatre. The practical aspects should be planned for, as well as identifying what equipment is required and communicating with other teams (e.g. in theatre, in ICU or in recovery as appropriate). **Using checklists** reduces the possibility of human error and their use in anaesthesia and surgery in veterinary practice is strongly encouraged. The Association of Veterinary Anaesthetists (https://ava.eu.com/) have examples of anaesthetic checklists.

In terms of drug protocols, **the anaesthetic triad consists of narcosis, muscle relaxation and analgesia** (or reflex suppression as technically unconscious animals cannot perceive pain). No single agent can produce all components of the triad, so multiple agents are used (usually in small doses compared to sole agent use); this is known as **balanced anaesthesia.** The importance of an effective analgesic protocol as part of the anaesthetic plan cannot be overemphasised.

Core Pharmacology

Pharmacokinetics

Pharmacokinetics is commonly thought of as what the body does to the drug, whereas pharmacodynamics is what the drug does to the body.

Pharmacokinetics describes the absorption, distribution, metabolism, and elimination of a drug as shown in Figure 1.

Administration and Absorption

Intravenous administration of a drug results in a rapid rise in plasma concentration and is reliable; the **drug is administered directly into the systemic circulation,** bypassing the absorption phase. From a practical perspective, the ease of administration of drugs by this route is variable; it may be straightforward in a well-handled, calm animal, but in some cases impossible due to the animal's temperament or size.

Bioavailability refers to the fraction of a dose that reaches the systemic circulation after administration (e.g. by intramuscular injection or oral dosing), compared to the same dose given by the intravenous route. Bioavailability is influenced by many

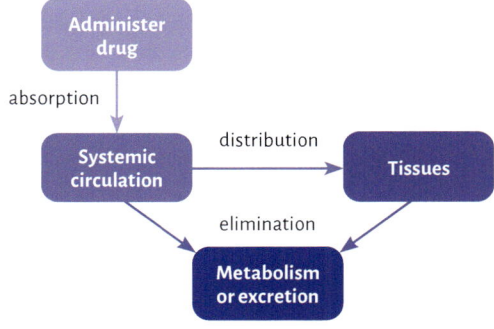

Figure 1. Diagrammatic representation of pharmacokinetics and the absorption, distribution, metabolism, and elimination of drugs.

factors including the properties of the drug itself, formulation, route of administration, interactions with other drugs, individual patient variation, and the patient's disease state.

Intramuscular injections are often used to administer premedication. The onset of effect is usually slower than after intravenous injection; with the speed of absorption depending not only on drug properties, but also the site of injection and muscle blood flow.

Subcutaneous injections can be used for the administration of premedication, although **absorption is unreliable** and influenced by local blood flow; this may be reduced in hypovolaemic animals. This route should be considered for large volumes of injectate. For example, in rabbits, if the calculated drug volume is large relative to the size of the muscle, then intramuscular administration can be painful, and it is often preferable to administer the drugs by subcutaneous injection for welfare reasons.

Oral and oral transmucosal administration of drugs can be considered in the context of anaesthesia for selected cases. There are some drugs with marketing authorisations for administration by these routes. Care should be taken when handling some of the drugs and syringe caps should never be removed with the mouth; ketamine, dexmedetomidine and some others can be absorbed well across mucous membranes posing a potential risk.

Drug Distribution

There are five important factors that determine drug distribution: protein binding, tissue binding, organ blood flow, membrane permeability, and drug solubility.

Albumin is the main plasma protein that binds drugs. The bound drug cannot elicit a response; it is the free or unbound fraction of drug that is available to interact with the drug target.

Hypoalbuminaemia influences the amount of plasma protein that is available to bind with drugs. For drugs that are highly protein bound, hypoalbuminaemia can increase the free fraction of drug and potentially increase the effect of the drug causing **a relative overdose.** Therefore, the dose of some drugs should be reduced or they should be administered slowly to effect in hypoalbuminaemic animals.

Drugs are initially distributed to organs with a high blood flow (e.g. the brain and heart), whereas tissues like fat and bone which are poorly perfused may take longer for the drug to reach equilibrium in.

It is worth assuming most drugs cross the placenta and are secreted into milk. Care should be taken in pregnant or lactating animals.

Drug Metabolism and Elimination

Most drugs are lipophilic and highly plasma protein bound so are not easily filtered by the kidney which excretes polar, water soluble compounds most easily. Therefore, most lipid soluble drugs are metabolised before renal excretion. The liver is the primary organ of metabolism although the gastrointestinal tract, lungs, kidney, skin, and plasma have some metabolic activity.

Within the liver:
- phase I reactions convert the drug to a more polar metabolite
- phase II reactions involve conjugation with substrates and consumption of energy:
    - conjugation may involve glucuronidation (not cats), acetylation (not dogs), methylation or conjugation with sulphate or glycine groups.

Drugs may be activated by metabolism (e.g. suxibuzone to phenylbutazone), have active metabolites (e.g. ketamine and norketamine) or have toxic metabolites (e.g. paracetamol).

Pharmacodynamics

Pharmacodynamics describes the effects the drug has on the animal or the body. There are the desired effects (the therapeutic effects), however there is also potential for undesired effects (Figure 2).

Within the body there are various targets for drugs to act on. These include:
- receptors (e.g. the μ-opioid receptor)
- enzymes (e.g. cyclooxygenase enzyme)
- transporters which carry molecules across a membrane
- ion channels
- nucleic acid
- miscellaneous targets.

Drugs such as opioids (e.g. methadone) and α-2 adrenoreceptor agonists (e.g. medetomidine) act on receptors. (Figures 3 and 4).

The Therapeutic Index

The therapeutic index is a crude measure of drug safety; it relates the maximum non-toxic dose to the minimum effective dose, or LD50/ED50. Therapeutic index is often based on data that is not clinically relevant and it is often difficult to determine what the effective dose is. For example, when treating pain there is a huge spectrum of pain severity and individual responses. In addition, it does not account for idiosyncratic drug reactions.

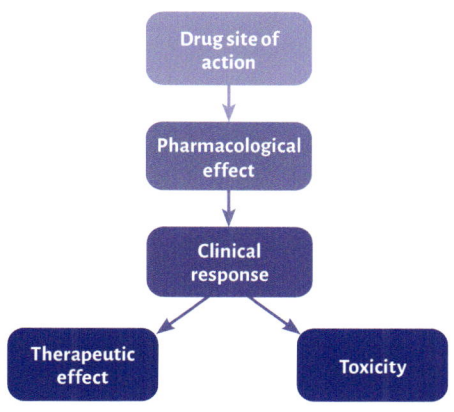

Figure 2. Diagram outlining what is meant by the term pharmacodynamics.

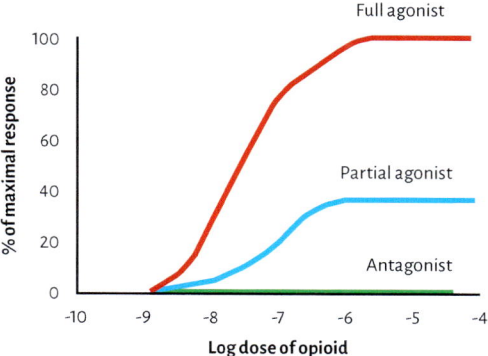

Figure 4. Log (dose) response curves for full and partial agonists and antagonists.

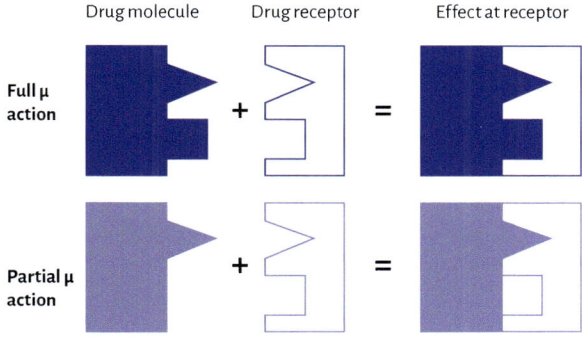

Figure 3. Diagram showing ligand – receptor binding of opioids, full and partial μ-agonists.

- **Affinity** describes how well or avidly a drug binds to its receptor.
- **Intrinsic activity or efficacy** describes the magnitude of effect once the drug is bound.
- **Potency** relates to the dose of drug required to produce a response.
- **A full agonist** can generate a maximal response after binding to its receptor.
- **A partial agonist** does not produce a maximal effect, even when the dose is increased.
- **An antagonist** has affinity for the receptor but does not produce an effect once bound. However, it can block the effect of an agonist, (e.g. atipamezole which antagonises the effects of the α-2 adrenoreceptor agonist (dex)medetomidine).

Principles of Premedication

Aims of Premedication

The aims of premedication are:
- to calm the animal through anxiolysis
- allow safer patient handing
- provide perioperative analgesia (however not all premedications have analgesic properties)
- contribute to balanced anaesthesia and reduce the doses of subsequently administered drugs
- smooth the recovery period.

In practice, combinations of drugs are often used for premedication. Opioids are frequently administered with a sedative. This has the advantage of:
- **synergistic effects:** a synergistic effect occurs when the interaction between two or more drugs causes the total effect of the drugs to be greater than the sum of the individual effects of each drug on their own
- improved reliability of sedation
- contributes to **pre-emptive analgesia**
- **reducing the dose** of subsequently administered anaesthetic agents.

Occasionally, opioids are administered as the only drug in the premedication. This is most common in very sick animals where there is concern over the haemodynamic effects of other sedatives.

Practical Aspects of Premedication

The timing of administration of the premedication should **ensure adequate time elapses for the maximum effect** before induction of anaesthesia. This depends not only on the drug used but also the route of administration. The animal's temperament and presence or absence of an existing intravenous catheter assists with the decision of which route to use for administration of the premedication.

To maximise the premedication's sedative effects, **the animal should be kept in a quiet area and handled in a calm manner.** Stress results in high levels of circulating catecholamines which interfere with the sedative effects of the drugs given and prevent adequate sedation.

The amount of monitoring required depends on the individual animal. For example, it may be appropriate to administer premedication to a healthy dog and then observe them intermittently. In contrast, some animals need direct, continuous observation as soon as drugs are administered with facilities for immediate induction of anaesthesia and endotracheal intubation prepared in advance of drug administration.

It is worth ensuring the area where the animal is kept after premedication is warm, and the animal has bedding to lie on to reduce heat loss by conduction. Although there is debate over the value of actively prewarming animals before anaesthesia, it seems sensible to **take measures to prevent hypothermia** from developing after the preanaesthetic medication is administered.

Sedation

This section focusses on premedication before anaesthesia, although the same drugs can be used for sedation. The preparation of the animal for sedation is like that for general anaesthesia and all animals should undergo a full clinical examination. When considering whether to perform a procedure under general anaesthesia or sedation, the following factors should be evaluated:
- the procedure to be performed:
    - duration
    - invasive or noninvasive
    - pain caused by the procedure or preexisting painful conditions
    - possibility of performing an effective local block
- the animal's temperament:
    - fearful or aggressive
- animal's health status
- whether consent exists for conversion to general anaesthesia if sedation is inadequate.

Important: it is important to remember even profoundly sedated animals can rouse, bite, and then become resedated. **Situational awareness is essential.**

Sedated animals should be monitored as carefully as those under general anaesthesia. In addition to evaluating the depth of sedation, **monitoring peripheral pulses, respiratory rate, rectal temperature, and oxygen saturation are recommended;** these help guide supportive therapies such as intravenous fluid therapy and inspired oxygen supplementation.

An effective plan for pain management should be implemented as appropriate and accurate, contemporaneous records kept.

Principles of Drug Selection

Legal Aspects

Drug selection should **follow the rules regarding the prescription of drugs** in the country where practicing. In many countries, **a veterinary licensed product** with a marketing authorisation for that indication in the species concerned (including dosing and route of administration) should be used. If this is not possible, the following sequence applies:
1. a veterinary medicine authorised for **use in another species** or by a different route in the same species (so called off label)
2. a medicine authorised in that country for **human use**
3. a medicine to be **made up on a one off basis** by a veterinary surgeon or a properly authorised person.

Although the selection and prescription of anaesthetic drugs is ultimately the veterinary surgeon's responsibility, input from the veterinary nurse working with them is important. It is therefore vital to have a **good understanding of each drug.**

Protocol Design

When selecting an anaesthetic protocol, it is important to consider the clinical examination and any anticipated complications during anaesthesia. The animal's temperament, desired level of sedation, and the feasibility of different routes of administration should also be evaluated.

The various drugs used for premedication produce different effects on the cardiorespiratory system, which impacts drug selection in animals with cardiorespiratory compromise or conditions such as hypovolaemia, dehydration, or anaemia. The metabolism and excretion of the drug influences the choice of protocol, particularly in animals with renal or hepatic dysfunction, along with drug dosages in cases of renal dysfunction or hypoalbuminaemia. **Overweight animals benefit from dosages based on their ideal lean weight** and dosage, and drug selection is influenced by age and breed (i.e. allometric scaling for giant breeds).

If the patient has other comorbidities, these should also be considered (e.g. a hypothyroid dog that is overweight may have peripheral neuropathies, such as undiagnosed laryngeal paralysis, and weakened respiratory muscles).

It is important **the animal rests in a quiet environment** and, although left undisturbed, they should be observed after premedication administration. For many cases there is more than one suitable premedication protocol, so **the advantages and disadvantages of different options should be considered** for that individual.

Individual Drugs

Acepromazine

Acepromazine belongs to the **phenothiazine class** of drugs and acts as a dopamine receptor antagonist. It produces **mild to moderate, long lasting sedation** in most dogs and cats. Increasing the dose administered does not necessarily increase the degree of sedation due to a **plateau effect seen at doses above 0.05 mg/kg,** or a total dose of approximately 1 mg.

KEY FEATURES
Acepromazine has a marketing authorisation for administration to dogs and cats at a dose range of **0.03–0.125 mg/kg IV, IM, or SC**, although lower doses appear effective in clinical practice. Lower doses should be used in older animals and giant breeds. **The onset of action is approximately 15 minutes (IV) or 30 minutes (IM)** and the duration of sedation is dose dependent, although it is **typically around six hours** which helps to smooth the recovery period. It is metabolised by the liver and cannot be antagonised.

Acepromazine has antihistamine effects so should be avoided in animals undergoing allergy testing procedures. It is also an α-1 adrenoreceptor antagonist, which results in an antiarrhythmic effect and vasodilation. Due to vasodilation, a decrease in blood pressure is often seen, **so acepromazine should be avoided in shocked animals** and used with care in those with cardiovascular disease. It can also reduce **the packed cell volume (PCV) by up to 20%** due to the splenic sequestration of red blood cells and has **antiemetic effects.**

Acepromazine is available in an injectable and a tablet form and has a MAC sparing effect when used as a premedication. The tablet formulation is rarely used in anaesthesia and experts in behaviour strongly oppose its prescription for the management of noise phobias in dogs.

CONTROVERSIES
Historically acepromazine administration to giant breeds of dogs has had a reputation for producing excessive amounts of sedation for prolonged periods. This may reflect the doses administered; with larger animals requiring relatively smaller doses. **An arbitrary maximum dose of 1–1.5 mg (total dose)** is now often used to reflect this (0.02 mg/kg dose for a 50 kg large breed dog).

There are anecdotal reports of fainting after administration of acepromazine to Boxers. Interestingly this appears to be a British phenomenon; it is unheard of in the USA, and maybe a feature of a specific breed line although this has not been investigated. In this breed, low doses with close monitoring are recommended. Care should be taken when administering acepromazine to other brachycephalic breeds and consideration given to using lower doses; these dogs have a high resting vagal tone which can result in syncope and as acepromazine is long acting, this can prolong the recovery period when it is desirable these patients have a rapid recovery with minimal drug hangover.

Acepromazine has a reputation for lowering the seizure threshold, although no evidence for this is found in the literature.

α-2 Adrenoceptor Agonists

Xylazine, medetomidine, and dexmedetomidine have marketing authorisations for administration to dogs and cats, although the more selective medetomidine and dexmedetomidine are most commonly used. They act as agonists at the α-2 adrenoreceptor although they also have some affinity for the α-1 adrenoreceptor.

Administration can produce **profound sedation and recumbency,** although this can be more unpredictable in aggressive dogs or excited dogs, as high levels of adrenaline can compete for the adrenoreceptors.

KEY FEATURES
α-2 adrenoceptor agonists have an onset of action within five minutes if given intravenously and within 15–20 minutes if given intramuscularly IM. They can be administered by continuous rate infusion and are well absorbed across mucous membranes. These drugs are metabolised by the liver and reduce hepatic blood flow. **Atipamezole is used to reverse the effects of α-2 adrenoceptor agonists.**

α-2 adrenoceptor agonists have significant cardiovascular effects; they cause initial vasoconstriction (peripheral vasoconstriction reduces heat loss), reflex bradycardia, and reduced cardiac output. A first or second degree AV block may be seen on an ECG trace.

This class of drug produces **good muscle relaxation** and is often administered alongside ketamine to counteract muscle rigidity. Vomiting may occur after IM or SC administration and xylazine is sometimes used to induce emesis in cats.

Other effects of the α-2 adrenoceptor agonists include **reduced gastrointestinal motility**, a reduction in antidiuretic hormone (ADH) and renin which **increases urine production,** and a reduction in insulin secretion resulting in **hyperglycaemia** (care should be taken when interpreting blood test results).

The analgesic effects of α-2 adrenoceptor agonists last a shorter time than their sedative effects, but they are **MAC sparing** (can decrease the use of volatile agent by up to 70%).

The profound effects the α-2 adrenoreceptor agonists have on the cardiovascular system should be considered when selecting a premedication protocol for an individual animal. At present, **(dex)medetomidine combinations are mainly reserved for use in healthy adult animals.** Their routine use in sick animals and those at extremes of age (except for the inclusion of dexmedetomidine in the kitten quad protocol), is not generally recommended.

In practice, there is often no need to routinely antagonise the effects of (dex)medetomidine during recovery from anaesthesia; in fact, after a long anaesthetic, given the relatively short duration of action of the drug they should only be reversed if the patient is excessively sedated, or a rapid recovery is required. Indeed, **some animals benefit from administration of a small dose (1–2 µg/kg IV) of (dex)medetomidine to smooth the recovery period.**

The management of bradycardia following administration of α-2 adrenoreceptor agonists can be challenging and the decision of when to intervene difficult. The animal's physiological status should be carefully evaluated to establish what impact the bradycardia is having; **often the bradycardia is a reflex and the patient's blood pressure remains normal or high.** The patient should be assessed for any other contributing factors (e.g. hypothermia or hyperkalaemia). The decision regarding how to approach the bradycardia is also influenced by the stage of anaesthesia; if bradycardia is problematic before the start of surgery, proceeding swiftly with the procedure may be appropriate to see what impact nociception has on heart rate, conversely, towards the end of surgery, administration of atipamezole should be considered.

There are several different interventions to consider, with each approach associated with positive and negative aspects:
- **administration of ketamine:** a low dose may increase heart rate, although responses are unpredictable and there is a delay between administration and the effect of up to five minutes;
- administration of a **partial dose of atipamezole:** this antagonises (dex)medetomidine and increases heart rate, although the plane of anaesthesia can suddenly lighten and subsequently it can be challenging to maintain a stable plane of anaesthesia;
- the administration of **an antimuscarinic is not recommended:** this can increase heart rate but risks exacerbating hypertension and increasing myocardial workload.

Ketamine

Ketamine is a phencyclidine derivative which can produce dissociative anaesthesia. **It is always administered in combination with other drugs for sedation or anaesthesia** since muscle rigidity and excitement is seen when used alone. Ketamine is an NMDA antagonist.

KEY FEATURES
In the UK, ketamine is a **Schedule 2 controlled drug,** which can be administered IM or IV, as a continuous rate infusion and is also absorbed well across mucous membranes. It is metabolised by the liver and the active metabolite (norketamine) is excreted by the kidney. It may therefore **accumulate in animals with renal dysfunction.** Often combined with an α-2 adrenoceptor agonist, the onset of action and duration of effect for ketamine depend on the combination and dose used, but the **onset of action is typically 3–10 minutes** and the **duration of effect lasts approximately 30–45 minutes.**

Ketamine maintains cardiovascular function; although ketamine itself produces myocardial depression, its administration results in catecholamine release which overall produces positive chronotropic effects. It is important to be aware that sick animals may not have this expected catecholamine response and a direct negative effect may be seen. It should be **avoided in cats with hypertrophic cardiomyopathy** as there may be inadequate myocardial perfusion due to the positive chronotropic effects.

Ketamine may **increase intraocular pressure and intracranial pressure.** It has antihyperalgesic effects which may contribute to analgesic protocols, and it provides **better somatic analgesia than visceral analgesia.** Somatic pain results from an injury to the body such as the skin, muscle, or bone and tends to be localised; whilst visceral pain refers to pain from the internal organs which is usually dull and diffuse.

Benzodiazepines

The benzodiazepines midazolam and diazepam are GABA (γ-aminobutyric acid) agonists. Administration may **produce sedation in young or sick animals,** especially when given with an opioid, but in contrast they can produce **excitement in healthy animals.** In the UK, diazepam has a marketing authorisation for administration to cats and dogs, whereas midazolam has a marketing authorisation for administration to horses.

KEY FEATURES
Benzodiazepines are metabolised in the liver. Midazolam is

water soluble and can be administered IM or IV and produces metabolites that are not active. **Diazepam is solubilised in propylene glycol, is painful on injection, poorly absorbed from IM injections, can produce thrombophlebitis if given IV, and has active metabolites. In cats, diazepam can result in idiosyncratic hepatic necrosis.** Both are usually given at a dose of 0.2–0.3 mg/kg and are often administered in combination with an opioid.

Benzodiazepines have minimal effects on the cardiorespiratory system and are therefore often used in critically ill patients. They produce good muscle relaxation and have anticonvulsant activity. Benzodiazepines can be antagonised with flumazenil (although in the UK this is not licenced).

Tiletamine and Zolazepam

Zoletil® or Telazol® contain tiletamine, a phencyclidine derivative and zolazepam, a benzodiazepine. The combination has similar effects to ketamine/benzodiazepine combinations. However, it is worth noting that in dogs, zolazepam is metabolised faster than the tiletamine, which can lead to rough recoveries from anaesthesia. There can also be accumulation if repeated doses are given.

Opioids and Other Drugs

Although some of the sedatives used for premedication have some analgesic properties, it is vital that **analgesics are incorporated into a robust plan** for anaesthesia rather than sedatives being relied on as sole analgesics.

The premedication protocol should include an opioid and in some instances the animal may receive an opioid alone for premedication.

Butorphanol, buprenorphine, fentanyl, methadone, and pethidine have UK marketing authorisations in dogs and cats. Butorphanol is a good sedative, but a poor analgesic and any analgesia is short lived. Morphine may be administered via the cascade if justified on an individual patient basis (e.g. as part of a continuous rate infusion technique). Fentanyl/fluanisone is often used to provide neuroleptanalgesia for rodents, guinea pigs, and rabbits.

Non-steroidal Anti-inflammatory Drugs (NSAIDs)

These do not contribute to sedation but may be administered preoperatively as part of the analgesic protocol in selected healthy animals. There are pros and cons to this approach.

The inclusion of **antimuscarinics (atropine or glycopyrrolate)** in premedication is controversial with a definite European/North American divide on the best approach. They were traditionally used to counteract salivation, produced by older anaesthetic agents. They can counteract bradycardia produced by drug administration or vagal stimulation but may produce a dramatic tachycardia which increases myocardial oxygen consumption. When administered with α-2 adrenoreceptor agonists they significantly increase myocardial workload, so this approach is not recommended.

Induction of Anaesthesia

Injection vs Inhalation

Anaesthesia can be induced by **injectable or inhalational anaesthetic agents.** Historically anaesthesia induction with inhalational agents was thought to be safer since the animal did not have to metabolise drugs. However, the CEPSAF study reported an increased risk of death in animals where anaesthesia was induced with an inhalational agent. In addition, this method exposes people to anaesthetic gases (undesirable from a health and safety perspective) and uses large amounts of inhalation anaesthetic agent; the negative impact of the release of these vapours into the environment has to be considered. Apart from anaesthesia in some exotic animal species **inhalation induction of anaesthesia is not recommended.**

Route of Administration

Injectable anaesthetic agents may be administered by **intramuscular, intravenous, or subcutaneous injection.**

Intramuscular Injection

- painful, so volume and site should be considered
- easier than IV in fearful or fractious animals
- calculated dose administered, difficult to predict what dose an individual animal requires
- slower onset time than IV administration
- important to ensure needle long enough in overweight animals
- requires drugs with good bioavailability
- can be administered after a premedication but most commonly the process in combined and a single injection given (e.g. triple combination of ketamine, medetomidine, and an opioid or the quad protocol, combination of medetomidine, ketamine, midazolam, and buprenorphine).

Intravenous Injection

When using drugs with a rapid onset of action it is relatively easy to dose to effect; this accounts for individual variability and potentially minimises adverse effects as dosing to effect rather than giving a precalculated dose.
- Requires adequate restraint/sedation for injection.
- Placement of an IV catheter before administration of drugs means there should be secure IV access in the event of an emergency during induction of anaesthesia.
- Most animals receive premedication before administration of IV drugs for induction of anaesthesia.

Subcutaneous Injection

- slow onset, unreliable absorption, particularly in shocked animals
- should be considered as an alternative to IM injection in small mammals (e.g. when the calculated drug volume is excessive for IM administration).

Inhalation Agent

- potentially stressful for the animal: if no other option feasible for induction of anaesthesia the judicious use of a premedication should be considered to reduce stress for the animal
- mask versus chamber
- a slow process with risk of regurgitation and aspiration during induction
- the anaesthetic agent must not be irritant to mucous membranes.

Neurotransmitters

Many of the injectable anaesthetic agents and sedatives **act on receptors within the central nervous system and other tissues.** Appreciating the role of the key neurotransmitters and receptors can help with understanding how the drugs work.
- **Acetylcholine (ACh):** found in the brain, spinal cord and peripheral nerves as well as some other cells. ACh acts on muscarinic and nicotinic receptors. All motor nerve fibres exciting the CNS release ACh which acts on nicotinic receptors. All postganglionic parasympathetic fibres release ACh which acts on muscarinic receptors.
- **Noradrenaline (norepinephrine):** found in many tissues of the body including the brain and sympathetic ganglia and acts on α and β-adrenoceptors.
- **Glutamate:** the principle excitatory neurotransmitter in the vertebrate central nervous system and acts on AMPA, NMDA, metabotropic glutamate, and kainite receptors.
- **γ-aminobutyric acid (GABA):** the principle inhibitory neurotransmitter in the adult CNS and acts on the GABA receptor to decrease excitability of neurones.
- **Histamine:** widely distributed afferent neurotransmitter which is involved in the senses of itching and pain.
- **Dopamine:** precursor of noradrenaline, involved in control of movement and behaviour.
- **Adrenaline:** produced by adrenal glands and neurones in the medulla oblongata and acts on α and β-adrenoceptors to increase cardiac output, increase muscle blood flow, increase blood glucose and dilate the pupils (fight or flight response).
- **Serotonin (5HT):** acts on 5HT receptors to regulate sensory pathways and control mood.

Injectable Anaesthetic Agents

Pharmacology

After administration **the plasma concentration of an intravenous anaesthetic agent rises rapidly to a maximum value.** The drug then redistributes to tissues and is metabolised and eliminated so when the drug plasma concentration is plotted against time it is seen to **decline in an exponential way** (assuming a one compartment model; in reality more complex compartmental models are needed for some drugs). There may be times when multiple doses or a constant infusion of an intravenous anaesthetic is required; therefore, it is important to know if the drug accumulates after multiple doses or an infusion. This is influenced by the half-life (time taken for plasma concentration to fall by 50%) of the drug. When an infusion, designed to maintain a constant plasma level of a drug is stopped the time taken for the plasma concentration to fall by 50% is known as **the context sensitive half-time:** the context refers to the duration of the infusion.

Ideal Properties of an Injection Anaesthetic Agent

The ideal injectable anaesthetic has the following properties:
- rapid onset: acts within one circulation time (one arm to brain time)
- non-irritant: either to the endothelium of the vein or if accidently injected perivascularly
- minimal cardiopulmonary effects
- rapidly metabolised and eliminated
- noncumulative so repeated doses or infusions do not unduly prolong the recovery time
- good analgesia: contribute to the analgesic plan for the animal
- good muscle relaxation: facilitate positioning for surgery and/or diagnostic procedures as well as surgery itself.

> The following have european marketing authorisations for administration to animals:
> - propofol: dogs, cats
> - alfaxalone: dogs, cats, rabbits
> - ketamine: horses, dogs, cats
> - tiletamine/zolazepam: dogs and cats.
>
> These agents are difficult to obtain or not licenced:
> - thiopental: horses, dogs, cats (difficult to obtain)
> - not licenced: etomidate, chloral hydrate, methohexitone.

Mode of Action

Barbiturates, propofol, alfaxalone, and etomidate are agonists at the gamma amino butyric acid (GABA) receptor in the CNS. When these drugs bind to the GABA receptor, they increase the frequency or duration of GABA dependent chloride channel opening. **The increase in chloride conductance causes hyperpolarisation and neuronal inhibition.**

Ketamine is a N-methyl-D-aspartate (NMDA) antagonist and antagonises the excitatory neurotransmitter glutamate at NMDA receptors in the CNS. It also has complex actions at opioid receptors. Tiletamine is also probably an NMDA antagonist and the benzodiazepine zolazepam is a GABA agonist.

Frequently Used Injectable Anaesthetic Agents

Propofol

There are two formulations of propofol; both presented as a milk coloured emulsion (egg protein/lipid). The original version is a single use vial which does not contain a bacteriostat and **must be discarded after the vial is broached.** Propofol with a benzyl alcohol preservative **(Propofol Plus/Propofol 28)** is also available. This product can be used for up to 28 days after the vial has been broached but, due to inclusion of benzyl alcohol, **should not be administered by infusion, particularly in cats.**

Key Features
- phenol
- GABA agonist
- may be mistaken for penicillin so syringes should be clearly labelled
- rapid onset of action
- administered IV
- rapidly metabolised in the liver and eliminated: cats lack glucuronidation pathway in liver so metabolism in cats is slower than in dogs
- possible extrahepatic metabolism: drug clearance is faster than hepatic blood flow
- noncumulative in dogs (not cats): used for TIVA (Total intravenous anaesthesia) in dogs
- postinduction apnoea common
- hypotension: myocardial depression and peripheral vasodilation
- no analgesia
- fair muscle relaxation though occasionally muscle twitching and muscle rigidity seen
- consecutive day use should be avoided in cats: oxidative damage to red blood cells (Heinz body formation) seen after three days and cats became generally unwell after 5–7 days of consecutive day administration
- non-irritant if injected perivascularly
- all formulations may produce an aversive response (attempted limb withdrawal) during injection: administration to people is reported to produce a burning sensation
- highly plasma protein bound 96–98% (Cockshot et al., 1992).

Alfaxalone

The anaesthetic molecule alfaxalone has been around for several decades, although it is not soluble in water which led to challenges in producing a solution for injection. It was originally solubilized in Cremophor EL® (along with the inactive isomer alphadalone) with the trade names Saffan® (veterinary product) and Althesin® (for people) though the Cremophor EL® induced clinically significant release of histamine. More recently, cyclodextrins have been used to solubilise alfaxalone. Cyclodextrins are ring sugar molecules which have the appearance of a donut. The interior is hydrophobic and the alfaxalone molecule sits in the middle while the exterior of the cyclodextrin is water soluble. The cyclodextrin has no pharmacological activity of its own and simply provides a way to make the insoluble alfaxalone molecule water soluble.

Key Features
- steroid anaesthetic
- clear solution: cyclodextrin
- high therapeutic index
- non-irritant
- administered IV
- marketing authorisation for IM use in Australia but not Europe. Injection volume can be large for IM use: often used for sedation/to facilitate IV catheterisation rather than full induction of anaesthesia due to the injection volume
- rapid onset
- rapid hepatic metabolism and elimination
- noncumulative
- respiratory depression and postinduction apnoea if given rapidly
- preserves baroreceptor tone: HR increases in response to reduced BP
- no analgesic effects.

KETAMINE

Ketamine is a versatile drug and in small animal practice is used in combination with other drugs as a sedative, anaesthetic, and as part of analgesic protocols. It is a Schedule 2 Controlled Drug. When used as an anaesthetic it produces a dissociative state and maintains many of the reflexes normally abolished during anaesthesia. The animal's eye may remain central with a brisk palpebral reflex, and pharyngeal and laryngeal reflexes are also maintained. Muscle tone is also maintained or increased so it is vital **ketamine is administered with other drugs with muscle relaxant properties** e.g. benzodiazepines, α-2 adrenoreceptor agonists.

Key Features
- administered IV or IM in small animals, also absorbed after SC or transmucosal administration
- quiet environment important: excitement if animal disturbed
- metabolised by the liver: active metabolite is norketamine
- plasma protein binding approximately 50%
- produces sympathetic stimulation and maintains cardiovascular and respiratory function
- should be used with care in animals with hypertrophic cardiomyopathy (increases myocardial workload)
- analgesia/antihyperalgesic effects can contribute to analgesic protocols but should not be relied on as a sole agent for analgesia
- slow onset
- noncumulative
- often used in horses IV
- potential to increase intraocular and intracranial pressure
- possible neuroprotective effects.

Less Commonly Used Injectable Anaesthetic Agents

THIOPENTAL

Thiopental is a barbiturate anaesthetic that is reconstituted from powder to form a 2.5 or 5% solution. This solution is very alkaline and can result in **perivascular tissue necrosis if accidently injected outside the vein.** If administering to cats and small dogs, diluting the 2.5% solution even further should be considered. Acquiring thiopental can be difficult.

Key Features
- administered IV only
- rapid onset with predictable effect, particularly in horses
- recovery from anaesthesia due to redistribution of the drug
- metabolism in liver
- prolonged recovery in Sighthounds due to lower capacity for metabolism of the drug in these species
- highly plasma protein bound: about 80%
- moderate cardiopulmonary depression with ventricular bigeminy seen in 40% of dogs
- predicable effect: especially in horses
- repeated dosing significantly prolongs anaesthetic recovery: not suitable for TIVA.

TILETAMINE AND ZOLAZEPAM
- tiletamine (phencyclidine family NMDA antagonist) and zolazepam (benzodiazepine)
- powder for reconstitution
- IM or IV administration
- reports of oral administration (e.g. hiding in meatballs) for capture of unhandleable dogs, though not licenced for use in this way
- in dogs the zolazepam is metabolised more rapidly than tiletamine which means that the tranquilisation wears off before the anaesthetic and the adverse effects of the tiletamine may be seen (muscle rigidity, poor quality of recovery)
- extensively metabolised
- abnormal respiratory patterns may be seen following administration.

Other Drugs

Other drugs used to induce anaesthesia include:
- **Etomidate:** minimal effects on the cardiovascular system. However, it produces adrenal suppression which has been associated with an increased death rate in people when used by infusion in ICU settings. In animals, induction of anaesthesia can be smooth in well sedated animals though in animals that received low doses of premedications (appropriate for most animals with significant cardiovascular disease) then induction of anaesthesia is unpleasant with vomiting, retching, myoclonus, and significant pain on injection. It does not have a marketing authorisation for administration to animals in Europe.
- **Chloral hydrate:** this anaesthetic agent is unusual in that it is administered orally. References may be seen in older textbooks though it is now obsolete.
- **Opioid/benzodiazepine:** induction of anaesthesia with a combination of a fentanyl and midazolam is reported in the literature. However, this only produces anaesthesia in very sick animals and an additional anaesthetic agent should be available in the event of failure to induce an adequate depth of anaesthesia.

Factors Influencing the Effects of Injectable Anaesthetic Agents

CARDIOVASCULAR FUNCTION

Injectable anaesthetic agents need to reach the brain. **In animals with low cardiac output** (either due to effects of drugs such as dexmedetomidine or pathological reasons) the onset of action of anaesthetic agents is slower and therefore **it is important to give them slowly and to effect.**

All the commonly used injectable anaesthetic agents have effects on the cardiovascular system. **Careful drug selection and slow administration are important,** particularly in sick animals, and **the animal's condition** should also be optimised before anaesthesia induction (e.g. using appropriate fluid therapy, analgesia and other treatments). Monitoring the cardiovascular system during induction of anaesthesia should be considered and in sick animals monitoring equipment should be attached before induction of anaesthesia. Healthy or fearful animals may not tolerate monitoring equipment attachment at this time so pulse palpation during induction of anaesthesia is a good idea until the airway is secured and equipment can be attached.

When the anaesthetic agent is administered by intramuscular injection, low cardiac output or reduced tissue perfusion can delay the onset of anaesthesia.

Recovery from anaesthesia is primarily due to redistribution of the injectable anaesthetic agents so may be lengthened if tissue perfusion is poor.

Plasma Protein Binding

Injectable anaesthetic agents bind to plasma proteins to a variable degree. Propofol is very highly plasma protein bound (~98%) whereas alfaxalone is much less so (~20%). The unbound fraction of the drug is free to cross the cell membrane and interact with the receptor. In hypoproteinaemic animals (e.g. those with liver renal or disease) there is a greater proportion of free, unbound drug compared to an animal with normal plasma protein levels. Therefore, it is important to **administer the anaesthetic agent slowly and to effect.**

Co-induction of Anaesthesia

Co-induction of anaesthesia is where more than one drug is administered to induce anaesthesia. Most commonly a benzodiazepine, ketamine, or short acting opioid is administered alongside either propofol or alfaxalone. The theory behind this approach is that it **reduces the dose of the induction agent and therefore the adverse physiological effects.**

Co-induction may be performed after a standard premedication (e.g. acepromazine or (dex)medetomidine plus an opioid). Alternatively, in animals with ASA scores of 3 or greater where there is a reason not to administer acepromazine or (dex)medetomidine the animal may receive only an opioid for premedication with subsequent induction of anaesthesia with a co-induction technique.

The timing of drug administration should be considered if a benzodiazepine is used as part of the protocol. Administration of a benzodiazepine in a conscious animal has the potential to induce excitement. To avoid this a small dose of the intravenous induction agent is administered first, then the benzodiazepine, then the rest of the intravenous induction agent is titrated slowly to effect.

There is conflicting evidence regarding the benefit of co-inductions in dogs and cats. Some studies report a decrease in dose of the anaesthetic agent though no improvement in the measured physiological variables. In other studies, the dose required of the anaesthetic agent is increased with a co-induction technique. An increase in the incidence of postinduction apnoea is reported in healthy dogs when anaesthesia was induced with midazolam and alfaxalone (Miller et al., 2019).

It is worth noting most studies have been conducted in healthy animals and more research is needed to determine the benefit (or otherwise) of the technique in sick animals.

Injectables for the Maintenance of Anaesthesia

The duration of anaesthesia obtained with injectable anaesthetics may be adequate to perform an entire procedure (e.g. the triple or quad combinations are often used for neutering procedures in cats).

It may also be possible to top up intravenous anaesthetic agents to prolong anaesthesia or to achieve immobility for procedures such as diagnostic imaging. The drug chosen should be suitable for topping up without accumulation in that species. It is also important to monitor the animal's airway patency (if not intubated), monitor the SpO_2 and the other variables normally monitored during full anaesthesia. In addition, supportive therapy (e.g. supplementing inspired oxygen and IV fluids) should be available and if IV anaesthetic agents are used for sedation rather than full general anaesthesia, the facilities for endotracheal intubation should be available.

Total intravenous anaesthesia (TIVA) is an option for maintaining anaesthesia with injectable agents. It is a useful technique particularly when administration of inhalational anaesthetics would expose people to excessive amounts of waste anaesthetic gases (e.g. during bronchoscopy). In its simplest form it involves topping up intermittently via IV injection, although this can result in a variable depth of anaesthesia which swings from too light to too deep.

A continuous rate infusion is a better way of achieving a stable plane of anaesthesia although the depth of anaesthesia should be assessed regularly, and the rate of infusion changed accordingly. A **syringe driver** ensures accurate delivery of the anaesthetic agent. The pharmacokinetic variables should be considered when calculating infusion rates and the context sensitive half-time used to determine if the drug is suitable for infusion for prolonged periods, without significantly increasing the recovery time from anaesthesia.

The context sensitive half-time of propofol and ketamine does not increase significantly as the duration of infusion increases, whereas it does for thiopental. Clinically, this means if thiopental was used to maintain anaesthesia there would be a very prolonged recovery from anaesthesia.

There are important species differences to note. Cats lack the metabolic capacity for glucuronidation which means that after infusion propofol can accumulate and cause prolonged recovery. **Propofol infusions are not generally recommended for maintenance of anaesthesia in cats.** However, they may be used in the intensive care unit. In this context, prolonged recovery is of less significance; there are facilities to monitor and support the cat during this period.

Alfaxalone can be used for TIVA in both dogs and cats. The dose rates are listed in the datasheet.

Regardless of the drug used for TIVA **careful monitoring is important.** Respiratory depression is common with injectable anaesthetics so respiratory function should always be monitored, ideally with capnography, and facilities should be available for intermittent positive pressure ventilation (IPPV).

Inhalational Anaesthetic Agents

Definition of Terms

Minimum Alveolar Concentration (MAC)

The minimum alveolar concentration (MAC) is the alveolar (end tidal) concentration of inhalant anaesthetic required to prevent purposeful movement in response to a supramaximal noxious stimulus in 50% of subjects. It is determined in a laboratory setting where the animal does not receive any drugs apart from the inhalational anaesthetic. After induction of anaesthesia with the inhalational anaesthetic, the anaesthetic concentration is varied. The supramaximal noxious stimulus is often a clamp or electrical stimulus applied to digits. During application of the stimulus whether the animal responds (or not) with a withdrawal of the limb is recorded as well as the inhalation anaesthetic percentage. MAC is then calculated.

There are limitations with MAC determination studies. The anaesthetic protocol does not reflect clinical practice and the equivalence of the stimulus to surgery is debatable; in addition, only a small number of animals are used in the studies. However, this standard method of measurement produces a measure of potency of the inhalational anaesthetic agents and enables the comparison of different volatile (inhalational) anaesthetic agents as well as guiding the anaesthetist as to appropriate vaporiser settings. Some anaesthesia practices may reduce the MAC, which is known as MAC sparing.

MAC is **decreased** by:
- sedatives: acepromazine, medetomidine (up to 70%)
- analgesics: opioids
- coadministered anaesthetic agents: midazolam
- hypothermia: decreased metabolic rate
- pregnancy: increase in endogenous endorphins and an increase in progesterone
- geriatric and neonatal animals less than two weeks of age: decreased metabolic rate, organ function reduced
- conditions such as hypothyroidism: decreased metabolic rate.

MAC may be **increased** in:
- young animals: increased metabolic rate
- hyperthermia: increased metabolic rate
- concurrent administration of catecholamines and sympathomimetics: ephedrine
- conditions such as hyperthyroidism: increased metabolic rate.

Note: **Volatile anaesthetics have no analgesic properties.**

Physical Properties

Most inhalational anaesthetics are **delivered as vapours; this is the gaseous state of a substance which is normally a liquid at an ambient temperature and pressure** (e.g. isoflurane and sevoflurane, which are stored as a liquid in a bottle, but delivered as a gas).

Nitrous oxide is a gas; it exists in gaseous form at room temperature at sea level.

Desflurane has some unique properties that differ to the common volatile agents used. Its boiling point is close to room temperature, so it remains as a liquid in the reservoir of a typical vaporiser and a specific desflurane vaporiser must be used.

Partial Pressure

The partial pressure of a gas is the pressure that the individual gas exerts in a mixture of gases. This is relevant to inhalational agents, since it is the partial pressure of the agent in the brain that determines its effects.

Partition Coefficient

A partition coefficient describes the ratio of the concentrations of a compound in two solvents at equilibrium (equal volume, pressure, and temperature). The blood gas partition coefficient (also known as blood gas solubility coefficient), describes the solubility of a gas in the blood. Agents with a low blood gas solubility exert a high partial pressure and a rapid induction and recovery from anaesthesia will occur. The more soluble the inhalant agent is in blood; the more inhalant agent is required to increase its partial pressure in the alveoli.

Potency

The potency of an inhalant agent is associated with its lipid solubility and **ability to cross the blood brain barrier** into the lipid tissues of the brain where it exerts its effect. This is measured by an inhalant agent's **oil gas partition coefficient.**

Mechanism of Action

In contrast to many of the drugs, the mechanism of action of inhalant anaesthetics has not been definitively determined. Proposed mechanisms include:
- disruption of the cell membrane lipid bilayer
- binding to proteins on ion channels and inhibiting synaptic transmission
- direct effects on specific receptors such as GABA, NMDA etc.

There is a link between the oil gas partition coefficient of an agent and its potency, known as **the Meyer-Overton Hypothesis.** The theory being the molecules of the inhalational anaesthetics dissolve in the lipid bilayer of cell membranes within the brain and when this happens in sufficient amounts, it induces a state of unconsciousness and anaesthesia. It is possible that the actual mechanism of action is a combination of the above suggestions.

Pharmacokinetics

Although inhalational anaesthetics are delivered via the lungs, the central nervous system is the site of action. The alveolar (end tidal) partial pressure of the anaesthetic reflects the partial pressure of the anaesthetic agent in the brain. Several factors influence the speed of uptake of the anaesthetic agent.

INSPIRED CONCENTRATION
The higher the setting is on the vaporiser, the higher the partial pressure of the agent is in the lungs, and thus the faster the onset of anaesthesia. Drugs also move down their concentration gradient from areas of high concentration to low concentration, so a high inspired percentage of inhalational agent facilitates this process and speeds it up.

ALVEOLAR VENTILATION
Increased alveolar ventilation increases the alveolar partial pressure of the inhalational agent, increasing the rate of uptake of the inhalational agent and the speed of induction of anaesthesia. How quickly the pulmonary circulation removes the anaesthetic gas from the alveoli is determined by how soluble the gas is in blood and the alveolar blood flow.

CARDIAC OUTPUT
A low cardiac output increases the speed of onset of anaesthesia, which is the opposite to what people normally expect. The reason being that with low cardiac output the uptake of anaesthetic agent from the alveoli to the pulmonary circulation is low, so the partial pressure of the agent in the alveoli rises rapidly. Since this reflects the partial pressure of the anaesthetic in the brain, the onset of anaesthesia is rapid.

BLOOD GAS PARTITION COEFFICIENT
Anaesthetics with a low blood gas solubility coefficient produce a rapid onset of anaesthesia and changes in anaesthetic depth are easy to control during anaesthesia. This is because these agents exert higher partial pressures within the alveolus, and it is this factor rather than the total amount of drug present in the body that is important.

The distribution of the anaesthetic agent depends on perfusion and the solubility of the agent in different tissues.

Recovery from anaesthesia depends on the reverse of the processes involved in uptake as elimination of the drugs is primarily via the lungs. There is a small amount of hepatic metabolism with some agents:
- halothane 20%
- sevoflurane 2–5%
- isoflurane 0.2%
- nitrous oxide is negligible (halothane 20%, isoflurane 0.2%, sevoflurane 2–5%, nitrous oxide.

Inhalational Anaesthetic Agents: Drugs

There are four different types of inhalant anaesthetic agents used in veterinary medicine, with varying advantages and disadvantages (Table 2).

Table 2. Summary of physicochemical characteristics of inhalation anaesthetic agents.

Agent	Boiling point (°C)	Saturated vapour pressure at 20 °C (kPa)	Blood gas solubility coefficient	Oil gas solubility coefficient	MAC (%) in dogs	MAC (%) in cats
Halothane	50.2	32	2.4	224	0.9	1.1
Isoflurane	48.5	33	1.4	99	1.3	1.6
Sevoflurane	58.5	21	0.7	53	2.1–2.3	2.6
Desflurane	23.5	89	0.45	19	7.2	9.8
Nitrous oxide	-90	—	0.47	1.9	>100	>100

The properties of the ideal inhalation anaesthetic include:
- non-irritant to mucous membranes
- minimal effects on cardiovascular and respiratory function
- low blood gas solubility: rapid uptake and elimination
- minimal metabolism
- non-toxic
- non-flammable and chemically stable
- easily vaporised
- good analgesia and muscle relaxation
- minimal environmental effects.

As with all drugs administered, there are dose dependant side effects whenever the dose (percentage) of inhalant anaesthetic delivery is increased.

Main Drugs Options

The main inhalational anaesthetic agents are listed below. There are some variations in availability of the drugs and in the marketing authorisations even between brands in the same country. For example, some brands of isoflurane include birds or horses in the licence, whereas others do not.

> The up to date information on licencing should be checked in the country in which the veterinary nurse is practicing.
> - Isoflurane: cats, dogs, some variations.
> - Sevoflurane: dogs and cats.
> - Desflurane: no veterinary product licences.
> - Halothane: no longer commercially available in Europe or the USA.
> - Nitrous oxide.
> - Ether, methoxyflurane, cyclopropane: historical use.

Isoflurane, sevoflurane, desflurane, halothane and nitrous oxide are greenhouse gases and have a negative effect on the environment.

Nitrous oxide and desflurane have the potential to have the worst environmental impact, and for this reason, many veterinary practices are phasing out the use of nitrous oxide. This also reduces the likelihood of desflurane obtaining a veterinary marketing authorisation as its use is currently off licence.

Isoflurane
Isoflurane is widely used in veterinary practice. It is a halogenated ethyl methyl ether which is presented without a preservative. There are some variations of the MAC depending on the species it is being used in, but typically it is reported to be between **1.3–1.6%**.

Dose dependant side effects include varying degrees of **hypotension due to myocardial depression (contractility) and peripheral vasodilation.** Hypoventilation due to respiratory depression may be seen in small animal anaesthesia and may be profound in horses. It also causes bronchodilation.

Isoflurane is excreted directly from the lungs during expiration, with only 0.2% metabolised by the liver. It has a low blood gas solubility coefficient of 1.4, which produces a rapid induction and a quick recovery from anaesthesia. The blood gas solubility coefficient describes how soluble a gas is in the blood.

It is irritant to mucous membranes and is not recommended as an induction inhalant. There are no analgesic properties in isoflurane.

Sevoflurane
Sevoflurane is also widely used in veterinary practice and is a polyfluorinated isopropyl methyl ether which is presented without a preservative. There are some variations of the MAC depending on the species it is being used in, but typically it is reported **between 2.1–2.6%**.

Dose dependant side effects include varying degrees of hypotension due to myocardial depression (contractility) and peripheral vasodilation. It may have less effects on cerebral blood flow than other inhalational anaesthetics and is sometimes referred to as being neuroprotective.

Sevoflurane is excreted directly from the lungs during expiration, but there is about 2–5% that is metabolised by the liver. **It reacts with soda lime** to produce the haloalkene Compound A. This is nephrotoxic in rats though clinically does not appear to be a concern in domestic species. A **minimum flow of 500–1000 ml/min** is recommended if using a circle system to limit accumulation.

Sevoflurane has a low blood gas solubility coefficient of 0.7, which produces an even more **rapid induction and a quicker recovery** from anaesthesia than isoflurane. If a gas is less soluble then it does not dissolve as readily in blood, therefore it moves quickly from the lungs to the tissues and does not linger in the blood.

It is **not irritant to mucous membranes** and therefore in the very few instances where inhalation induction is required, sevoflurane could be considered. There are no analgesic properties in sevoflurane.

Desflurane

Desflurane is a fluorinated ethyl methyl ether. The reported MAC of desflurane is **between 7.6–9.8%,** and only 0.02% is metabolised by the liver.

It requires a **special vaporiser** as the boiling point is close to room temperature making it difficult to vaporise safely. Although it has a very low blood gas coefficient of 0.45, it is irritant to mucous membranes and can **cause airway hyperreactivity.**

Hypotension from desflurane is typically associated with a decrease in myocardial contractility. It has minimal effect on the respiratory system. **Sympathetic storms** have also been reported with its use in human medicine, with two cases reported in horses. A sympathetic storm is an increase in heart rate and arterial blood pressure due to an increase of sympathetic tone and activity of the renin angiotensin system.

Halothane

Halothane is a halogenated hydrocarbon which requires a preservative (0.01% thymol) as it is unstable in the presence of light. Although now almost obsolete, halothane revolutionised anaesthesia in both people and animals and there are more publications relating to its use than for any other drug.

The MAC of halothane has been reported as **0.8–1.1%** in dogs and cats with a blood gas coefficient of 2.5, the most soluble of all the inhalants mentioned in this chapter.

Hypotension is common due to myocardial contractility depression, and it also sensitises the heart to catecholamine induced arrhythmias. Halothane has also been associated with **hepatitis** in humans, however it is not convincingly documented in animals. It has no analgesic properties.

Nitrous Oxide

Nitrous oxide (N_2O) is manufactured by heating ammonium nitrate to 250 °C. It is stored as a liquid in cylinders and administered as a gas. Its MAC is greater than 100% so it cannot be used as a sole anaesthetic agent. N_2O has analgesic effects so is used to supplement other anaesthetics. It has a blood gas coefficient similar to desflurane.

It is not commonly used in general practice due to the use of other analgesics, and the negative impact on the environment. There are however some specific considerations with its use:

Case Selection
Nitrous oxide is very insoluble and **diffuses into air filled cavities in the body.** Therefore, it should be avoided in animals with (or at risk of developing) pneumothorax and air embolism. Since it is administered concurrently with oxygen it reduces the inspired fraction of oxygen so should also be avoided in animals that are predisposed to hypoxia.

Concentration and Second Gas Effect
Nitrous oxide is administered in high concentrations (>50%) and this, combined with the low blood gas solubility means that it is rapidly taken up from the alveolus during induction of anaesthesia (making the alveoli smaller), this increases the partial pressure (and therefore concentration) of the inhalation agent in the alveolus (e.g. sevoflurane/isoflurane), which enhances uptake of the inhalation agent, speeding up induction of anaesthesia.

Diffusion Hypoxia
At the end of anaesthesia when N_2O administration is stopped, the low blood gas solubility coefficient means that it rapidly enters the alveoli from the blood and dilutes the alveolar gases (likely room air during recovery) and this can lead to hypoxia. This explains why supplemental oxygen is administered for five minutes after N_2O is turned off at the end of anaesthesia.

Actual values are for reference, although explain the effects which are seen clinically (e.g. halothane has a higher blood gas solubility than sevoflurane or isoflurane, which means uptake and elimination are slower with halothane).

Maintenance of Anaesthesia

Physiological Effects of Inhalational Anaesthesia

The options for maintenance of anaesthesia include **inhalation anaesthesia** (via facemask or endotracheal intubation), or **injectable anaesthesia** (IM, IV, or infusion).

Anaesthetic equipment, facilities and monitoring equipment are required when delivering inhalational anaesthesia maintenance. These are common in small animal practice, however their use may be difficult or unavailable in field situations, although some mobile sets of equipment are available.

The advantage of inhalational anaesthetics (isoflurane, sevoflurane) is that it is relatively easy to adjust the depth of anaesthesia and they can be administered for long procedures without side effects (such as toxicities or prolonged recoveries). Recovery from volatile agent anaesthesia is primarily dependent on exhalation rather than metabolism.

However, atmospheric pollution is a concern, especially when it is difficult to scavenge the waste anaesthetic gases, and they also have profound physiological effects on the patient. One of the most common negative physiological effects and changes seen during inhalational anaesthesia is hypotension, respiratory depression, and cerebral metabolism. It is important to minimise the percentage of inhalant anaesthetic used during anaesthesia to reduce these dose dependant negative side effects. This can be achieved by:
- **careful planning** of anaesthetic protocols for individual animals. Using appropriate premedication and administering intravenous induction agents;
- incorporating **robust analgesic protocols** into the plan for anaesthesia;
- **monitoring depth of anaesthesia** closely and adjusting the vaporiser setting as appropriate to ensure depth of anaesthesia is adequate though not excessive;
- considering administration of additional analgesia or neuromuscular blocking drugs if high percentages of inhalational agent are required either in response to nociception or to produce muscle relaxation for surgery;
- considering the use of partial intravenous anaesthesia to supplement the inhalational anaesthetic agent in appropriate cases.

Hypotension

Hypotension is defined as a Mean Arterial Pressure (MAP) of <60 mmHg where tissue perfusion and oxygen delivery to tissues becomes compromised. Measurement of arterial blood pressure during anaesthesia is recommended so that hypotension can be identified and managed.

The preoperative preparation of patients predicted to be vulnerable to hypotension during anaesthesia should be considered, and the animal's physiological status optimised before attempting anaesthesia. Preexisting hypovolaemia or dehydration can compound anaesthetic induced hypotension. Additionally, sevoflurane, and isoflurane contribute to hypotension by decreasing cardiac output (via myocardial depression) and decreasing systemic vascular resistance (vasodilation).

It is worth noting that renal or hepatic blood flow can be reduced by hypotension, increasing the risk of acute kidney injury and/or prolonging the recovery from anaesthesia.

Respiratory Depression

As with some of the injectable anaesthetic agents, inhalational anaesthetic agents can result in some respiratory depression. Monitoring the respiratory system during anaesthesia is important. In addition to visual monitoring of the reservoir bag and thoracic wall movements, capnography is useful to determine the degree of hypoventilation. Intermittent positive pressure ventilation (IPPV) may be indicated in some cases to maintain the end tidal carbon dioxide between 35–45 mmHg. Pulse oximetry should also be monitored.

Cerebral Perfusion

Isoflurane and sevoflurane **decrease cerebral metabolism** and therefore oxygen consumption though cerebral vasodilation, resulting in an increase in cerebral blood flow. For this reason, care should be taken in animals with neurological disease. If an inhalation agent is planned to maintain anaesthesia, it should be taken into consideration that cerebral perfusion may be better maintained with sevoflurane. However, other parts of anaesthetic management which will be discussed in subsequent chapters are arguably more important and have more of an impact than deciding whether to use isoflurane or sevoflurane.

Other Considerations

Successful anaesthesia relies on more than drug selection. **An individual plan** is important, which takes a holistic view and is based on the findings of the preoperative clinical exam. It is also important to be adaptable and **respond to the patient's changing needs** during anaesthesia and to **anticipate problems.** Situational awareness and excellent patient monitoring are important skills for the veterinary nurse.

Ocular Lubrication

Many of the drugs used during anaesthesia and perioperatively **reduce tear formation,** and during anaesthesia and the recovery period blinking may be reduced. **The patient's eyes are therefore vulnerable to desiccation and ulcer formation.** Bland ophthalmic ointment should be applied regularly during anaesthesia and also postoperatively, preferably with a product with a long corneal duration time. Tear production can be reduced for up to 36 hours after anaesthesia, therefore dispensation of eye lubrication for the owner to take home with the patient (e.g. in brachycephalic breeds) should be considered. Cats receiving opioids for analgesia should have lubricant applied regularly whilst hospitalised.

Positioning

Careful positioning minimises the potential for muscle or nerve damage during anaesthesia. It can also reduce postoperative pain since many animals which are anaesthetised have degenerative joint disease.

There is scope to optimise ventilation during anaesthesia through careful positioning. For example, by adopting a head up tilt to the table in animals with increased intraabdominal pressure (e.g. pregnant or ascitic animals). Conversely, it is easy to compromise ventilation through pressure on the thorax or abdomen caused by positioning.

Thermoregulation

Hypothermia is common in animals under general anaesthesia or sedation. Patients should have their **temperature monitored during the entire anaesthesia period and in recovery,** until they are normothermic. **Small patients are particularly susceptible to hypothermia** due to their high surface area to volume ratio, as are those with a low metabolic rate (e.g. hypothyroid dogs).

Moderate perioperative hypothermia (36.49–34.0 °C) is tolerated by healthy animals, but in sick patients it can result in increased morbidity and mortality.

Hypothermia can lead to:
- **reduced anaesthetic requirement:** with each 1 °C decrease in body temperature the MAC of volatile anaesthetic agents decreases by 5%;
- shivering can significantly increase oxygen requirements: this should be considered in the recovery phase as **supplemental oxygen** may be required;
- bradycardia that is often not responsive to antimuscarinics (like atropine and glycopyrrolate);
- cardiac arrythmias: there is an increased risk of atrial fibrillation at about 30 °C, ventricular fibrillation and death occur at temperatures between 24 °C and 28 °C;
- **impaired coagulation and wound healing,** which impact surgical procedures;
- decreased enzyme activity which can slow hepatic biotransformation of drugs and **prolong their duration of action;**
- decreased renal plasma flow which can **affect drug excretion and fluid balance.**

Hypothermia can be minimised by:
- minimal clipping and avoiding excessive wetting of an animal during skin preparation
- heat pads, hot water circulating blankets, and hot air blankets; care should be taken not to burn the animal's skin
- warm environmental temperature
- insulating the animal with booties and blankets
- warm IV and irrigation fluids
- heat and moisture exchanger or rebreathing systems.

Animals suffering from hypothermia and shock should be warmed very carefully, with active methods of **warming stopped at 37 °C.** Warming peripheral tissues may result in vasodilation which worsens hypotension, so attention to fluid balance and appropriate fluid therapy is important.

REFERENCES

- Brodbelt, D.C., Blissitt, K.J., Hammond, R.A., Neath, P.J., Young, L.E., Pfeiffer, D.U. and Wood, J.L. (2008) The risk of death: the confidential enquiry into perioperative small animal fatalities. *Veterinary anaesthesia and analgesia*, 35(5), pp.365–373.

Self-assessment

Test

Answers on page 60

1. You do the preanaesthetic examination of a 6-month-old Dwarf Lop Rabbit who is scheduled to be neutered. The owner reports that he is in good health and his physical examination is normal. What ASA category would you assign?
   a. I.
   b. I E.
   c. II.
   d. II E.

2. How long should adult, healthy dogs be fasted for (food only) before anaesthesia?
   a. 1–2 hours.
   b. 4–6 hours.
   c. 8–10 hours.
   d. 12–16 hours.

3. Which route of drug administration results in the most rapid rise in plasma concentrations?
   a. Intravenous.
   b. Oral.
   c. Subcutaneous.
   d. Transdermal.

4. When describing an analgesic as very potent what does this mean?
   a. The magnitude of effect is large.
   b. A small dose is required to produce the effect.
   c. The drug is unsafe.
   d. The drug enhances the effects of other drugs.

5. You are monitoring an anaesthetic and the cat is mildly hypotensive. You believe that this is, in part, due to α-1 adrenoreceptor blockade and vasodilation caused by the sedative in the premedication. What drug is most likely to have been administered to produce this effect?
   a. Acepromazine.
   b. Diazepam.
   c. Dexmedetomidine.
   d. Ketamine.

6. What is the principal excitatory neurotransmitter in the vertebrate central nervous system that acts on NMDA receptors?
   a. Acetylcholine.
   b. Adrenaline.
   c. Glutamate.
   d. γ-aminobutyric acid (GABA).

7. Which receptor does propofol and alfaxalone act on to produce their effects?
   a. γ-aminobutyric acid (GABA).
   b. N-methyl-D-aspartate (NMDA).
   c. α-2 adrenoreceptors.
   d. Metabotropic glutamate receptors.

8. Which injectable anaesthetic agent may contribute to analgesic protocols?
   a. Alfaxalone.
   b. Ketamine.
   c. Thiopental.
   d. Propofol.

9. Which combination of factors (alveolar ventilation, blood gas partition coefficient, cardiac output) will result in the fastest onset of action when using an inhalant anaesthetic agent?
   a. High alveolar ventilation, high blood gas partition coefficient, high cardiac output.
   b. High alveolar ventilation, low blood gas partition coefficient, high cardiac output.
   c. Low alveolar ventilation, high blood gas partition coefficient, low cardiac output.
   d. High alveolar ventilation, low blood gas partition coefficient, low cardiac output.

10. What effects does hypothermia have on inhalant anaesthetic requirements and metabolism of drugs?
    a. Increase inhalant anaesthetic requirements and increase rate of metabolism of drugs.
    b. Decrease inhalant anaesthetic requirements and decrease rate of metabolism of drugs.
    c. Increase inhalant anaesthetic requirements and decrease rate of metabolism of drugs.
    d. Decrease inhalant anaesthetic requirements and increase rate of metabolism of drugs.

Notes

Self-assessment

CORRECT ANSWERS:

1. a
2. b
3. a
4. b
5. a
6. c
7. a
8. b
9. d
10. b

Notes

CPR and Emergencies

Pamela Murison

> **Chapter Summary:**
> - How to identify common complications in anaesthesia.
> - Causes and treatment of respiratory and cardiac arrest.
> - How to manage an arrest, basic cardiopulmonary resuscitation, ventilation and artificial circulation.

Introduction

When complications occur during anaesthesia, early recognition and a confident, appropriate response undoubtedly improve the chances of a successful outcome. This chapter covers how to reduce the risk of respiratory or cardiac arrest, and what to do should cardiopulmonary resuscitation be required.

Respiratory Arrest

The dictionary definition of a **respiratory arrest is a sudden complete cessation of respiratory movement.**

Although the definition of apnoea (absence of respiration) is similar to that of respiratory arrest, the difference is that in **apnoea regaining respiration is expected, but in an arrest respiration is unlikely to spontaneously resolve.**

Although it might seem obvious to identify if an animal is not breathing, very small tidal volumes and very inefficient breaths are difficult to see. However, it should be remembered that **if the respiratory function is ineffective then intervention is required, regardless of whether this is truly respiratory arrest.**

Another point to consider is **agonal gasping.** Agonal gasps are produced by a brainstem reflex and should not be mistaken for true respiration. In agonal gasps, there is a jerking movement, which can be dramatic. The mouth is open wide and the movement vigorous enough to move the body, however there is little if any actual gas passage into the lungs.

The following should be observed:
- **movement in the ribcage/abdomen/both:** it is important not to be distracted by jaw or limb movement; and
- **airflow through the nose:** or bag movement on the breathing system during anaesthesia.

Cardiac Arrest

Cardiac arrest is defined as a sudden and often unexpected stoppage of effective heart action.

A key point here is the word effective as there may be some heart activity (e.g. electrical activity in the myocardium) but if this is not effective at pumping blood around the body, it is classed as an arrest.

Although the definition states **sudden and often unexpected** this varies considerably between individual situations. Some arrests are preceded by events which indicate an arrest is imminent, giving a potential opportunity to act and prevent the arrest from occurring.

> In cardiac arrest, there are a number of signs which may help **identify an arrest has occurred:**
> - no heart sounds
> - ECG shows asystole or arrhythmia (e.g. ventricular fibrillation)
> - no palpable pulse
> - absence of breathing or agonal gasps
> - blood at surgical site looks thick, dark, and is not flowing freely
> - mucous membranes are dull, grey-white or blueish
> - prolonged capillary refill time (>2 seconds)
> - no cranial nerve reflexes
> - eye central with a dilated pupil
> - dry cornea.

Many of these signs do not appear instantly after an arrest, e.g. mucous membrane colour takes time to change (depending on the cause of the arrest). It can be difficult to differentiate between a stopped heart and poor circulation. **Use of an ECG helps** show the electrical activity of the heart but **does**

not indicate output. Sometimes if the circulating volume is poor, the heart can be working but have nothing to pump, this inevitably leads to an arrest unless the circulatory problem is detected and treated.

The presence or absence of reflexes and the eye (e.g. pupil size and responsiveness) is also useful to differentiate between arrest and a severely collapsed circulatory status.

Causes of Arrest

Causes of **respiratory arrest** are numerous and many seem obvious.
- **Excessive anaesthetic drugs:** cause apnoea and possibly arrest.
- **Airway obstruction:** initially the animal attempts to ventilate but later this develops into an arrest.
- **Muscle fatigue:** may lead to arrest, related to a disease process in the animal causing weakness or excessive effort causing normal muscles to weaken.

Cardiac arrest may follow respiratory arrest (causes above) or occur simultaneously. Other causes include extreme pH changes, electrolyte imbalances, other toxaemias, and extreme changes in temperature.

- **Excessive drug administration**/other toxicity:
    - When pentobarbital (or other drugs) is given for euthanasia, this causes cardiac arrest due to excessive drug administration; hence arrest can also occur through inadvertent anaesthetic overdose. Although not usually thought of as toxins, essentially this is what drugs are. Other poisons can also cause arrest, directly or indirectly via some other mechanisms.
- **Prevention of adequate respiration:**
    - Cardiac arrest may be preceded by respiratory arrest if ventilation/respiration is not corrected adequately. The various ways that respiration may be compromised are discussed in the emergencies section, as treatment at this stage may prevent development to cardiac arrest. Cardiac arrest ensues as the heart/brain receive inadequate oxygen.
- **Hypovolaemia:**
    - Technically many arrests are due to a failure in adequate amounts of oxygenated blood reaching the heart itself. One of the main reasons for this in animals is severe hypotension where blood pressure is inadequate to collect oxygen from the lungs and then to circulate around the body, delivering oxygen to the tissues including the heart/brain. In cases with loss of blood volume (e.g. in haemorrhage) then there is also a lack of red blood cells to carry oxygen to the tissues. Poor circulation and blood pressure are discussed in the emergencies sections.
- Other causes
    - Temperature extremes (profound hyperthermia or hypothermia) lead to arrest.
    - Extremes of pH (acidic or alkaline) also lead to arrest. The pH change with carbon dioxide accumulation is another reason why respiratory arrest may lead to cardiac arrest.

Survival after Cardiac Arrest and Resuscitation

Although more is now known about resuscitation than years ago, the chances of success remain slim. Kass and Haskins published a report on survival after CPR in dogs and cats. Although old, this paper (from 1992) is still relevant. In this retrospective study, the authors reported **only 28% of dogs and 42% cats were successfully resuscitated.** This figure refers to initial (short term) success. However, in the longer term, only five dogs and one cat were alive three days after CPR and only four dogs plus one cat discharged from the hospital (out of 135 dogs and 43 cats in total).

There are many reasons for the difference in figures between the initial success and final outcome. If the animal had a poor prognosis long term, owners may have opted for euthanasia; however many of the animals in this study died within three hours of the initial resuscitation. Of particular note is that all of the animals who successfully left the hospital had arrests associated with drug use (e.g. anaesthesia). This is a relevant factor when deciding how long to continue with resuscitation attempts.

In a more recent study from 2009, Hofmeister et al. reported an initial success rate with CPR of 35% in dogs, 44% in cats. However, the survival to discharge from the hospital was much lower, only 6% of animals overall. Like the previous older study, the authors found arrest associated with anaesthesia was more likely to have a successful outcome.

Despite improved guidelines and recommendations for CPR, more recent reports of survival rates to hospital discharge remain unchanged in dogs (7%) but may be somewhat improved in cats (Hoehne et al., 2019).

There are many reasons why arrest associated with anaesthesia is more likely to be successful as it is correctable:
- when an adequate circulation is maintained, the drug is distributed to the liver where it can be eliminated;
- an anaesthetic associated reduction in body temperature may be protective to the brain; and

— an endotracheal tube in situ and an intravenous cannula reduce the delay to starting resuscitation, with fewer interruptions or problems in providing efficient CPR. There is good evidence that delays to commencing CPR (and interruptions to the resuscitation) decreases survival rates.

Whatever the cause for arrest, **success is unlikely unless the reason for the arrest is corrected.** So, an animal which arrests due to the effects of an invasive tumour affecting respiration (for example) is much less likely to have a positive long-term outcome.

It is important staff have a realistic view of the likelihood of success. Staff should not feel like failures, but rather celebrate the rare success. Good communication with clients is needed to ensure reasonable expectations.

Arrests may be preceded by accidents or emergencies, so before discussing the treatment, it is relevant to look at prevention of arrest by considering how to treat accidents and emergencies.

Accidents and Emergencies

An anaesthetic emergency is a situation which puts the animal's life at serious risk; this may be a series of smaller complications or one big event. **Incidents** are events which could cause severe risk to staff or patient, and **an accident** is such an incident which could have been avoided. This section looks at accidents and emergency situations affecting the animal (rather than staff).

Whilst key causes of emergencies are often respiratory or cardiovascular, it is important to consider other incidents and problems such as ocular, nerve compression, arrhythmias, and delayed recovery.

Respiratory Complications

Respiratory complications include apnoea (or respiratory arrest), respiratory obstruction, or hypoventilation.

Mechanisms of Ventilation

As the **diaphragm muscle contracts,** this causes it to flatten, which pushes abdominal contents caudally and is seen as an **outward movement of the abdomen.** The intercostal muscles contract, pulling **the ribs up and out.** These movements create a **subatmospheric pressure within the thoracic cavity,** which causes air to be drawn into the trachea and lungs. In a normal situation (in mammals), **expiration is a passive process** whereby relaxation of the muscles causes the restoration of normal positioning of rib/diaphragm, causing gas to be exhaled and the volume of the lung to decrease. When there is a failure of these mechanisms the animal may not be able to breathe or have severely impaired breathing.

The phrenic nerve supplies the diaphragm. Although the diaphragm is a strong muscle which is rarely affected by disease processes, it is possible for diaphragmatic function to become impaired, e.g. in cervical spinal disease which may affect ventilation. This is potentially a very serious condition.

The **intercostal muscles** are weaker than the diaphragm. The function of the intercostals and rib cage movement is affected by disease processes affecting the muscle and/or the nerves.

The initiating signal to start a breath comes from the **brain stem** and is not usually a conscious activity. Various factors influence the brain signals to the muscles affecting ventilation. The main physiological signal to take a breath is usually **build-up of carbon dioxide,** which is detected by chemoreceptors in the blood. This indicates to the brain that a breath is required.

Apnoea may arise as a sudden event or due to progressively poorer ventilation.

> Respiratory complications or failure which lead to arrest are broadly characterised into **five groups:**
> - ventilatory drive
> - mechanical ability to breath
> - obstruction (upper/lower airway)
> - restriction
> - absorption of oxygen.

Ventilatory Drive

If an animal has reduced carbon dioxide in the body, there is reduced drive to breathe.

Hyperventilation reduces body CO_2; this may be iatrogenic e.g. overenthusiastic ventilation to treat postinduction apnoea. Sometimes the hyperventilation is associated with stress, and carbon dioxide being eliminated (blown off) prior to anaesthetic induction and then contributing to postinduction apnoea.

Some **drugs affect the brain's sensitivity** to increasing CO_2, for example opioids cause the animal to allow more carbon dioxide to accumulate before signalling to breathe, which is known as an increased tolerance to carbon dioxide.

Hypothermia reduces the drive to breathe (but also has many other effects in the body).

Physical Ability to Take a Breath

Interference with the nervous system or muscles, may affect the ability of the animal to achieve movement of muscles from the brain signal.

The **phrenic nerve** originates from the cervical vertebrae. Cervical spinal damage may damage the phrenic outflow and affect ventilation. This is serious.

Spinal damage more caudally in the spinal column may affect intercostal nerves, however the animal is more likely to cope with this.

Muscular disease or neuromuscular disease may affect the function of the ribcage by affecting the strength of the muscles controlling rib movement.

Obstruction (upper airway)

Upper respiratory tract (URT) obstruction is commonly seen around anaesthesia in veterinary species, especially dogs.

Brachycephalic dog breeds have multiple reasons for airway obstruction such as narrow nares, a long soft palate, and everted laryngeal saccules. Although the presence of an endotracheal tube abolishes the URT obstruction, **obstruction is common during induction or at recovery after extubation.**

It is important to remember that brachycephalic breeds may have a narrower airway and the trachea may be more difficult to intubate. A range of tubes should be available as well as a good laryngoscope to help visualisation.

Other causes of URT obstruction include:
- **Pharyngeal tissue/tongue:** relaxation of the pharynx and tongue causes partial obstruction, especially in sedated dogs or during recovery from anaesthesia. The presence of a thick tongue increases obstruction, so pulling the tongue forward can help.
- **Head position:** often related to relaxation of pharyngeal tissue, a flexed head position increases the likelihood of obstruction in recovery, due to the poorer airflow.
- **Bandaging:** head and neck bandaging can cause severe obstruction. Extreme care should be taken when bandaging around the head and neck.
- **Congestion:** nasal turbinate congestion reduces airflow through the nasal passages; this can happen when the head is positioned lower than the body for a prolonged period of time. Gravity causes blood and fluid to accumulate. Drips of clear fluid from the nares can be an indication of congestion.
- **Inflammation/swelling:** if there is swelling of any part of the airway (e.g. larynx) this impedes airflow and causes obstruction. Inflammation and swelling is most likely when there has been trauma. This could be related to surgery e.g. of the larynx/palate or unintentional trauma e.g. rough intubation. Both can cause damage to the mucous membranes and lead to postoperative swelling.
- **Laryngeal paralysis:** in this medical condition, there is damage to the nerve(s) controlling the opening of the glottis in the larynx, which results in a passive larynx causing obstruction (which becomes more dramatic when there is significant negative pressure drawing the edges of the glottis together). Often, this condition is known to be present before anaesthesia, however in rare situations it could develop during anaesthesia and only become apparent postoperatively in recovery. On laryngeal examination, there is no active opening of the larynx, with a distinctive stridor sound associated with breathing before intubation.
- **Other causes** of upper airway obstruction. Tumours, blood clots etc., which can cause airway obstruction.
- **Endotracheal tube obstruction:** endotracheal tubes become obstructed by material such as blood clots, foreign material e.g. tape, respiratory secretions, overuse of lubricant gels (especially in small tubes). Dried material is particularly difficult to detect, as it can produce a flap which is not easy to remove with suction.
Endotracheal tubes can also be obstructed by partial or complete kinking e.g. when the head is flexed. The degree of kinking depends on the degree of flexion and also on the type of material, with some materials (e.g. red rubber) more likely to kink.

Upper Airway Complications

When checking for upper airway obstruction, respiratory sounds (especially before/after intubation), respiratory pattern, and alterations in the capnogram (when under anaesthesia) should be considered.

The sounds made by breathing past partial upper airway obstruction are quite distinctive and useful when identifying the location of the obstruction. It is helpful to distinguish between **stertor** (caused by pharyngeal/nasal obstructions) and **stridor** (more likely to be a laryngeal obstruction). Stertor is a typical snoring type of noise. Stridor is a wheeze coming from the URT rather than the thorax.

> **No sound at all can indicate total obstruction.**
> **If ventilation is noisy, there is some air flow. If there is no sound at all, there could be total obstruction.**

During airway obstruction, **paradoxical ventilation (or paradoxical breathing)** is common. This is where the normal mechanical means to inflate the lungs are employed: the diaphragm contracts and a subatmospheric pressure is created in the thorax. However, due to airway obstruction it is not possible to draw air in to fill the lungs (which normally helps to push the ribcage outwards). Instead, **the negative pressure causes the rib cage to be sucked in on inspiration.** Close observations show **the abdomen moving out on inspiration, and the thorax moving in.** It is important to be aware that these movements can happen with a complete obstruction, with no air entry to the lungs.

Treatment

Treatment of airway obstruction depends on the timing and situation.
- **Pull tongue out:** this is a useful technique when monitoring animals in recovery and helps encourage the dog to breathe through the mouth (important in nasal obstruction), as well as removing bulk from the pharyngeal area.
- **Straighten neck position:** a flexed neck tends to cramp space in the pharyngeal airway and increase turbulent gas flow. Straightening the head and neck position allows a better airway. During anaesthesia, straightening minimises chances of ETT kinking and also of the tube bevel being occluded e.g. pressing against the tracheal mucosa.
- **Remove cause if possible:** remove bandages that are restricting the airway and any foreign material.
- **Suction:** suction is particularly useful for clearing liquid and secretions from the airway, but sometimes if there is a dry crust of material it is possible to push a flap aside (which then returns to cause an obstruction when the suction catheter is removed).
- **Intubate:** if the animal cannot maintain its own airway then one should be provided, usually by intubation. If the trachea is already intubated, replacement of the endotracheal tube may be needed (if there is an obstruction which cannot be cleared using suction). If intubation is not possible, bypassing the upper airway surgically may be necessary, using a tracheostomy tube. As a temporary measure, oxygen should be supplied using narrow tubing (e.g. dog urinary catheter connected to oxygen) through the larynx or even a needle or IV catheter inserted between the tracheal rings to supply oxygen below an obstruction (this is an emergency procedure and transtracheal oxygen should rarely be needed).

ADDITIONAL TREATMENTS
If there is airway swelling, the veterinary surgeon may prescribe steroids. Drugs such as dexamethasone are effective at reducing swelling and improving the airway, but do not act instantly.

- Some conditions may require surgery, e.g. laryngeal paralysis.
- Supplying supplementary oxygen is useful to prevent hypoxaemia (e.g. by mask, nasal prongs or nasal catheter).

> Delivering oxygen to a dog e.g. by mask, is only effective if the dog is breathing and the oxygen can get into the lungs.

- **Sedation** is useful for animals, particularly if they are stressed. A stressed or excited animal has a sharp inspiratory pattern. This large negative pressure tends to draw soft tissue inwards and make any dynamic obstruction (i.e. a moving obstruction rather than a fixed foreign body etc.) worse. As the animal is sedated it slows the rate of inspiration, reducing dynamic obstruction and also reducing turbulent gas flow, which is less effective. A **calm environment** also helps. **Excessive sedation is not helpful in cases of respiratory obstruction,** particularly if it increases relaxation of tissues or reduces the ability of the animal to manage its own airway.
- Many animals with airway obstruction are **hyperthermic**. If possible (without causing distress), the animal's temperature should be taken and cooling mechanisms e.g. fans provided.

Lower Airway Complications

Lower Airway Obstruction

Narrowing of lower airways can occur as a result of bronchoconstriction, e.g. in response to manipulation of the airways (e.g. during bronchoscopy) or disease processes. One relatively common situation is **feline asthma**. Although this is not quite the same as in people, there are some similarities. Affected cats have narrowed lower airways (bronchioles etc.). **This can appear to affect expiration as much if not more than inspiration,** resulting in what is known as gas trapping. **Gas trapping is where there is residual gas after a normal expiration, which remains in the lungs.**

Recognising Lower Airway Narrowing

- **Capnogram:** a typical bronchoconstriction capnogram has a curved upstroke, showing there is a delayed exhalation of alveolar carbon dioxide. (Figure 1).

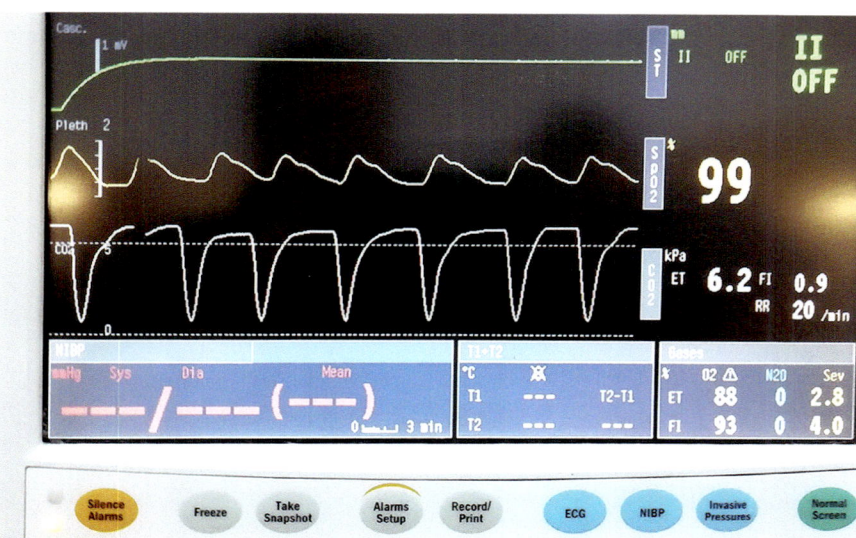

Figure 1. Bronchoconstriction capnogram.

- **Resistance on the bag:** narrowed airways mean it is more difficult to expand/allow lungs to deflate when artificially manipulated. This translates as the bag on an anaesthetic machine feeling tighter and a higher pressure being needed. It is important to be aware that other causes could also give a tighter feel e.g. endobronchial intubation.
- **Lower tidal volume:** this may be measurable with the appropriate equipment or suspected e.g. from smaller movements of the reservoir bag during anaesthesia or a less distinct difference between the volume of the thorax at inspiration and expirations.
- **Oxygen saturation:** oxygen saturation is affected by many factors, one of which is lower airway narrowing.

Treatment of Lower Airway Narrowing

Suspected airway narrowing should be reported immediately to the veterinary surgeon. It may be possible to avoid/reduce a stimulus to the airways to constrict (e.g. remove a bronchoscope temporarily). Most volatile anaesthetics produce a little bronchodilation. There are medical treatments available, e.g. terbutaline, however these may be difficult to administer or can have dramatic side effects, and so should be used with care.
- **Lung restriction:** lungs may fail to inflate due to restriction which prevents full expansion; this may be external to the thorax or internal.
  a) **Simple external restrictions:** for example, restraint aids where sandbags are squeezed onto the thorax or a restrictive fibreglass cradle. Using warm fluid bags for patient warmth can cause a problem if these press on the body and restrict thoracic movement. During surgery, a surgical assistant leaning on the thorax (e.g. when holding a retractor in place) can cause a marked limitation to thoracic expansion. The animal is likely to have a reduced tidal volume and become hypercapnic.
  b) **Abdominal distension:** a large, tense abdomen reduces the ability of the diaphragm to push backwards, restricting tidal volume. This presents as a rapid respiratory rate (to compensate) but the ventilatory pattern is inefficient. There may problems with uptake of volatile anaesthetic, resulting in a light plane of anaesthesia, ineffective elimination of carbon dioxide (seen as a larger carbon dioxide value when a large manual breath administered), and potentially hypoxaemia due to ineffective, small tidal volumes.
  It is important to be alert for distension developing during anaesthesia (e.g. if the stomach is inflated during endoscopy). This should be brought to the attention of the vet, who may recommend passing a stomach tube.

Internal Lung Restriction

Lung restriction within the thorax can also recur. Examples include **pneumothorax or haemothorax,** where air or blood respectively are in the pleural space outside the lung, this restricts the ability of the lungs to expand.

Diaphragmatic rupture affects the ability to move gas (as the diaphragm is non-functional), and also restricts lung movement if abdominal contents enter the thorax. In most cases this is identified before anaesthesia, but rarely an animal may have a chronic condition which was previously undiagnosed.

Recognising internal lung restrictive conditions:
- small tidal volume: should be assessed by watching bag movements;
- respiratory pattern: alterations in rate may indicate an attempt to compensate;
- reduced SpO_2 especially in marked restriction, however a mild restriction may not produce hypoxaemia if the animal is breathing 100% oxygen during anaesthesia. It may be more significant at recovery when the animal breathes air;
- diagnostics e.g. radiography, to identify changes within the thorax.

Treatment of internal lung restriction requires veterinary intervention, such as chest drainage. A one-off drainage in an emergency can be done using an IV cannula with a three-way tap and syringe. For longer term management, chest drain placement is required. These are acts of veterinary surgery and should be performed by a veterinary surgeon under current UK legislation, as they enter a body cavity.

Other Causes of Respiratory Complications

Equipment

An **empty reservoir bag** can cause a change in respiratory pattern and lead to lung trauma and pneumothorax. There is also other equipment related causes of problems, e.g. hypercapnia when soda lime is exhausted or by faulty valves.

Inadvertent intubation of one bronchus, means the animal is only breathing through one lung. The tidal volume is reduced, and oxygen saturation may be decreased (though in healthy lungs may not be hypoxaemic).

This is identified by auscultating both sides of the thorax; if one side sounds dull this may indicate it is not being aerated. If undecided, a radiograph should be taken to confirm the position of the end of the tube.

Lung Disease

Alveolar pathology causing thickening of the structures causes a reduction in oxygen take-up, and hence lower oxygen saturation. This is likely to be due to preexisting respiratory disease rather than developing during anaesthesia, but an important exception is if **pulmonary oedema develops during anaesthesia,** which is related to fluid overload. In this situation fluid accumulates elsewhere, such as chemosis (swelling of eyelids) or facial oedema. It can be confirmed with radiography and treatment includes diuretics to reduce pulmonary oedema. Intermittent positive pressure ventilation ensures good lung inflation and may reduce the formation of pulmonary oedema or even correct it due to positive pressure within the lung.

It is wise to provide supplementary oxygen to patients in recovery, with lung disease or pulmonary oedema. Although the animal may maintain reasonable oxygen saturation when breathing 100% oxygen during anaesthesia, difficulty is anticipated when transferring to air (21% oxygen). As respiratory function improves during the recovery period, the oxygen supplement may be discontinued.

Hypoxaemia

Normal oxygen saturation is above 95% and it is definitely of concern if levels fall below 90%; however, this is a non-specific sign and it should be remembered that for many ventilatory abnormalities, (see below) the oxygen saturation remains normal. Lung disease, causing decreased oxygen absorption into the blood, is a common reason for a low SpO_2 during anaesthesia.

Hypercapnia

Hypercapnia is when end-tidal carbon dioxide is greater than the normal value of approximately 40 mmHg (5.3 kPa). Minor elevations are not unusual during anaesthesia and not too concerning, although investigation and possibly instigating preventative measures to halt progression may be warranted. **Hypercapnia is of most concern when greater than approximately 60 mmHg (8 kPa) and definitely when above 70 mmHg (9.3 kPa).**

Hypercapnia has widespread effects in the body and the response is complicated. A small to moderate increase in carbon dioxide increases sympathetic stimulation (increasing heart rate, blood pressure, etc.) whereas a greater increase in hypercapnia produces vasodilation and decreasing blood pressure, with reddening of the mucous membranes and deepening anaesthesia.

Hypercapnia increases the likelihood of other, potentially dangerous, abnormalities such as cardiac dysrhythmias (e.g. ventricular premature complexes) and alters the pH of the blood. In extreme cases it is a genuine emergency, with risk of seizure activity and cardiac arrest, however this is uncommon, with most occurrences of hypercapnia being mild to moderate.

CAUSES OF HYPERCAPNIA
Hypercapnia is usually caused by hypoventilation, where the minute volume of the animal is too low to eliminate the carbon dioxide produced in the body.

There are several causes of hypoventilation:
- **Depth of anaesthesia:** deepening anaesthesia causes increasing depression of the ventilatory centres, which means minute ventilation decreases.
- **Drug induced:** drugs such as opioids, decrease the sensitivity of the respiratory centres in the brain to increasing carbon dioxide, so the body tolerates rising carbon dioxide more than usual. The respiratory rate is likely to decrease, during anaesthesia this may be partly associated with the depth of anaesthesia as more drug is given. This occurs particularly when opioids e.g. fentanyl, are given during anaesthesia.
- **Physical limitations:** if the animal cannot effectively expand its thorax/abdomen to breathe, it fails to eliminate adequate carbon dioxide. An example is when using restraining aids e.g. a rigid cradle or cross-tying limbs.
- **Rebreathing:** rebreathing is where there is a significant inhaled fraction of carbon dioxide, so over time the body carbon dioxide increases (Figure 2). It is abnormal to have any significant amount of carbon dioxide in the inspired gas during anaesthesia. This is usually equipment related:
    - if using a non-rebreathing system, e.g. a Bain, inadequate gas flow and inadequate elimination means carbon dioxide rebreathing will occur;
    - if using a circle breathing system, rebreathing is related to exhausted soda lime or faulty one-way valves allowing reinhalation of expired gases which contain carbon dioxide; or
    - rebreathing can be identified on the capnogram, as the baseline does not return to zero.

The appearance of the animal is different with rebreathing associated hypercapnia rather than hypoventilation hypercapnia. The animal takes very large tidal volumes with an increasing respiratory rate in an attempt to eliminate carbon dioxide (this is not seen in hypoventilation). Indeed, these movements can look dramatic and mimic light anaesthesia (although without other changes such as with jaw tone, with palpebral reflexes etc.).

Correction of rebreathing is dependent on the cause.

Hypocapnia

Hypocapnia is where end-tidal carbon dioxide is abnormally low (e.g. <30 mmHg or 4 kPa), and is fairly unusual. **The causes are related to hyperventilation** e.g. with light anaesthesia, or iatrogenic if the lungs are overventilated during anaesthesia.

Low carbon dioxide affects vessel diameter and perfusion, and body pH. Although a moderate decrease is not too harmful, excessive or prolonged hypocapnia is undesirable.

However, an important aspect to be aware of is **a sudden drop in end-tidal carbon** dioxide as this is significant and may warn of an impending cardiac arrest. It indicates a sudden change in the circulation, which is no longer delivering blood (and hence carbon dioxide) to the lungs. Causes include massive haemorrhage or something preventing blood flow return to the heart, but if seen it is important to notify the other members of the team and thoroughly investigate.

Hypotension

Blood pressure is widely measured during anaesthesia and values that are markedly different from normal can indicate risk for the animal. Blood pressure may be abnormally low (hypotension) or abnormally high (hypertension). **Hypotension is an abnormally low blood pressure,** often taken to be a mean arterial pressure less than 60 mmHg or a systolic arterial pressure under 80 mmHg.

Hypotension is a specific definition of abnormally low blood pressure. A decreasing trend of blood pressure or a value which is somewhat lower than normal does not necessarily indicate hypotension.

Hypotension is important as it governs organ and tissue perfusion, and oxygen delivery to those tissues. The blood pressure is the force pushing the blood around the circulation.

Blood pressure is not the only factor controlling perfusion and oxygen delivery. If there is marked vasoconstriction, high blood pressure may be present but perfusion to peripheral tissues is poor.

SIGNS OF HYPOTENSION
Low blood pressure is <60 mmHg mean arterial pressure

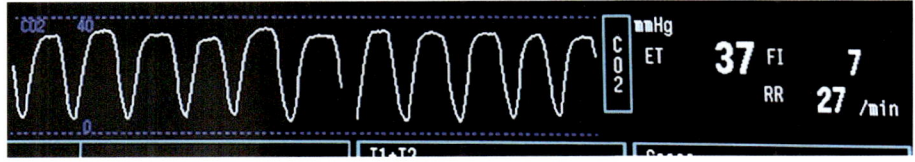

Figure 2. Rebreathing capnogram.

(MAP), or 80 mmHg systolic arterial pressure (SAP). If measuring using Doppler, the SAP value should be used, if oscillometric measurement is used, MAP should be used.

- **Pulse:** how obvious the pulse is depending on many factors, such as presence of vasoconstriction and the difference between systolic/diastolic pressures. A normal, full artery feels firm and tubular, and in hypotension feels softer and less turgid. Evaluation of how much pressure is required to occlude the vessel (preventing a palpable pulse) is helpful. In most cases, a femoral pulse does not feel poor until hypotension is very serious.
- **Slow capillary refill time (>2 seconds):** indicates poor peripheral perfusion, with hypotension likely to be a factor.
- **End-tidal carbon dioxide:** a sudden drop of end-tidal CO_2 can indicate a severe circulatory problem, as carbon dioxide is not being transported to the lungs. This is a useful indicator when there is an intraoperative problem.
- **Urinary output** is related to renal perfusion, if a urinary catheter is in place then this can be useful.
- The presence of **factors known to lead to hypotension** (e.g. preexisting dehydration or observed haemorrhage) should increase the level of suspicion.

CAUSES OF HYPOTENSION

The main causes of hypotension can be classified as hypovolaemia, low cardiac output, and systemic vasodilation.

Hypovolaemia

Hypovolaemia means a low circulating blood volume. This can occur for a variety of reasons, the most obvious being **haemorrhage** where the circulating volume is decreased due to the loss of blood.

However this is not the only cause. **Dehydration** can also cause a decrease in circulating volume. Water loss may be pure water loss (e.g. a dog in a hot car, absence of water) or losses of water and electrolytes (e.g. vomiting, diarrhoea). Water is lost from all compartments of the body, so there is a decrease in systemic circulating volume but water is also lost from the tissues, causing other signs e.g. skin tent, sunken eyes etc.

Ideally, hydration deficits should be corrected before anaesthesia (see Chapter 5 fluid therapy). In emergencies, deficits may not be fully corrected before anaesthesia and so become relevant.

In haemorrhage, there is loss of volume from the circulation. It should be borne in mind that **initially after an acute haemorrhage, the packed cell volume is unchanged.** In time, fluid shifts replace volume, so the PCV decreases as remaining cells become diluted. Over an even longer period of time there will be cells added to replace the cells lost.

Compensatory Mechanisms

The body compensates for losses in the circulatory volume. **Vasoconstriction** occurs and the **heart rate increases** to increase cardiac output. There is a limit to the ability to compensate.

Recognising Volume Depletion

Signs of dehydration include **skin tenting and sunken eyes.** In volume depletion due to haemorrhage, visible blood loss may be apparent or there may be a history consistent with haemorrhage. It is important to be aware of **internal blood losses,** for example, blood lost into the space around a femoral fracture, or into the abdomen due to rupture of a splenic haemangiosarcoma. Although the blood is not lost from the body as a whole, it is no longer within the circulation so hypovolaemia is present.

Patient history can provide clues to different causes of hypotension, so this should be used along with observations under anaesthesia to determine the best course of corrective action.

Treatment of Hypovolaemia

Generally, a deficit which **developed slowly is replaced slowly** (e.g. gradual losses with diarrhoea) and one which **develops quickly needs rapid replacement** (e.g. sudden significant haemorrhage). Ideally, the type of fluid lost is replaced as closely as possible.

Crystalloids e.g. 0.9% saline or Hartmann's solution, are good choices to replace water and electrolytes. The fluids only remain within the circulation for a short period of time and then distribute throughout the fluid compartments of the body to replace losses.

In most cases, **hypotonic fluids,** such as 5% glucose or 0.18% saline, are **not suitable to treat hypotension.**

Colloids contain larger molecules which stay within the circulatory space for a longer period than crystalloids. This is beneficial to support the circulatory volume for longer and in cases where there is hypovolaemia but without dehydration affecting other fluid compartments. Although colloids are more restricted in availability in the UK now, most practices can obtain Gelofusin, a gelatine based colloid.

Blood products can be used, especially to treat haemorrhage. Common blood products are packed red cells and whole blood. Banked packed red cells are available in the UK and several other countries. Remember these help with oxygen carrying capacity but often do not provide clotting factors (depending on the time since they were taken and storage). Other blood products such as fresh frozen plasma are used in some situations.

It is important to think about what needs to be replaced. As a rough guide, a 10% of blood volume loss should be replaced with crystalloids, 10–20% with colloids, and over 20% with blood products (however this is only an approximate guide). An animal with a low PCV before the haemorrhage may need transfusion earlier, whilst a healthy young animal may cope without blood products even after a large haemorrhage.

Low Cardiac Output
Cardiac output is the product of heart rate and stroke volume. If the heart rate is decreased, this significantly affects output and causes lower the blood pressure.

The **stroke volume** is the amount of blood ejected each time the heart contracts. Poor filling of the heart or poor contraction of the muscle cause poor output. In most cases, poor contractility is related to cardiac disease, which is beyond the scope of this chapter. The heart fails to fill effectively when there is severe volume depletion, but there are other possibilities.

Poor filling of the heart can be related to **factors affecting flow of blood in the vena cava,** for example pressure of a large tumour on the caudal vena cava or twisting of a blood vessel causing occlusion, e.g. during surgical manipulation of the liver. In these examples this may develop suddenly or start during surgery and pose a risk to life. Extreme abdominal gas distension can also press on the vena cava.

The surgeon should be alerted to the problem so they can try moving their hands/instruments. If large abdominal structures are reducing cardiac output when the animal is put into dorsal recumbency, efforts to clip/prepare as much as possible in lateral recumbency should be made to minimise the time in dorsal recumbency. **The animal should be tilted ever so slightly off vertical,** as this may be enough to move the pressure off the vena cava and improve venous return.

Vasodilation
Vasodilation is an important reason for hypotension, produced with modern volatile anaesthetic agents. In vasodilation, the mucous membranes appear redder (as there is more blood present in the peripheral tissues) and diastolic blood pressure readings may be low.

Response to Hypotension
Ideally, treatment targets the cause, where possible. In mild cases, the depth of anaesthesia should be checked and **decreasing the isoflurane** delivered often corrects mild hypotension. Large amounts of **circulating carbon dioxide** cause vasodilation and lower blood pressure too, so checking ventilation may help.

A **fluid bolus** is often a good first level response after checking depth of anaesthesia. In cases of vasodilation, this helps to fill the space to increase the blood pressure. Approximately 10 ml/kg of crystalloid fluid over 10 minutes is a good rate for most dogs, perhaps 5 ml/kg for cats. **Caution is warranted in cats which are more easily overloaded,** and fluid boluses avoided if disease processes (such as hypertrophic cardiomyopathy) make this inappropriate.

Unless it is confirmed that hypovolaemia is the cause of hypotension, repeating fluid boluses if no beneficial response is seen, may not be helpful. Alternatives should be considered and the cause of hypotension evaluated.

If there is a lack of response to simple measures, drugs may be prescribed to help.

Drugs Used to Treat Hypotension
- **Parasympatholytics:** atropine or glycopyrrolate is used but **only** if the hypotension is associated with a bradycardia. These drugs block the parasympathetic input to the heart, which tends to slow the heart down (and therefore increase heart rate).
    - Suggested doses: 0.02–0.04 mg/kg IV atropine or 5–10 µg/kg IV glycopyrrolate.
- **Ephedrine:** ephedrine is an unusual drug. It causes release of endogenous stores of catecholamines. It is useful and can be given as a bolus, unlike many of the drugs listed here. However, it is less likely to be effective if endogenous stores of drug have been exhausted (e.g. in sick animals, where the condition has been ongoing for some time).
    - Suggested dose: 0.1–0.2 mg/kg IV.
- **Dopamine:** dopamine acts on cardiac β-adrenoreceptors to increase cardiac output, but its effects are also different with different dose rates, so it can be difficult to predict its action precisely. Lower doses actually cause vasodilation and may not increase blood pressure, medium doses increase cardiac output, larger doses cause some vasoconstriction. Individual animals may respond differently.
    - Suggested dose: 2–15 µg/kg/minute IV.
- **Dobutamine:** this is the best choice to increase contraction of the heart, if it is suspected as the cause of hypotension (although poor contractility is not common in dogs and cats). It acts on β-adrenoreceptors.
    - Suggested dose: 1–5 µg/kg/minute IV.
- **Noradrenaline:** noradrenaline produces vasoconstriction via α-adrenoreceptor action, and also has some β-effects. It is used in intensive care to support blood pressure. It is useful in vasodilated animals, e.g. in sepsis.
    - Suggested dose: 0.05–0.4 µg/kg/minute IV.
- **Phenylephrine:** phenylephrine acts on α-adrenoreceptors to produce vasoconstriction. It can have a profound effect and may cause a decrease in heart rate due to a reflex response to the increasing systemic vascular resistance. It is not used as commonly as the other drugs listed here.

Hypertension

The definition of hypertension is an abnormally high blood pressure, >100–120 mmHg mean arterial pressure. If the excessive blood pressure is caused by vasoconstriction, this also results in poor tissue perfusion. Prolonged hypertension is damaging to organs, e.g. the retina.

Causes of high blood pressure include:
 – nociception/pain and inadequate analgesia
 – carbon dioxide
 – inadequate depth of anaesthesia
 – increased intracranial pressure.

Hypertension is associated with chronic renal diseases or endocrinopathies, but treatment of these is out with the scope of this chapter.

The main focus of treatment is to identify and eliminate the cause of hypertension. A good starting point is to **check the depth of anaesthesia** and increase if required. If depth of anaesthesia is adequate this suggests another cause. **More analgesia** may be required particularly if an association with a surgical stimulus is identified. It is useful to determine heart rate, as a high heart rate may indicate depth of anaesthesia or inadequate analgesia as the cause; whilst bradycardia could suggest elevated intracranial pressure. Hypoventilation increasing carbon dioxide may increase blood pressure. In persistent severe hypertension, a vasodilating drug could be used.

Arrhythmias

Arrhythmias are abnormalities of the heart rate or rhythm, and can result from heart disease or arise due to anaesthesia. For the latter, it is important to identify the cause, since removal of the inciting cause may correct the problem without further treatment.

Heart rate and rhythm disturbances are of concern as they affect cardiac output and blood pressure. Some arrhythmias precede more serious rhythm disturbances, and possibly even arrest.

Tachycardia

Tachycardia is an excessively elevated heart rate, usually considered to be >180 bpm in the dog, >200–210 bpm in the cat. It is important to differentiate between an elevated heart rate or an increasing heart rate and tachycardia. In a true tachycardia other concerns arise, not just the change in heart rate.

As the heart rate increases, the cardiac work increases. The energy required by the heart and its oxygen usage increases with the muscle activity as the heart contracts more frequently. However, **the heart is a unique muscle in the body; it cannot rest.**

The heart muscle itself (myocardium) is supplied by the coronary vessels. These vessels are vital to provide the myocardium with a constant supply of oxygen and glucose etc. However, the **coronary vessels can only deliver oxygen to the heart during diastole.** During systole, when the heart is contracting, the vessels are compressed and no blood can flow through them. This results in an intermittent supply of oxygen to the heart muscle, which has little inactive time.

As the heart rate increases, the duration of systole decreases to an extent but there is a limit to how much this phase can shorten: the heart needs a certain amount of time to contract. This means that an increased heart rate disproportionately affects diastolic time, the gap between heart beats becoming reduced.

Therefore, the time in diastole shortens. However, as oxygen delivery to the heart can only happen in diastole, a situation with increased cardiac work and increased oxygen demand occurs, but there is a reduced ability to deliver oxygen to the heart muscle itself. This means the heart develops an oxygen deficit known as **myocardial hypoxia.** This is a local effect and can occur even if the animal is not systemically hypoxic, as it refers to a lack of oxygen relative to the needs of the heart muscle.

In myocardial hypoxia changes occur in the ST segment of the ECG. Either the trace does not return to the same level as the baseline (known as ST segment depression) or slurring/coving occur where there is a curved part between the S and T waves. (Figure 3)

It is important that ST changes are not overinterpreted. In people, these are quite diagnostic e.g. for coronary heart disease and used in exercise testing. However animals often have more variation in their normal ECG. If seen from the start of the anaesthetic, this may be normal for this individual, however if ST segments are normal then become depressed e.g. in tachycardia, this is significant as a change in that animal.

Myocardial hypoxia can increase the risks of developing serious arrhythmias.

There is another reason to be wary of very high heart rates. Cardiac filling can only happen in diastole; this is when blood fills the ventricle ahead of the next contraction. **Shortened time in diastole limits the time for filling,** so the amount of blood pushed out per contraction (the stroke volume) decreases.

Causes of Tachycardia
 – **Sympathetic stimulation:** likely to be due to inadequate depth of anaesthesia or inadequate analgesia. On rare occasions caused by excessive use of sympathomimetic or parasympatholytics drugs.

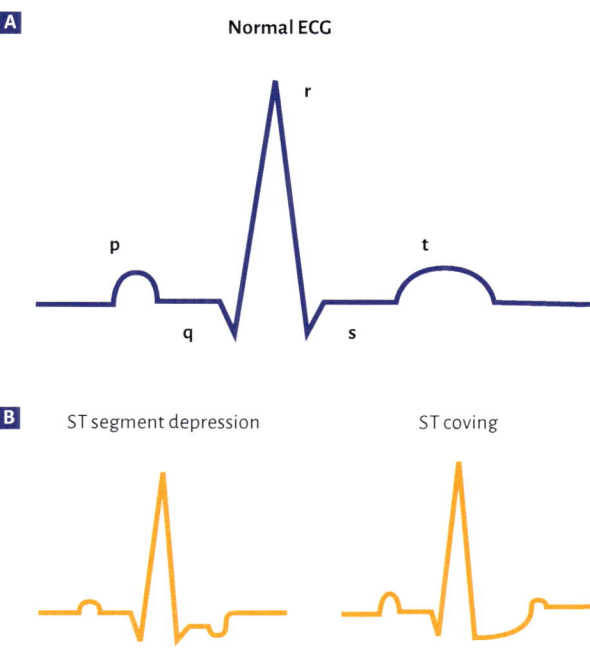

Figure 3. **A.** Normal ECG with ST segment level with baseline; **B.** Changes in ST segment which may be seen in myocardial hypoxia.

> **Action in tachycardia:**
>
> - **Depth of anaesthesia** should be checked and increased if appropriate.
> - Does stage of surgery imply nociception/**inadequate analgesia?** Simple factors which may help should be considered, e.g. if the position of the animal might be causing pain (arthritic joints).
> - **Blood pressure and CO_2** should be measured, if possible, to help distinguish causes.
> - A **fluid bolus** is a useful response if there is low blood pressure or sometimes if there is a relatively normal blood pressure despite a high heart rate, and the animal requires the fast heart rate to maintain blood pressure.
> - Checks for **myocardial or systemic hypoxia** should be carried out.
> - Oxygen supply should be ensured, as **supplementing oxygen** may be beneficial if the animal is in recovery and adequate ventilation should be ensured.

- **Hypercapnia:** can increase the heart rate, although often needs the addition of other factors to produce a genuine tachycardia, rather than just an increased heart rate.
- **Hypovolaemia/hypotension:** a high heart rate may be a response to increase cardiac output to compensate for other factors decreasing blood pressure. Care should be taken not to decrease the heart too much in these cases, but instead respond to the hypovolaemia.
- **Hypoxia:** can cause an increased heart rate in an effort to increase blood supply to the lungs, picking up oxygen and to deliver oxygen to tissues.
- **Hyperglycaemia** has been quoted as a cause of tachycardia, however tachycardia is not always seen.

A rapid onset full agonist opioid e.g. fentanyl, may be helpful as it brings down the heart rate directly and improves analgesia. The actions listed above will regain control in most situations, but **β-blocker drugs** (e.g. esmolol) can be used to reduce the rate in a persistent tachycardia.

Bradycardia

Bradycardia (excessively low heart rate) is defined as under about 60 bpm for a dog, or under about 100–110 bpm for a cat. However, interpretation of heart rate is somewhat situation dependent.

It is helpful to check the blood pressure. A dog/cat who received an α-2 agonist may have a low heart rate but a normal/high blood pressure, and this is of less concern than if it was also hypotensive (except in elevated intracranial pressure, see later).

Cardiac output = rate x stroke volume

If the heart rate decreases, there may be an increase in stroke volume but cardiac output falls overall. This is likely to cause a decrease in blood pressure and perfusion throughout the body.

CAUSES OF BRADYCARDIA
There are many factors which may be associated with bradycardia:
- drugs
- hypoxia
- electrolyte abnormalities
- vagal stimulation
- hypothermia
- hypoglycaemia
- Cushing's reflex in raised intracranial pressure.

Depth of Anaesthesia
Heart rate tends to decrease with increasing depth of anaesthesia. This may not become a true bradycardia, but may be significant when combined with other factors listed below.

Drugs

Several types of drugs associated with anaesthesia cause a decreased heart rate, which may become bradycardia. Examples include **opioids, especially mu-agonist opioids.** α-2 agonists used for sedation also produce marked decreases of heart rate.

Electrolyte Abnormalities

Hyperkalaemia in particular causes a bradycardia, which causes distinctive T wave changes (often described as spikey). (Figure 4).

This type of bradycardia is treated by correcting the electrolyte abnormality. In minor cases, fluid therapy with **glucose supplemented fluids** may be enough to correct hyperkalaemia (glucose encourages the uptake of potassium into cells). More severe cases benefit from **insulin administration alongside the glucose,** again to encourage cellular uptake of potassium. With serious, life threatening arrhythmias associated with hyperkalaemia, calcium reduces the effect of the ions on the myocardium, although this is rarely required.

Conditions linked to hyperkalaemia include urinary obstruction or urinary rupture, in particular. Ideally, it is sensible to correct, or at least reduce, potassium levels before anaesthesia.

Hyperkalaemia occasionally develops in previously healthy animals (and people) when under anaesthesia; this is particularly recognised in **Greyhounds**. Although the mechanism of this is uncertain, effects of drug administration associated with anaesthesia and shifts of ions in the body are likely to be the cause. If a suspicious ECG is seen, it is worth checking electrolyte levels.

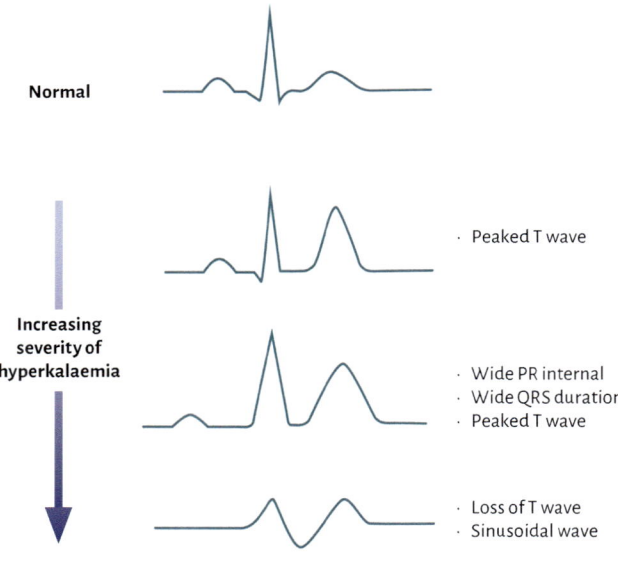

Figure 4. ECG with bradycardia/hyperkalaemia.

Vagal Stimulation or Vagally Mediated Reflexes

The vagus nerve carries parasympathetic nerve fibres to the heart. **Stimulating the vagus nerve increases parasympathetic outflow, which decreases heart rate.** Essentially virtually all situations which cause a decreased heart rate have vagal stimulation, but the terms are usually used to refer to a specific response.

Certain types of stimulation produce a marked vagal response (vagally mediated reflexes). A classic one is the **oculocardiac reflex** where pressure on the eye or traction can cause a significant heart rate decrease. Alternatively, bradycardia is seen with visceral tractions (e.g. ovary or testis), an increased heart rate is more common, but the reverse is also possible.

The vagus nerve may increase its discharge rate (sending more signals to the heart) when handled/stimulated directly. The vagus nerve runs through the neck, and an example of direct stimulation is where surgical retractors in the neck pull on the nerve itself. This causes a massive stimulation of the nerve and a dramatic decrease in heart rate, even to the point of cardiac arrest.

Hypothermia

Hypothermia promotes a decreased heart rate, with the cold effectively slowing everything down. It is also notable that a bradycardia with hypothermia is less responsive to treatments.

Hypoglycaemia

Hypoglycaemic animals may present with bradycardia, so it is worth checking glucose, particularly if hypotension is not responding to treatment as expected.

Raised Intracranial Pressure (Cushing's reflex)

When animals have brain pathology, such as a tumour, the intracranial pressure (ICP) may become elevated.

In a conscious animal, signs of increasing ICP include alterations of behaviour, nausea et.c. Under anaesthesia, those signs are not seen. Changes in the appearance of the optic disc under ophthalmic examination have been reported, but the reliability of this has been questioned.

When monitoring anaesthesia, an elevation in intracranial pressure can lead to a Cushing's triad of signs (also known as **Cushing's reflex**):
- decreased heart rate
- increased blood pressure
- irregular respiratory pattern.

Care should be taken as α-2 agonists can cause similar cardiovascular signs, albeit with different timing. Also if mechanical ventilation is employed, respiratory changes will not be seen.

It is important to take into account the animal's history and the reason for anaesthesia. If there are previous neurological signs, this increases suspicion of raised ICP as the cause.

It is theoretically possible to measure intracranial pressure, but this is not a readily available technique. However, these cases are frequently animals anaesthetised for imaging, for example MRI (for investigation of their neurological signs). This gives the opportunity to see inside the skull, the imaging team can report on visible changes within the brain which may be associated with raised intracranial pressure.

The skull is a rigid structure and cannot swell like other areas of the body with a large increase in ICP. This means the brain gets pushed backwards, towards the start of the spinal canal (the only opening). This may sometimes be termed **coning** as the caudal areas of the brain protrude into the top of the spinal canal. **This is an emergency.** As the brain is pushed backwards into the spinal canal, it becomes compressed and this affects brain function. The location of the pressure means parts such as the respiratory centre are affected, leading to respiratory arrest and death. **Any suspected signs should be reported immediately.**

Hypoxia

Whether hypoxia causes increases or decreases of heart rate **depends on the severity of the hypoxia and duration of the problem.** A mild or short term hypoxia is likely to cause an increase in heart rate, once the hypoxia worsens or is longer lived, there is more direct depression of function and resultant bradycardia.

> ### Actions in bradycardia:
>
> - The **ECG** should be checked to confirm if it is sinus bradycardia (a slow heart rate of normal complexes) or another arrhythmia. If an ECG is not available, the regularity of the heart rate/pulse should be examined.
> - **Blood pressure should be checked:** identifying hypotension, normotension, or hypertension are helpful in distinguishing causes.
> - **History:** is there any history to lead to suspicions towards certain causes, e.g. ocular surgery, neurological signs, or urinary obstruction.

A low heart rate but with suitable blood pressure and no suspicion of any other abnormalities may be tolerable, particularly if the cause is known (e.g. after α-2 agonists). If there are other abnormalities (most usually linked with hypotension) then this is more likely to warrant treatment.

The mainstay in **treating bradycardias is the use of anticholinergics e.g. atropine or glycopyrrolate.** The veterinary surgeon may prescribe these to bring the heart rate up quickly, atropine takes effect more quickly than glycopyrrolate.

Atropine sometimes causes an initial decrease in heart rate or produces second degree atrioventricular block (see below) immediately after administration and may produce a temporary high heart rate later. These changes are short-lived. If the heart rate decreases or atrioventricular block is marked, it may be appropriate to give more anticholinergic, depending on the dose and time since first administration. Glycopyrrolate is said to have less of these effects than atropine, however it can occur with glycopyrrolate too.

In animals that received **α-2 agonists, care should be taken with anticholinergics.** There is a risk the heart rate increases whilst there is vasoconstriction from the α-2 effect. One option is to antagonise the α-2 first (which may adequately correct heart rate in itself) and only give an anticholinergic after if required.

If the cause of the hypotension is an elevation in intracranial pressure, specific treatment to reduce the pressure is required.

Initially, commencing lung ventilation to reduce carbon dioxide can help (while other treatments are prepared). Slight hypocapnia (e.g. 4 kPa/30 mmHg) should be aimed for if raised ICP is confirmed. In situations where there is a possibility of raised intracranial pressure, ventilation to prevent hypercapnia may be employed without hyperventilation.

The main treatments use solutions with an osmotic effect to reduce the intracranial pressure by drawing fluid away. The most commonly used is **mannitol,** an osmotic diuretic. Doses of 0.5–1 g/kg may be prescribed by the veterinary surgeon. Another option is hypertonic saline, which has similar effects.

Arrhythmias

The Normal ECG

A variety of arrhythmias are seen in dogs and cats, of which those most likely to develop during anaesthesia are discussed in this text.

When evaluating an ECG, it should be ensured there is **good contact** with pads/clips and the skin, and ideally the leads should be in a normal position. If suspicious of an arrhythmia, it is worth pausing any movement (e.g. clipping or preparation) for a clear view without any interference.

Atrioventricular Block

Of the different types of atrioventricular (AV) block, the one most commonly associated with anaesthesia is **second degree AV block** (Figure 5). In this condition, an electrical signal originates at the sinoatrial node, spreads across the atria to produce the P wave on the ECG; but not all of the signals are conducted through the AV node. This means there are P waves visible on the ECG without an associated QRS. The rhythm is irregular, but may appear **regularly irregular** as there are a few beats with a normal rhythm, then a missed beat.

There are two variations of second degree AV block, Mobitz type 1 and Mobitz type 2. In a type 1 block, there is a gradual prolongation of the P-R interval (sometimes known as Wenckebach phenomenon) until one fails to conduct, causing a missed QRS. In type 2 blocks, the P-R interval is consistent.

Atrioventricular blocks can be thought of like bradycardia, related to parasympathetic predominance on the heart, so they are usually **associated with a low heart rate.** The block is commonly seen with apha-2 agonists.

This arrhythmia should be approached the same as a bradycardia; antagonising α-2 agonists should be considered, or treatment with atropine or glycopyrrolate. A small amount of AV blockade may be tolerable if the blood pressure is normal and the complexes are unconducted.

Some blood pressure devices may struggle to achieve a reliable result if the pulse rate is highly irregular. Although second degree is the main type of AV block, it is worth considering differentiation with first degree or third degree blocks.

In first degree AV block (Figure 6), the P-R interval is prolonged. Although it may be suspected from a monitor, strictly speaking diagnosis requires measurements taken from a printed ECG, rather than judging from a screen. The arrhythmia is unlikely to cause any clinical effect on the animal and is not usually treated. It may be worth recording in case of further development later in the animal's life.

In third degree AV block, P waves are visible on the ECG which are regularly spaced, e.g. at a rate of 120/minute. There are also regular QRS complexes at a much slower rate (e.g. 36/minute). Importantly there is **no association between the two.** On close examination, P waves are seen either close to or far from the QRS. Occasionally a P wave appears to be followed by a QRS, however this is merely coincidental. Sometimes a P wave may overlie another wave on the ECG, e.g. the T wave, producing something rather larger and different in shape. The key is identifying the two separate but regular rhythms. (Figure 7).

Atropine may be used as a treatment but is often ineffective. This arrhythmia is often due to cardiac disease and the animal requires **specialist interventions e.g. a pacemaker.**

This condition is likely to be identified prior to anaesthesia or in response to investigation after collapsing episodes, rather than develop during anaesthesia, but is included here to differentiate with second degree block, which is more common and more easily treated.

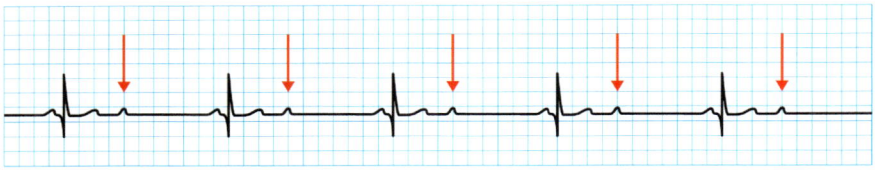

Figure 5. Second degree AV block.

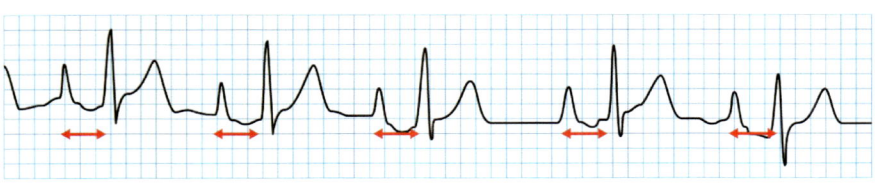

Figure 6. First degree AV block.

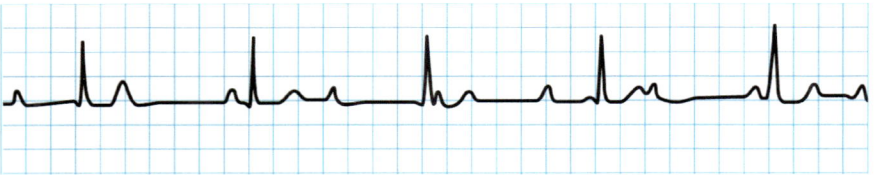

Figure 7. Third degree AV block.

Ventricular Premature Complexes (VPCs)

Figure 8 shows an ECG with some normal complexes with clearly identifiable P, QRS, and T waves; **there is a large and bizarre complex which is the VPC.** The normal shape of the QRS complex is due to the rapid spread of the electrical activity through the specialised conduction channels (rapid spread = narrow width). The VPC is wide, as it does not travel in those specific channels and is a different shape as it is originating in a different place (in the ventricle). This complex clearly arises earlier than expected from intervals between normal complexes. Therefore, it is a **ventricular (originating in the ventricles) premature complex.**

Some people use the term ventricular premature contraction, however as they are not always associated with contraction this can be confusing. The term complex retains the awareness that an electrical signal does not always indicate mechanical activity in the heart.

If a complex which looks like a VPC arises after a long pause (with no electrical activity) rather than earlier than expected, this is what is known as a **ventricular escape complex.** They are a safety mechanism in the absence of a normal complex fired from the usual pacemaker routes. This is quite an important differentiation, because the escape is likely to come with a slower heart rate (or at least long gaps) and these rescue complexes should not be stopped.

CAUSES OF VPCs

VPCs are usually related to sympathetic stimulation so the depth of anaesthesia and analgesia should be checked to ensure it is adequate. They are also more likely to occur with elevated carbon dioxide or with hypoxia.

An occasional VPC is usually of no concern. There are a few situations which would cause more concern, however:
- **Runs:** when several complexes are seen following one another.
- **Polymorphic complexes:** usually all the VPCs are a similar shape. If several different shapes are seen, this is termed polymorphic and is of more concern as it indicates several sources of abnormal electrical activity within the ventricles.
- **Regular patterns,** e.g. one normal/one abnormal/one normal/one abnormal etc. (termed ventricular bigeminy) and this is of a concern.
- **R-on-T phenomen:** if the VPC is so close on top of a previous complex that the T wave is still present when the VPC starts this is known as the R-on-T phenomenon. This is important, as the T wave is associated with repolarisation of the heart. If the membranes/electrolyte movements have not returned to their normal resting stage when a new depolarisation occurs, this can trigger a dangerous arrhythmia e.g. ventricular fibrillation.

A rhythm where every complex is a VPC is termed **ventricular tachycardia.** There is very little space between the complexes and the heart rate is likely to be >180 bpm. In the case of a pattern of ventricular complexes but at a slower rate (e.g. 120–160 bpm) this is termed an **accelerated idioventricular rhythm,** but is of less concern than a ventricular tachycardia due to the recovery time between complexes which permits oxygenation and cardiac filling.

INVESTIGATION WITH VPCs
If VPCs are seen, more information should be sought:
- Is there a pulse for every complex?
- Do all the pulses feel consistent?
- Are they affecting the pulse?
- Is there a lot of sympathetic stimulation, e.g. light anaesthesia, pain, inadequate analgesia?
- Is ventilation (CO_2) and oxygenation adequate?

This is particularly important if there are runs of abnormal complexes. Measuring blood pressure is useful to determine how significant this arrhythmia is in terms of affecting cardiovascular function (bearing in mind some devices struggle with an irregular heartbeat).

TREATMENT OF VPCs
As mentioned above, occasional VPCs do not warrant treatment. If they do need treatment, after normal correction of depth/analgesia/ventilation/supplemental oxygen, the mainstay is **lidocaine.** It can be used with a bolus first (e.g. 1–2 mg/kg) and then followed by an infusion (2–4 mg/kg/hr).

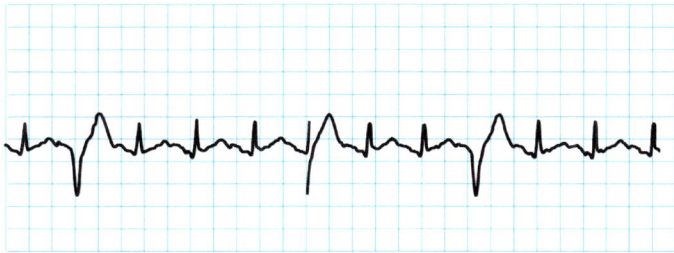

Figure 8. Ventricular premature complexes.

Miscellaneous Accidents and Emergencies

There are a variety of other accidents and emergencies which may occur in the perianaesthetic period, including recovery; some are more serious than others:
- histamine release
- seizures
- delayed recovery
- hypothermia
- hyperthermia
- ocular injuries
- neuropathies
- postoperative blindness in cats
- regurgitation
- perivascular injection
- incorrect drug administration.

Histamine Release

Histamine release occurs for two main reasons:
- **anaphylactic reactions** to drugs (e.g. imaging contrast media) are rare but do occur; and
- **degranulation of a mast cell tumour.**

The histamine has widespread effects on the body:
- skin redness
- urticaria (where multiple small, raised areas of the skin develop, sometimes known as "hives")
- vasodilation and decrease in blood pressure
- elevation of heart rate (in response to the decrease in blood pressure).

The increase in heart rate may be noted first if blood pressure is being measured intermittently.

Histamine release should be suspected if the signs occur shortly after drug administration or manipulation of a suspected mast cell tumour.

Antihistamines are the main treatment, and may be **given pre-emptively to high-risk animals** (e.g. with a mast cell tumour). **Chlorphenamine is commonly used,** but other antihistamines are available. Chlorphenamine and most common antihistamines act to block the H_1 receptor. Histamine acting at this receptor causes the signs listed above. Chlorphenamine may be administered at the time of premedication or IV just after induction of anaesthesia, but it is preferable for the drug to be active before manipulation of any suspected mast cell tumour. Nurses clipping and preparing the site should be aware of the fact that it is a mast cell tumour and treat the mass with appropriate gentle care and not scrub vigorously.

However, histamine may also act at H_2 receptors, particularly in the stomach, associated with ulceration. Specific H_2 receptor antagonists are available, although ranitidine, the most commonly used, was removed from the market due to concerns about a small quantity of a potentially carcinogenic compound being found in ranitidine products. There is evidence that dogs with mast cell tumours may suffer **chronic low grade gastric ulceration,** related to histamine actions at the H_2 receptor. A veterinary licensed H_2 blocker (cimetidine) is available in oral tablet form and could be used for treatment before and/or after procedures. Some veterinary surgeons use alternative medications suitable for gastric ulceration.

If histamine release occurs, apart from antihistamine therapy, treatment is symptomatic. A fluid bolus is a useful early treatment due to the vasodilation produced.

Seizures

Most anaesthetics decrease seizure activity, with the time most likely for seizures to occur being after premedication or in recovery (when drug effects wane). Specific treatment depends on the causes, and treatment in the first instance includes **benzodiazepines IV or rectally.** Propofol infusions may be used for persistent seizures.

General nursing care should be remembered, ensuring neither the animal nor staff are hurt.

Delayed Recovery

There are a number of reasons for a slow recovery from anaesthesia, which are often interrelated.

Hypothermia
This is the **major cause of slow recoveries in small animals.** If an animal is recovering slowly from anaesthesia, their temperature should be checked.

Hypoglycaemia
Hypoglycaemia may occur in expected cases (e.g. **pups/kittens, diabetics**), but also unexpectedly in other patients. So again, it may be useful to check glucose in slow recoveries, e.g. cats.

Electrolyte Disturbances
These have wide ranging effects, possibly including delayed recovery as they may affect circulation and other factors.

Impaired Circulation
Poor circulation affects the delivery of the anaesthetic agent to whichever organ is responsible for its biotransformation or excretion, meaning it is eliminated more slowly.

Nursing Anaesthesia

IMPAIRED VENTILATION
In the case of volatile agents, anaesthetic recovery is related to the circulation delivering the drug to the lungs and the action of the lungs to eliminate the agent. An animal which is not ventilating effectively struggles to eliminate the volatile agents (assuming these were effectively taken up previously).

DRUGS (E.G. OPIOIDS)
Drugs, for example opioids, given close to recovery may slow the recovery. This is not necessarily a problem. **A slow but pain-free recovery is preferable** to an animal recovering quickly, but in pain and distress.

MEDICAL (E.G. HORMONAL)
Poor organ function (e.g. liver) affects the ability of the body to process and eliminate drugs. Hypothyroidism affects general metabolic processes in the body and drug elimination, plus makes hypothermia more likely to develop.

Hypothermia

Hypothermia is defined as a core body temperature less than 37 °C; a normal temperature in a dog is around 38–38.5 °C, so 37 °C is not normal.

Hypothermia causes delayed recovery but is also of concern for other reasons:
- increased risk of arrhythmias or bradycardia
- clotting dysfunction
- affects enzymes
- decreased biotransformation of drugs
- decreased renal blood flow
- left shift of oxyhaemoglobin dissociation curve: this means haemoglobin holds on to the oxygen at lower oxygen partial pressures which affects the ability to oxygenate tissues, however is not something evident clinically.

Action in hypothermia:
- **insulation:** blankets, bubble wrap etc. to retain heat
- **external warming:**
  - heat pads
  - wheaties/microwave pads
  - warm air blower e.g. Bair hugger™, etc.
- internal warming:
  - warm saline lavage of the bladder or enemas to warm a cold animal
- prevention is definitely best as it can be difficult to regain the normal body temperature once lost.

Skin is easily burnt if the dog/cat is unable to move away from the heat source. This is particularly problematic during anaesthesia or in the immediate recovery period. Warming the skin may also cause vasodilation in the area, which increases blood flow to the skin causing a decrease in blood pressure. **Therefore external warming should be used with caution in hypovolaemic or shocked patients.**

Hyperthermia

In general hyperthermia is rarer than hypothermia, as many of the heat producing mechanisms are lost with anaesthesia. When seen, it is often related to warm conditions and dogs with very dense thick coats, e.g. Newfoundlands. **Hyperthermia is dangerous as enzymes may cease to function and body systems become damaged.**

Monitoring temperature during anaesthesia allows early detection of an increasing temperature and instigation of control measures as soon as possible.

Action in hyperthermia:
- **fans** are useful in recovery, but less useful during anaesthesia;
- **cool packs** placed against the skin. Icepacks should be avoided as vasoconstriction can return warm blood to the central compartment and maintain core temperature higher for longer;
- **wetting the skin** for evaporative heat loss is highly effective. Bear in mind any wetting of the coat must actually reach the skin, this can be tricky to do in some very densely coated breeds;
- cool internal lavage, e.g. bladder lavage or enemas are only likely to be considered in extreme cases; and
- high gas flows (under anaesthesia) to allow more respiratory heat loss.

When cooling rapidly, care should be taken not to overshoot the desired temperature.

MALIGNANT HYPERTHERMIA
Malignant hyperthermia (MH) is a very rare cause of an increased body temperature. It is caused by a **genetic mutation** in a very specific part of the muscle. When the condition is triggered (stress can trigger it, but importantly for anaesthetists volatile anaesthetics may do so) **persistent muscle contraction** develops. This is visible as muscle rigidity and poor relaxation during anaesthesia; the ears may appear pulled back on the head or the digits splayed.

This consistent contraction uses more oxygen and produces more CO_2 so another relatively early sign is an **increase in end-tidal CO_2.** Increase in body temperature occurs later in the disease time course.

This is a very rare condition and generally increasing body temperature is more likely to be related to a failure to lose heat, but it is important to be aware of it as a possibility.

If it is suspected, the main aim is to decrease temperature as much as possible, using symptomatic means. If it is necessary to continue anaesthesia, **administration of volatile anaesthetics should be ceased, and anaesthesia continued using injectable drugs** e.g. propofol. An older volatile agent, halothane had a reputation for causing MH but the more modern agents can trigger it too.

Testing for MH includes tests on muscles fibres obtained from biopsies or genetic testing; neither are quick processes. As it is a genetic inherited condition, testing is recommended if a breeder has had a suspected case.

Ocular Injuries

More of an accident rather than necessarily an emergency, this also depends on the severity of the injury. The surface of the cornea is readily damaged with foreign material. Surgical scrub solutions in particular may cause damage to the delicate surface of the eye. During anaesthesia the animal is unable to blink, so **desiccation (drying) of the corneal surface** can develop as there is reduced tear production and a failure to spread the tear film over the cornea. This drying can cause **ulceration and corneal damage.**

Prevention is better than cure, so **ocular lubricant** should be used and care should be taken to protect eyes from spirit and scrub solutions (e.g. using swabs, covering and protecting the eye). Spray bottles of spirit/alcohol cause a widespread distribution which can reach the eye from a surprising distance.

Ocular lubricant can sink over time and still allow damage to occur. It is a good idea to **redistribute the tear film/lubricant when the eye is checked for monitoring** purposes e.g. to check eye position/reflexes, then blink the eye gently by moving the eyelid over the top. This ensures an even distribution of lubricant. If the eyes are not readily accessible during anaesthesia (e.g. in MRI or when covered in drapes) the eyelids should be taped shut.

It is important to ensure there is no contamination of lubricant tubes, as this can spread infection between patients.

Neuropraxis

Neuropraxis is a temporary paralysis which usually recovers after 24–48 hours, caused by pressure on the nerve. An example is where a heavy dog has had limbs extending off the edge of a hard table which presses on the nerve. It can take a remarkably short period of time to develop. There is no real treatment apart from time. Ultimately, this is an accident best avoided with careful patient positioning and padding especially on edges.

Postoperative Blindness in Cats

An unusual condition is when a cat recovers from anaesthesia and over the first few hours of recovery it becomes apparent the cat cannot see. Usually, the vision recovers within 24–48 hours however in rare cases it is permanent.

Although many drug combinations have historically been blamed for this condition, specific drugs are unlikely to be the cause. The blindness occurs after **a period of poor blood flow or oxygenation to the relevant area of the brain.** Blindness may be associated with a cardiac arrest where it is easy to understand how a part of the brain could be starved of oxygen. In other situations, it could be related to marked **hypotension or hypoxaemia** during anaesthesia, although many people report having seen this condition even when monitoring appeared totally normal.

It has been demonstrated that opening the jaw excessively (e.g. with a spring-loaded mouth gag) affects blood flow via the maxillary artery. This occurs in some cats but not in others.

Although not all reported blindness cases have had a gag or **wide opening of the mouth, this is something to avoid.** If extreme opening of the mouth is essential (e.g. for some dental procedures) the time spent with the mouth wide open should be kept to a minimum, with short bursts of open mouth activity then return to actions which can be performed with a more neutral mouth position (e.g. some simple scaling further rostrally).

There is no specific treatment available, a good physiological status should be ensured with blood pressure and oxygenation, and any symptomatic therapy which is warranted.

Vomiting/Regurgitation

Vomiting is an active process, accompanied by retching and muscle contraction. Unlike vomiting, **regurgitation is passive** and the more likely occurrence during anaesthesia. Regurgitation is more likely in some species, and there are reported associations with pain and some procedures. It may be particularly common when there is considerable patient movement (e.g. for radiography/orthopaedic procedures).

The main risk is at induction and recovery, as regurgitated material could be aspirated. This leads to immediate physical obstruction of airways, a bronchoconstrictive and inflammatory response to the acidic nature of stomach contents, and later pneumonia is likely to develop.

The main aim is to prevent aspiration:
- For high risk animals, anaesthesia should be induced with the animal in a sternal position, with the head elevated.

The cuff on the ETT should be checked to ensure it is inflated before the head is lowered. Any stomach contents within the oesophagus are therefore less likely to reach the pharynx.
- If regurgitation occurs during anaesthesia, the head should be positioned downwards to drain, and suction used to remove the stomach contents. If the material is very acidic, flushing the oesophagus should be considered to reduce the acidity.
- Drug treatments such as omeprazole are commonly used. **Omeprazole is best used prior to anaesthesia** to allow it time to work, and this is a good plan for high-risk animals or those known to regurgitate.

Reflux Oesophagitis

In some animals, **stomach contents are released from the stomach and sit in the oesophagus without any visible regurgitation.** The acidic material causes inflammation and discomfort in the oesophagus. The acidic damage leads to scarring over time, which causes a stricture, reducing the ability of the animal to pass food down the oesophagus. This is more likely with abdominal procedures or high abdominal pressure.

Treatment, in the early stages, includes symptomatic treatment to reduce discomfort. If a stricture develops, this can require an endoscopic procedure to dilate the narrow part.

Injection Associated Accidents

Although not discussed here, needle stick injuries and other accidents to personnel are relevant.

Perivascular Injection

Older agents (e.g. thiopental) cause sloughing if injected outside the vein, but most modern agents do not cause such damage. However, a more likely outcome of **perivascular injection is a lack of the desired effects** of the drugs administered. Injection of a saline flush through the cannula before starting the drug administration is advisable. Even if there is failure of action of a sedative or induction agent after confirming a flush, the possibility that a catheter has moved/come out of the vein should be considered.

Incorrect Drug Administration

There are situations where the wrong drug is given to the animal. **Syringes should always be clearly labelled** to reduce the chance of inappropriate administration.

The action taken depends on the drug administered and when, for example if the induction agent was given instead of flush at the start of anaesthesia, continuing to induce anaesthesia is the best option.

If lots of these accidents occur in the practice, the reason should be investigated. It could be related to staff under pressure, short staffing e.g. overnight, or unclear instructions.

Cardiopulmonary Resuscitation

Cardiopulmonary resuscitation is often abbreviated to CPR. Some authors use the term cerebro-cardiopulmonary resuscitation (CCPR, or CPCR) to indicate clearly that the aim is to maintain oxygenation and perfusion of the brain as well. Once a cardiopulmonary arrest (CPA) is identified, CPR should start as soon as possible.

Cardiopulmonary arrest occurs when the heart stops beating and the patient stops breathing. This is either caused by a primary cardiac arrest or by a primary respiratory arrest, which develops to a full cardiopulmonary arrest.

> The process of CPR is broken down into various tasks. Classically these are categorised using the A-B-C mnemonic. These tasks are not necessarily always performed in this order:
> - Airway
> - Breathing
> - Circulation
> - Drugs (defibrillation may also be seen here)
> - ECG/Electrical defibrillation
> - Follow up.

It is important to remember CPR is **unlikely to be successful unless the cause of the arrest is correctable.** For example, in the case of a patient with a large tumour, it may be possible to regain breathing and circulation, however without removal of the original problem, recurring arrest is almost inevitable.

It is important to consider **the extent to which resuscitation is pursued.** It is increasingly common for hospitals, which have busy intensive care units and emergency teams, to ask owners how far they wish to go when the animal is admitted; in the unlikely circumstance the animal suffers a CPA.

This may seem a difficult topic to raise, however recent research shows **owners do value discussions surrounding resuscitation.** It may also mean the owner does not feel pressurised into a decision, as they might do if they receive a phone call at the time of an arrest where there is less time available to make a decision.

Resuscitation can also be broken down into **basic and advanced life support,** with some overlap.

Basic Life Support Tasks

Basic life support is usually taken to encompass **airway-breathing-circulation.**

A = Airway

If there is an airway obstruction, this prevents effective ventilation and oxygenation. Checking the airway involves manual palpation in some instances and **visual examination of the pharynx and larynx.** If the trachea is already intubated, it is important to remember there could be a tube obstruction.

If an airway is required, the first step is **to insert an endotracheal tube or to replace the one present** if there is doubt over patency. ETT position should also be checked, for accidental extubation when moving the patient or oesophageal intubation.

If it is not possible to intubate, oxygen should be supplied via a smaller tube (e.g. dog urinary catheter) passed into the larynx, but in complete obstruction of the upper airway, a tracheostomy could be required.

B = Breathing

After CPA, there will be no breathing movements or alternatively there may be agonal gasping.

CHECKING FOR BREATHING:
- Is there visible thoracic movement? Beware of paradoxical ventilation.
- Is any respiratory movement palpable with a hand gently on the thorax?
- The chest should be auscultated for lung sounds.

Primary respiratory arrest easily leads to a cardiac arrest, therefore ventilation should be provided. The endotracheal tube should be attached to a breathing system connected to 100% oxygen.

If the arrest occurs during anaesthesia, it is important to remember to **turn off the volatile agents and stop any drug infusions.**

If it is not possible to use a breathing system and oxygen, a self-inflating bag (e.g. Ambu) with room air can be used. These bags have a one-way valve preventing reinhalation of expired air. There is a tube to allow oxygen supplementation to the bag, if available. These reinflating bags can be large (human sized); it is important to ensure **lungs of small animals are not overinflated.**

Guidelines for CPR state provision of a tidal volume of 10 ml/kg. However, this is not always useful information, as in many situations it is not possible to measure the tidal volume being administered.

Visible expansion of the lungs should be the aim; the cranial abdomen should just rise to the level of the ribs. Small variations in tidal volume are not important provided there is lung inflation.

It can be difficult to determine degree of thoracic inflation during simultaneous cardiac compressions.

To inflate the lungs the APL valve of the breathing system should be closed, the bag squeezed to the desired inflation levels, and then released, opening the valve as swiftly as possible.

When providing breaths, some people are taught not to close the valve fully. There is logic in this in reducing overinflation or risks during normal ventilation, however it is possible in CPR, when there is considerable thoracic pressure with the cardiac compressions, there may be inadequate lung inflation. The valve should be opened fully as soon as possible, to prevent pressure build up in the lungs. Although specific appropriate breathing systems are recommended for long term ventilation, this is less important during CPR as there is less exhaled carbon dioxide. It is useful to use a high gas flow in case of leaks and losses.

Maintaining positive pressure in the thorax is not helpful to producing circulation as it discourages venous return to the heart. An inspiratory time of approximately one second should be used. The valve should be released, and five seconds allowed for expiration before the next breath. This gives a rate of 10 breaths per minute, allowing time without the positive pressure being applied. A consistent rate should be ensured, without speeding up over time.

> ### C = Circulation
>
> As soon as arrest is suspected, **the presence or absence of circulation should be checked for.** The assessment of circulation should take no longer than 5–10 seconds to complete.
>
> **CHECKING THE CIRCULATION:**
> - pulses
> - apex beat
> - auscultation.
>
> When checking the pulse, a peripheral pulse (such as the dorsal pedal) should be used during anaesthesia to give more information on circulation, however in this case, using the **femoral pulse is more appropriate** for a rapid check of pulse presence/absence. If in doubt, auscultation is useful, but the overall check must be very brief.
>
> Assuming there is no circulation generated by the animal itself, cardiac compression should be used to generate circulation. In basic life support, these are external cardiac compressions. This is where the thorax is compressed to generate some blood flow. There are two different forms of external compressions; **the cardiac pump and thoracic pump techniques.**
>
> A delay in the start of compressions decreases the likelihood of the patient's survival.

CARDIAC PUMP TECHNIQUE
This technique is **appropriate for small dogs (<15 kg), or medium and large breed dogs with narrow chests, such as Greyhounds.** If compressions are provided over the heart area itself, it is known as the cardiac pump:
- the dog should be placed in lateral recumbency;
- the 3rd–6th intercostal space should be located, compressions are performed over the heart (at the site of auscultation/apex beat);
- the hands should be locked together; one over the other or with fingers interlocked;
- straight arms should be used with locked elbows to provide rigidity. It is important to ensure the table is low enough to permit using bodyweight downwards during the compression. If the table height is not adjustable, a small step might be required for some operators. Alternatively, large dogs can be resuscitated on the floor;
- the thorax should be compressed at least one third of its depth;
- the movement should push down over the heart area and release, allowing the rib cage to recover totally to its original position. It is very important there is full recoil of the thorax. With downwards pressure, blood is pushed from the thorax. The recoil allows the vessels to fill again. Without this step, it is not possible to generate an effective circulation;
- a **compression rate of 100–120 per minute** should be aimed for; and
- it can be helpful to perform compressions with the patient's back against the compressor's body. This prevents the dog being pushed off the table.

For **very small animals** (such as a rabbit, cat or very small dog), the same area should be compressed but only **using a thumb and two fingers** on either side of the chest. Using the same rates, at least a third of the depth of the thorax should be compressed, remembering to allow the recoil.

Performing adequate chest compressions is tiring (even on small animals) so personnel should be swapped around to ensure continuing effective compressions.

THORACIC PUMP TECHNIQUE
When choosing which cardiac compressions are most appropriate not only the weight of the dog should be considered, but **the shape of the thorax** too. For large dogs (those over 15 kg) or barrel shaped dogs (like French Bulldogs), a better technique for external cardiac compressions is the thoracic pump method. The exception are very narrow chested dogs such as Greyhounds where the cardiac pump technique is better.

For the thoracic pump, the dog is also in lateral recumbency and compressions are performed at the same rate, similarly compressing the thorax at least 1/3 of depth and allowing complete recoil. **The difference between the two techniques is the focus point of the compression.** In the thoracic pump technique, the highest point of the chest when the dog is in lateral recumbency should be used. This widest portion of the chest is usually dorso-caudal to the heart.

DORSAL POSITION FOR COMPRESSIONS
In some breeds, such as the English Bulldog, compressions can be performed with the dog in dorsal recumbency (the thorax in these dogs is flattened dorsoventrally). The thoracic pump may also work well.

Don't worry too much about which CPR technique to use; the important point is to start compressions quickly and evaluate if they are working. If compressions are not providing a circulation, change the technique.

EVALUATING EFFICACY OF COMPRESSIONS
During cardiac compressions, it is important to **evaluate if they are generating blood circulation.**

Carbon Dioxide on Capnography
- this is the best way to determine if compressions are

generating a circulation. The higher the end tidal CO_2 the better the circulation generated, with a value >15–18 mmHg (2–2.5 kPa) indicating the prognosis is improved; and
- carbon dioxide indicates there is blood circulation, perfusion to tissues for blood to collect carbon dioxide, and then adequate circulation to deliver it to the lungs.

Palpable Pulse
- a femoral artery should be used; and
- as movement of blood around the body is generated, a pulse is felt for each thoracic compression.

Audible Sound When a Doppler Probe is Placed on the Cornea
- a generous application of lubricant gel on the surface of the eye should be used;
- the probe should be applied to the cornea; in most dogs it will remain in position if tucked under the upper eyelid;
- as cardiac compressions are performed, an audible flow sound should be heard;
- this method is controversial, as some authors say this is not indicative of retinal/optic blood flow but related to movement of the aqueous humour in the eye. However, this is an audible indicator for when staff performing compressions are tiring and is helpful when performing CPR with limited numbers of personnel or if end-tidal CO_2 monitoring is not available.

Advanced Life Support

After basic airway, breathing, circulation (using external cardiac massage/compressions) provision, advanced life support includes an alternative to external cardiac compressions and when to use it, monitoring use (particularly to identify arrest rhythms), and the drugs used to treat arrests.

Internal Cardiac Massage

As well as compressing the outside of the thorax to generate cardiac output, it is also possible to enter the thorax and manipulate the heart directly to generate circulation; **this is termed internal cardiac compressions.**

Internal cardiac compressions are best performed by a veterinarian familiar with surgery, preferably thoracic surgery. They are able to enter the thorax more rapidly and with confidence. The nurse's role is supportive, but it is important to understand what is required.

Internal cardiac massage is more technically challenging than external methods, and rather fiddly to perform in small dogs or cats.

Performing Internal Cardiac Massage
- a rapid clip should be performed between the 3–6th intercostal spaces (point of the elbow at 90 degrees);
- during expiration, an incision should be made over the 5th intercostal space;
- rib retractors should be inserted;
- the pleura and pericardium should be opened;
- the ventricles should be milked into the arteries; and
- as the thorax is open, it is very important ventilation is continued.

There is no time for a neat, clean preparation. One strip of the clippers is adequate, perhaps a spray of spirit, but the procedure should not be delayed with a full surgical preparation.

When to Use Internal Compressions
One of the main times internal compressions are used is **during surgery;** if the thorax is already open then this method is essential. It could be considered in large dogs, where external cardiac massage is not producing an effective circulation. It is an important method when the **disease leading to arrest is such that external compressions are not likely to be effective** e.g. if a dog has a pericardial effusion with tamponade (where fluid has accumulated in the pericardial sac and prevents the heart from expanding).

It is worth considering internal massage during abdominal surgery too, depending on the size of the patient, the surgeon may be able to enter the thorax via the diaphragm should an animal arrest. This should allow a very rapid start to compressions with much less delay and risk than trying to turn the animal to lateral recumbency for external compressions.

Using internal compressions is more likely to generate a good circulation during CPR and it is possible to directly evaluate cardiac activity. However, this is a **major procedure and requires considerable aftercare** (e.g. drainage of the thorax, analgesia, monitoring ventilation). Performing internal cardiac compressions in CPR is a major decision and many hospitals do not automatically go to this stage. Suitable surgical kits, rib retractors and a surgeon who can boldly and rapidly open the thorax to gain access need to be available.

Fluids

The approach to fluids in CPR is not the same in every case:
- administration of fluids is part of attempting to maintain the circulation;
- if hypovolaemia contributed to the arrest, rapid intravenous fluids should be provided; and
- administering some fluid (intravenous flushing) helps push drugs from the injection site into the central circulation.

Drugs

How drugs are administered is important, to ensure the drugs reach the target organs. **The most effective route is via jugular injection** (not necessarily via a central line, but given in the large vessel close to the heart), however a peripheral site (e.g. the cephalic vein) is often used. **An appropriate quantity of flush should be used if drugs are injected from a cephalic catheter, in order to reach the heart: 3–5 ml in cats, 5–10 ml in small to medium dogs, 10–15 ml in large and giant breeds.**

If intravenous access is not possible (it can be difficult to locate or distend veins without a good circulation) there is an alternative. Drugs may be administered by **the transtracheal route**. A dog urinary catheter or similar long structure is passed down the endotracheal tube to sit at the carina and deposit drugs there. The carina is located at approximately the level of the sixth rib. **A dose two to three times what might be given IV is required, but reasonable absorption is possible. Adrenaline and atropine are the only drugs generally used in this way. Drugs should be diluted to a total volume of 5–10 ml with sterile water.** Ventilation of the lungs with a few breaths after administration ensures drug distribution.

Intracardiac injections are not generally used. Myocardial damage is common and injections into the wall of the myocardium are not effective. Intracardiac injections may be the only possible option in some situations though, e.g. in some small exotic species.

Drugs Used in CPR

There are three main drugs used in CPR:
- adrenaline (N.B. adrenaline and epinephrine are the same drug)
- atropine
- lidocaine.

Other drugs may be required in specific situations (e.g. antagonists) or for follow-up.

Adrenaline
Adrenaline is **used in asystole,** where its main action is to increase systemic vascular resistance and return blood to the central circulation. It also increases the force of contraction (if there is contraction of the heart). If ventricular fibrillation is present, adrenaline may coarsen a fine VF, making it easier to convert to a normal rhythm.

A dose of 0.01 mg/kg IV is recommended, but 0.1 mg/kg (high dose) may be used after a prolonged arrest. Adrenaline is often presented in vials labelled with a concentration of 1:1000 rather than mg/ml. A 1 ml vial of 1:1000 adrenaline (epinephrine) contains 1 mg, so a low dose would be 0.01 ml/kg, a high dose 0.1 ml/kg.

Atropine
Atropine is used where **bradycardia precedes the arrest,** e.g. in vagal reflexes, or in the presence of an atrioventricular block. After resuscitation, the regained cardiac rhythm may be bradycardic, so atropine is helpful.

A dose of 0.04 mg/kg IV is recommended. Lower doses may be adequate for treatment in other situations, but during arrest it should be ensured the full amount is given.

Lidocaine
Lidocaine is used to **treat ventricular arrhythmias such as ventricular tachycardia.** Again, this may not be the instigating rhythm of an arrest but could occur on regaining some cardiac function. An infusion may be used but usually a bolus to convert the rhythm first is beneficial.

Doses:
- 1–4 mg/kg (as a bolus) IV
- 25–75 µg/kg/minute as an infusion.

In the absence of a defibrillator, lidocaine may be used to attempt to convert ventricular fibrillation.

Vasopressin
Vasopressin can be used instead of adrenaline and in the same manner. It is thought to confer advantages in human CPR (especially with some causes of arrest), but so far studies in dogs have not shown significant benefits. In the UK, vasopressin is considerably more expensive, so it is not widely used.

ECG

Monitoring the ECG is helpful in an arrest. It helps to identify the electrical activity of the heart (or the arrest rhythm) which in CPR allows direct treatment of the cause

There are three main arrest rhythms and one other ECG trace to be aware of:
- **Asystole:** assuming there is good contact and a working ECG, this should be easy to identify. It is a flat line with no discernible complexes. (Figure 9).
- **Ventricular fibrillation:** in ventricular fibrillation, there is **totally irregular electrical activity.** There are no clearly defined waves and no clear baseline. Ventricular fibrillation (VF) can be further described as coarse (when there is a large variation, large movements of the trace) and fine (when the zig zags are really small). Coarse VF is reported to be easier to correct. (Figure 10).
- **Ventricular tachycardia:** this is not usually defined as an

arrest rhythm. However, it can be pulseless, and if there are no pulses associated with the complexes then this would be considered an arrest. (Figure 11).

Pulseless Electrical Activity

Pulseless electrical activity (PEA) was previously known as electromechanical dissociation (EMD). This ECG rhythm is more difficult to describe. Essentially the rhythm looks normal or near-to-normal and identifiable complexes with P, QRS, and T waves are visible, although complexes may be somewhat wider than usual. Over time they become increasingly abnormal but for a short time this can **look superficially like a normal ECG, but there are no pulses associated with it** and no audible heartbeat. This rhythm may often be seen during euthanasia with pentobarbital.

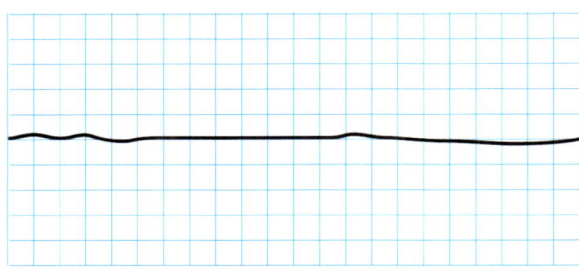

Figure 9. Asystole.

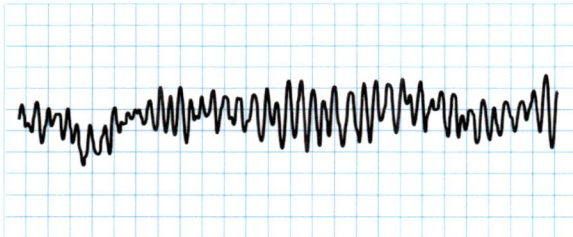

Figure 10. Ventricular fibrillation.

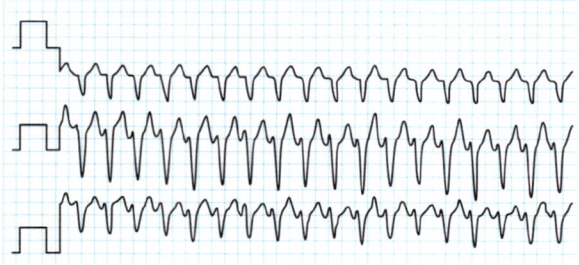

Figure 11. Ventricular tachycardia.

It is important to remember the ECG does not indicate output from the heart: a trace may be visible on ECG with no cardiac output and no pulses.

Whilst compressions are performed, there is considerable interference on an ECG so it can be difficult to identify fine detail. Brief evaluation pauses should be used to clearly see the ECG rhythm.

Electrical Defibrillation

Electrical defibrillation is used extensively in human CPR and is very successful. However, dogs and cats are more likely to exhibit asystole (most common) or PEA as their arrest rhythms, which **do not respond well to this treatment.** Most people place the dog in dorsal recumbency for defibrillation.

> Using a defibrillator:
> - the device should be charged
> - conducting gel should be applied to the paddles and to the patient
> - current should be applied across the heart, with one paddle on each side of the thorax
> - stand clear
> - 1–5 joules/kg.

It is important to remember that saline can conduct electricity, and **it is important that staff do not make contact with the table or other equipment during the charge.** Gel which has slipped down onto hands and arms could cause a shock.

If using a monophasic defibrillator, the higher end of the energy range should be used, and the lower end for biphasic defibrillators. If uncertain of the type of defibrillator initially low current should be used and then the energy increased. Only old defibrillators are monophasic, and many newer devices are labelled as biphasic.

Internal paddles are available for use e.g. when the thorax in open during surgery. These paddles are used in direct contact with the heart. **Much lower energy settings** are required (0.1–0.5 joules/kg).

Actions in Arrest

The A-B-C mnemonic is a useful way to remember CPR tasks; however this is not necessarily the best order of events.

When an arrest occurs, **a quick check for respiration and pulse should take no more than 10 seconds.** It is important to also **call for help and note this time.** When there is no cardiac activity present, the priority is to **start immediate cardiac compressions** (e.g. while waiting for assistance). **When help arrives, the trachea should be intubated and ventilation started.** Once monitoring is in place (e.g. ECG, capnography) a pause should be made to briefly evaluate the effectiveness of resuscitation This facilitates the correct next step (adrenaline, defibrillation).

The RECOVER guidelines advise **two-minute cycles of CPR,** repeating adrenaline every three to five minutes. The person performing compressions should be changed frequently (at least every two-minute cycle, sooner if needed). It can be difficult to keep track of time with an arrest, so if someone can keep records these can be referred to later. (Figure 12).

After the return of spontaneous circulation (ROSC), when the animal generates a pulse itself, follow up care is required.

Task Distribution

Ideally three to four people are involved in CPR, with **each person designated a role** and the various tasks distributed among the team.

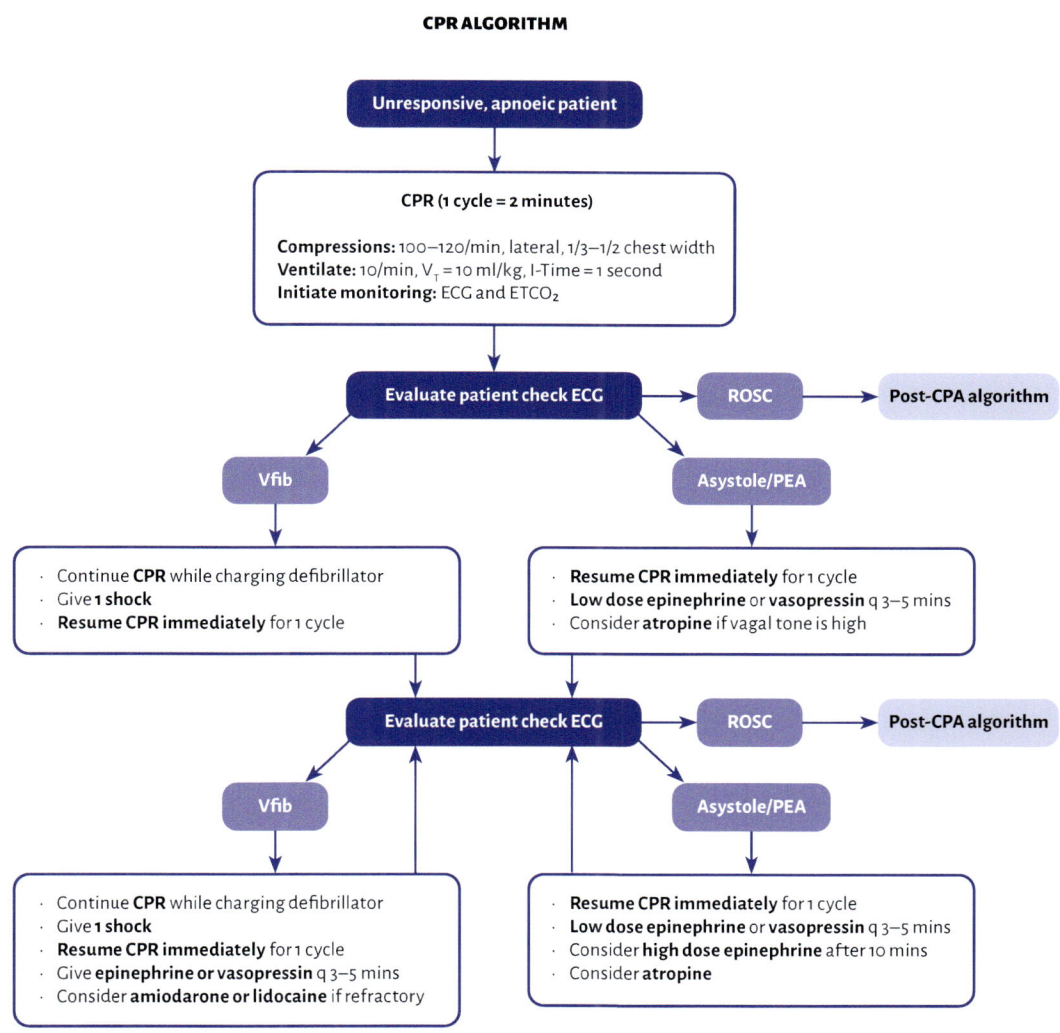

Figure 12. CPR algorithm. CPR: Cardiopulmonary Resuscitation; ROSC: Return of Spontaneous Circulation; Vfib: Ventricular fibrillation; PEA: Pulseless Electrical Activity.

An example of distributing tasks is outlined below, but other options are equally valid, provided all tasks are covered.
1) Directing situation, making decisions, assessing patient.
2) Ventilation.
3) Compressions.
4) Drawing up drugs, attaching ECG, keeping records.

It is important there is a clear direction for the arrest, with **one person taking charge.** Although discussions are useful in management, during an arrest is rarely an appropriate time to start thinking about pros and cons of various actions.

If fewer people are present, multitasking is required; however, it is important that compressions are interrupted as little as possible, so this person should not be given other tasks.

Other Actions Which May Help in CPR

One proposal to improve the circulation during CPR is to use **two people and interpose abdominal compressions.** One person performs compressions using the thoracic or cardiac pump technique, and one person compresses the abdomen each time the thorax is released. This is difficult to coordinate, particularly at speed, but it may be attempted. The theory is that the abdominal compression pushes blood into the thorax before the next thoracic compression.

Some years ago, it was recommended for someone to tightly bandage the hindlimbs, starting at the paws and working upwards, tightly bandaging to push blood towards the central compartment. Although this has logic in pushing blood to where it is most required, the disadvantages are that it takes considerable time and reduces the ability to use femoral pulses for monitoring, so is rarely contemplated.

A rather controversial addition to CPR is the **precordial thump.** This is only remotely likely to be of benefit in specific circumstances. If the arrest is witnessed, particularly going into fibrillation, a short, sharp forceful thump over the heart could reset the rhythm. There is little evidence available for this apart from anecdotal instances of success. The key points being this must happen instantly after the arrest. Any delay and this technique is useless.

Stopping CPR

How long resuscitation attempts continue is a difficult question to answer. There are always examples of animals who have successfully recovered after a long arrest; however these are few and far between.

It is relevant to think **why this animal arrested and what the likely prognosis is.** From the published evidence, **an animal that has arrested due to drug use/anaesthesia is more likely to survive,** and so in these cases it is likely to be worth continuing CPR for longer.

If the animal has obvious pathology, which is likely to be untreatable (e.g. a massive, inoperable tumour around the pharynx/tonsils), then even if the CPR is successful, a positive outcome is unlikely for this animal.

How well the circulation of the animal is managed is relevant. If effective pulses are generated and a reasonable end tidal carbon dioxide on capnography obtained (indicting a fair circulation), it may be worth maintaining resuscitation attempts for a longer to see if the animal responds. If CPR is not generating a good circulation, then firstly the technique should be amended (e.g. change staff on compressions and/or change technique); and secondly, if the end tidal carbon dioxide is decreasing, this indicates a poor prognosis and further CPR attempts should be abandoned.

As a guide, **20 minutes is appropriate for most animals** to give a reasonable chance of success.

Equipment for CPR

Equipment for resuscitation may be available at a specific CPR area and/or in basic crash boxes located in different areas within the practice. Many hospitals have an extensively stocked trolley available to take where required during an arrest or in preparation (e.g. moved into theatre prior to a high-risk procedure). To ensure readiness for emergencies, these trolleys/kits should be **checked regularly,** to ensure drugs are in date and replaced after use.

Training for an Arrest

It is vital **all staff are aware of CPR protocols** and the actions they should take. This can be part of new start training and **regularly revisited** as reminders for existing staff. Some centres allocate a role to specific personnel groups e.g. the veterinary care assistant is the record keeper. If the practice has a defibrillator, it is important that staff know how to use it and the safety precautions necessary.

Teamwork is vital for an effective response to an arrest. One way to develop this is to have mock crashes where the alarm is called. Although staff may resent this type of role play approach, it is useful to clarify any gaps in knowledge or anything that can be improved on. It is important people take this seriously. **An observer,** for the mock crash, can provide useful feedback. This person is not directly involved in managing the mock arrest but takes an overview to see what could be improved.

Debriefing

After an actual arrest it is useful to have a **debriefing session** afterwards to think about what happened, why, and how it could be managed differently next time. These sessions need to be handled sensitively; as many staff feel fragile after an arrest.

It is important these sessions are **not associated with blame.** The point is to identify any shortcomings for future situations, not to blame an individual for their actions or responses. Good CPR depends on a team approach.

Signs of Recovery After CPR

When monitoring recovery after CPR, the first aim after ensuring compressions are generating an effective circulation, is to establish when/if the animal will be able to generate its own circulation (i.e. can generate cardiac output and pulses are palpable heralding the return of spontaneous circulation (ROSC)).

Ongoing signs of further recovery include:
- improvement in colour of mucous membranes
- ECG changes to a more normal rhythm
- lacrimation
- pupillary constriction
- return of cranial nerve reflexes
- return of spontaneous ventilation
- return of other neurological functions, e.g. response to sound, righting reflexes etc.

Follow Up After an Arrest

After ROSC, i.e. a pulse and heartbeat are detectable, there is a need to continue postresuscitation care.

Over 50% of dogs that arrested will suffer a second arrest, so monitoring is also particularly important.

Many animals need continued ongoing support, which includes treatment for the inciting cause of the arrest.

Respiratory System

Is the animal breathing spontaneously? If not, continuing ventilation is required. This may be a limiting factor as few hospitals have the facilities for longer term ventilation if the animal does not start to breathe again.

Capnography and pulse oximetry are essential to evaluate the efficacy of respiration once spontaneous ventilation is seen. It may be acceptable to permit a slightly higher than normal end tidal carbon dioxide, but failure to maintain acceptable carbon dioxide is not a good long-term sign. Is a normal oxygen saturation being maintained? It may be necessary to supplement oxygen for a period of time.

Cardiovascular System

Is the cardiac rhythm normal? Sometimes a pulsatile rhythm is obtained but with an abnormal rate/rhythm. This may require veterinary intervention for resolution.

What is the blood pressure? Many animals have low blood pressure just after an arrest and may require pharmacological or fluid interventions. If the animal is hypovolaemic, fluid therapy is required. This may involve crystalloids (in the case of widespread dehydration), colloids (if retention within the circulation is required), or blood products.

Using a pressor drug to vasoconstrict may be useful in animals with vasodilation. Vasodilation may be identifiable if diastolic pressures are very low. In vasodilation, the mucous membranes are darker as there is more blood present (redder, assuming oxygen saturation is adequate). Some suitable agents may include dopamine, noradrenaline or phenylephrine.

If the myocardial contractility is poor, this leads to a failure of cardiac output and maintenance of the circulation. In these cases, a drug like dobutamine may be beneficial to increase contractility and cardiac output. An example of this may be in a dog with dilated cardiomyopathy.

Occasionally animals are hypertensive on recovery. This may be the case if a pressor/inotrope has been used but is no longer required at the same dose. The veterinary surgeon should be consulted about dose reduction.

Other reasons for higher blood pressure include pain; cardiac compressions cause trauma to the thorax and bruising at the very least. There may also be preexisting causes of pain which related to the arrest. Using drugs to reduce blood pressure (e.g. a vasodilator) is rarely required.

Neurological System

Some animals regain a spontaneous circulation and possibly ventilation too, but without regaining consciousness or normal neurological function.

A patient's neurological function is assessed by checking their reflexes; in some cases there is a lack of reflexes, such as an absent palpebral reflex or an absent righting reflex.

General Care

Nursing care is also important, such as ensuring the animal's comfort and speaking to the veterinary surgeon if there is uncontrolled pain. A recumbent animal will benefit from turning. Care of urination and defaecation is useful and placing a urinary catheter helps monitor urine output, as an to aid determination of fluids and other therapies.

References

The RECOVER initiative was undertaken some years ago, where experts studied the evidence for our actions in CPR to produce a set of guidelines. These are the guidelines followed in this chapter. All the work was published in an open access edition of the Journal of Veterinary Emergency and Critical Care. Part 7 includes the clinical guidelines and immediate follow up care. The link below is included for more information.
https://onlinelibrary.wiley.com/toc/14764431/2012/22/s1

At the time of writing, a large multinational team of experts are again studying the evidence associated with CPR in animals, including other species as well as dogs and cats on this occasion. This may lead to revised guidelines.

- Hoehne, S.N., Hopper, K. and Epstein, S.E. (2019) Prospective evaluation of cardiopulmonary resuscitation performed in dogs and cats according to the recover guidelines. Part 2: Patient outcomes and cpr practice since guideline implementation. *Frontiers in veterinary science*, 6, p. 439. https://www.frontiersin.org/article/10.3389/fvets.2019.00439
- Hofmeister, E.H., Brainard, B.M., Egger, C.M. and Kang, S. (2009) Prognostic indicators for dogs and cats with cardiopulmonary arrest treated by cardiopulmonary cerebral resuscitation at a university teaching hospital. *Journal of the American Veterinary Medical Association*, 235(1), 50–57.
- Kass, P.H. and Haskins, S.C. (1992) Survival following cardiopulmonary resuscitation in dogs and cats. *Journal of Veterinary Emergency and Critical Care*, 2(2), 57–65.

Test

1. Which group of drugs are most commonly used to treat bradycardias?
    a. Anticholinergics.
    b. Catecholamines.
    c. Vasoconstrictors.
    d. Positive inotropes.

2. Cardiac compressions during resuscitation should be performed at which rate?
    a. 60/minute.
    b. 90/minute.
    c. 120/minute.
    d. 150/minute.

3. Lung inflation during resuscitation should be performed at which rate?
    a. 6 breaths per minute.
    b. 10 breaths per minute.
    c. 12 breaths per minute.
    d. 20 breaths per minute.

4. Why are small dogs and cats more prone to hypothermia?
    a. Considerably smaller muscle mass.
    b. Larger surface area to volume ratio.
    c. Lower metabolic rate compared to larger animals.
    d. More likely to have peripheral vasodilation, increasing heat loss.

5. What are the cardiovascular sings of the Cushing's reflex (or triad) seen with increased intracranial pressure?
    a. Bradycardia, hypertension.
    b. Bradycardia, hypotension.
    c. Tachycardia, hypertension.
    d. Tachycardia, hypotension.

6. How can rebreathing be determined on capnography?
    a. A curved upstroke on exhalation.
    b. A notch in the plateau of the capnogram.
    c. A sloping downstroke on inhalation.
    d. Not returning to baseline between breaths.

7. A 10 kg whippet with no preexisting thoracic pathology has suffered a cardiac arrest. Which method of cardiac compressions would be your first choice?
    a. Cardiac pump (with thumb and two fingers over the heart).
    b. Cardiac pump (with 2 hands over the heart).
    c. Thoracic pump (with 2 hands over the highest point of thorax).
    d. Internal cardiac massage.

Answers on page 94

8. Which drug is the most commonly used to treat ventricular arrhythmias such as runs of ventricular tachycardia?
    a. Adrenaline.
    b. Atropine.
    c. Dobutamine.
    d. Lidocaine.

9. Second degree atrioventricular block may be associated with the administration of which sedative drug?
    a. Acepromazine.
    b. Butorphanol.
    c. Ketamine.
    d. Medetomidine.

10. How do the currents required for a biphasic defibrillator usage compare to that of a monophasic device?
    a. A higher current is needed for external use but the same for internal use.
    b. Biphasic defibrillators require a higher current.
    c. Biphasic defibrillators require a lower current.
    d. The requirements are the same.

Clinical Case 1

An 8-year-old female neutered Boxer presented with vomiting. She requires anaesthesia for surgery (exploratory laparotomy and gastrotomy) due to pyloric obstruction. At induction, copious liquid is regurgitated.

1. What immediate action should be taken?

2. What are priorities for early recovery management in this case?

3. Thinking about the risks for this particular case, are there particular signs to look out for in the postoperative period?

4. After regurgitation, one risk is the development of aspiration pneumonia. What signs might indicate this is developing?

5. The presence of acidic material in the oesophagus could cause an oesophagitis (strictures, however would only form over a long period of several weeks). What signs might be seen with oesophagitis?

Self-assessment

Clinical Case 2

A 9-year-old Staffordshire bull terrier crossbred dog is anaesthetised for removal of a mast cell tumour on the flank (side of abdomen). During preparation of the site, the heart rate increases from 76 to 148. What may be causing the increase in heart rate?

This is very likely to be histamine release from the mast cell tumour. Other causes of increasing heart rate (e.g. nociception) seems unlikely at this stage of the procedure, however it is always worth checking depth of anaesthesia and any other changes.

> Histamine release from mast cell tumours can occur during preparation perhaps more frequently than during the actual surgery. It is the manipulation of the tumour itself which causes the problem, and harsh rubbing with scrub solutions in particular can stimulate release of histamine.

1. What other signs should be looked for?
2. What action should be taken?
3. Are any other organ systems that affected by histamine release?

Nursing Anaesthesia

Notes

Self-assessment

Correct Answers:

Test

1. a
2. c
3. b
4. b
5. a
6. d
7. b
8. d
9. d
10. c

Clinical Case 1

1. What immediate action should be taken?

In this situation, it would be wise to quickly move the dog to the edge of the table to allow the head to drop down to drain material from oesophagus. Although a head up position is recommended during induction to try to prevent regurgitation, once there is material at the pharynx, draining downwards is preferable, to use to gravity to remove as much material as possible as rapidly as possible.

Ensure a secure airway. If the ETT is already in position, check the cuff is adequately inflated to prevent any aspiration of regurgitated material. If the tube has not yet been placed, as much regurgitant material should be removed from the pharynx as possible whilst preventing (as much as possible) its entry to the trachea. In addition to drainage, suction is very important. Flushing the oesophagus using a dog urinary catheter and water or saline could be performed, however in this actual case the stomach was so dilated there was little acidity in the contents.

2. What are priorities for early recovery management in this case?

It is important to ensure the dog has fully regained swallowing reflexes and can maintain its own airway before removal of the ETT, although it is usual to wait for swallowing before extubation; in this case it might be wise to see more than one good, clear swallowing action before extubation if at all possible.

It is sometimes advised to withdraw the ETT with the cuff still partly inflated. This is to draw up any foreign material around the ETT. It is a risky strategy however, as it can cause damage to the larynx. It should probably only be considered where it is likely material remains around the ETT (in the trachea) despite suction/drainage.

3. Are there particular signs to look out for in the postoperative period?

There are a few concerns here. Pain is always a postoperative priority, but in this case example the focus is on the specific management for this situation. More regurgitation or vomiting could occur, and there may be a need balance fluid intake and check electrolytes.

4. What signs might indicate this is developing?

Signs of aspiration pneumonia (not all animals may show all signs):
- depressed
- high respiratory rate
- poorer oxygen saturation
- pyrexia.

5. What signs might be seen with oesophagitis?

Discomfort, excessive swallowing, salivation, reluctance to eat (bear in mind many of these signs might be present in this particular animal anyway, but these would be more indicative of oesophagitis in an animal which did not present with in this way but had developed acid reflux during anaesthesia.

Clinical Case 2

1. What other signs should be looked for?

There may be redness in the skin, with local swelling at the site or urticaria (hives).

The blood pressure is likely to be reduced (the heart rate is trying to compensate, but as blood pressure is often measured intermittently e.g. every 3–5 minutes, the heart rate rise may be seen first).

Bronchoconstriction is theoretically possible after histamine release from mast cell tumours, probably related to an enzyme called tryptase. This is rare. In this case, a smaller tidal volume may be seen, there would be more difficulty in inflating the lungs when a breath is given, slower emptying of the lungs means the capnogram is likely to have a distinctive curved upstroke indicating a slower exhalation.

2. What action should be taken?
Antihistamines are appropriate, such as an H1 antagonist such as chlorphenamine. Immediate cardiovascular support can be provided by giving a fluid bolus to fill that vasodilated space.

3. Are any other organ systems that affected by histamine release?
The effects above are due to histamine acting at H1 receptors. There are also H_2 receptors in the stomach so ulceration can be seen. There is evidence of low grade stomach ulceration in dogs presenting with mast cell tumours. It would be logical to treat or pretreat with an H_2 antagonist. Ranitidine was commonly used but has recently been removed from the market in many countries. Cimetidine has a similar action, also some vets have used famotidine.

Be careful with cimetidine though as it can affect the cytochrome p450 enzyme systems (so slowing metabolism of drugs which rely on this system for elimination). This is a licensed veterinary product in oral form, so could be given for a few days before surgery, but is not available in an injectable form. How effective these treatments are is somewhat controversial, but some form of treatment for gastrointestinal ulceration is probably beneficial.

Anaesthesia of Exotics and the Horse

Pamela Murison

Chapter Summary:

- Principles of anaesthesia in exotic species.
- Equine anaesthesia: the horse as an anaesthetic candidate. Drugs and anaesthetic techniques including monitoring and complications in equine anaesthesia.
- Special considerations, techniques and advice for anaesthesia in other species including birds, reptiles, ferrets, rabbits and other small mammals.

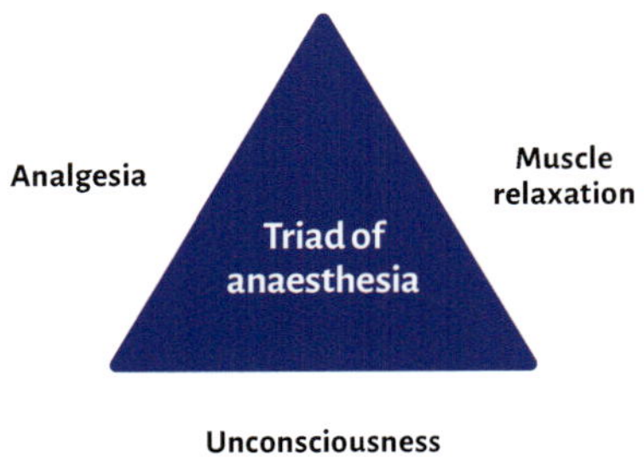

Figure 1. The principles of the triad of anaesthesia remain the same regardless of species.

OUTLINE AND PRINCIPLES

Anaesthetising an unfamiliar species may appear daunting, but it is reassuring to recognise **the principles of anaesthesia are the same** be it for a mouse or an elephant, a budgerigar, or a Beagle. Although it is important to address the differences between species **the aims remain the same, which are to maintain good circulation and effective ventilation, whilst ensuring a lack of awareness and sensation during the procedure.**

Regardless of species, the drugs used aim to provide:
- **Unconsciousness:** by suppressing brain activity and awareness.
- **Analgesia:** reduced nociceptive reflex responses to pain, rather than just a lack of awareness of the stimuli.
- **Muscle relaxation:** to facilitate surgery and aid positioning for imaging.

Whilst there are differences when assessing unconsciousness in different species, the similarities of anaesthesia outweigh the differences. **The aim during anaesthesia being to maintain the patient's physiology with as little deviation from normal as possible**, whatever the normal for that species is (Figure 1).

Key points which should be considered:
- Is the airway patent?
- Is effective breathing present?
- Are the mucous membranes pink?
- Are pulses of a good rate, rhythm, and quality?

Risks

Various studies have examined the mortality rates associated with anaesthesia in different species. The most wide ranging studies are the Confidential Enquiry into Perioperative Equine Fatalities (CEPEF) and Confidential Enquiry into Perioperative Small Animal Fatalities (CEPSAF). Although now considered somewhat aged, they remain the best overall indicator of risks and mortalities (Table 1).

Table 1. The risk of death associated with anaesthesia in dogs, cats, and horses, summarised from the CEPEF and CEPSAF studies.

Species	Risk of death		
	Overall	Healthy	Sick
Dog	0.16%	0.05%	1.33%
Cat	0.24%	0.11%	0.01%
Horses	1.9%	10%	Up to 8%

Data was collected from many different specialist and general veterinary practices, and this spread differentiates these studies from many others which are often associated with individual centres or a narrower population. This means the data is more generally applicable.

Dogs, Cats, and Horses

The overall death rate in dogs is fairly low, although higher than figures in people, which give mortality rates of 0.01–0.02%.

However, direct comparisons should be made with care as veterinary studies tend to **include a longer period after anaesthesia as an anaesthesia related death** (in the figures quoted above, 48 hours postanaesthetic for dogs and cats and 7 days for horses), which may not be equivalent to the human figures. Additionally, **if euthanasia was performed electively, this counts as a death** in veterinary studies such as the CEPEF (e.g. an inoperable tumour found at exploratory laparotomy).

Note that cats are a higher anaesthetic risk than dogs, with more deaths, particularly for healthy animals. Interestingly, the death rate in sick dogs and cats (e.g. ASA III–V) is similar. The timing of deaths varies somewhat between dogs and cats, with almost **two thirds of cats that die doing so in recovery,** whereas with dogs this is just over half.

For horses, the death rate is higher than in dogs or cats; notice the particularly high death rate with sick horses and emergencies. Of course, quite a few of these are euthanised due to a poor prognosis, not just actual anaesthetic deaths, but it remains clear that **horses are a higher anaesthetic risk than common small animal species.** The ASA categorisation was not used in the same way in the equine study, hence use of the terms sick and healthy.

Rabbits, Guinea Pigs, and Hamsters

In rabbits, anaesthesia is high risk, less so than compared to horses but more so than in dogs and cats (Table 2). Again, note **the large difference between healthy and sick animals,** with a sick rabbit being a very high risk anaesthesia.

In rabbits, death associated with anaesthesia is again predominantly during the recovery period, with nearly two thirds of deaths after, rather than during, anaesthesia. This highlights the importance of careful monitoring in recovery.

Table 2. The risk of death associated with anaesthesia in rabbits, guinea pigs and hamsters, summarised from the CEPEF and CEPSAF studies.

Species	Risk of death		
	Overall	Healthy	Sick
Rabbits	1.39%	0.73%	7.14%
Guinea pigs	3.85%		
Hamsters	3.7%		

In other species e.g. small rodents, the CEPSAF study did not have adequate numbers to draw valid conclusions when divided into healthy and sick animals, so these figures are overall only. Guinea pigs and hamsters are at a much higher risk of anaesthetic death (as were other small rodents), which is important to understand especially when discussing risk with the owner.

Birds

Birds generally have a high mortality rate, although slightly better than in small rodents. However, it is notable that the **budgerigar specifically appears to have a much higher risk;** but the reason for this is unclear.
- Budgerigar: 16.67%.
- Other birds: 2.44%.

Different species may cause specific concerns in several areas during anaesthesia.

Drugs

Many of the same anaesthetic drugs are used across species, although there are drugs (e.g. guaiphenesin in horses) which are not used in other species, so user familiarity may be lower. However, what does differ is how the animal deals with the drug, including uptake, distribution, or biotransformation. The dog and cat being good examples of this; for example, cats efficiently absorb buprenorphine via the transmucosal route, whereas dogs do not; and paracetamol is a useful analgesic in dogs but very toxic to cats due to reduced biotransformation and elimination (and should ever be used in cats).

Drug dosages also differ between species, and do not necessarily remain proportional to the differing size (a concept known as allometric scaling). This means that although a small rodent requires a much smaller total dose compared to a dog, the dose per kilogram is considerably greater. On the other hand, in larger species doses per kilogram are often reduced e.g buprenorphine in horses. Again, this phenomenon is observed even in small animal practice, such as in dogs that vary considerably in body size. **Doses of some drugs, in particular α-2 agonists, are more correctly calculated based on body surface area** and so proportionately less is given to bigger dogs. Of course, many people use per kilogram doses, though in this case it is wise to administer a slightly lower dose per kilogram to larger dogs.

Drug receptor sites may be different between species, for example some bird species have been shown to have a greater distribution of kappa (κ) opioid receptors, which may alter their responses to different opioid drugs.

Direct toxicity is possible but in fact is rare, and even the classic example of penicillin in guinea pigs is probably more likely to be because of the effect on the gastrointestinal flora rather than a true direct toxicity.

Equipment

There are **many similarities in equipment** used across species, for example a mask or endotracheal tube, an oxygen supply, volatile agent, and a breathing system. Obviously, specialised endotracheal tubes are needed to deal with a 600 kg horse, whilst it is difficult to intubate in a 300 g rat.

Likewise, the **breathing systems must be appropriate for the patient's size,** taking into account their ability to cope with factors such as resistance in the breathing circuit and there must be sufficient oxygen reserve, e.g. a mouse is not able to overcome resistance in the breathing system, whilst a large soda lime canister and a large reservoir bag are needed for a horse.

Perhaps less obviously, **equipment for veterinary anaesthesia was often originally designed for use on people** (bear in mind equipment marketed for veterinary use may have bought in technology from human monitors), which has limitations. Many human ECGs only count a heart rate between 30–250 bpm, whilst a horse may have a slower heart rate and small mammals a considerably higher heart rate outside this range.

Anatomy and Physiology

Anatomical variations between species can affect equipment, for example how well a mask fits on the face or how difficult certain techniques are, e.g. intubation.

Species size is also relevant, since the smaller the patient the trickier it is to obtain intravenous access. **Species related variations in physiology** can also affect anaesthesia, for example the cardiovascular system in reptiles, the respiratory system in birds, or the gastrointestinal system in horses or cattle. However, despite a wide range of differences between species, it is important not to lose sight of the similarities.

EQUINE ANAESTHESIA

Risks and Complications

Horse anaesthesia poses many challenges, which contribute to the overall high risk of death associated with anaesthesia. **An understanding of these risks and challenges and how to prevent them (if possible) is important before considering the practical steps in anaesthesia.**

Size

The majority of horses are large (400–600 kg) with some larger still, e.g. a Shire, Clydesdale, or other heavy horse breed of over 900 kg. However, in contrast a young horse of a miniature breed might only weigh 30–35 kg.

The size is relevant for anaesthesia as it affects the equipment required and is a factor for both human and animal safety. A large horse that falls onto a person can cause serious injury and must always be considered. A large, heavy horse may also be at greater risk of complications (e.g. myopathies or ventilation derangements).

> **A practical concern is that horses are frequently anaesthetised in the field,** where there is no equipment to weigh horses (which requires a specialist weighbridge). Weigh bands may be used, which wrap around the horse's girth, but these are not always accurate.

Temperament

Most horses are used to being handled and are nice natured, if nervous at times. However, if the horse is totally unhandled this poses real risks to handlers, because of the animal's size. As in small animals, the temperament affects ease of sedation, with an excited or aggressive patient often not responding to sedative agents as effectively as a calm animal. In horses it is usual to use intravenous (IV) injection of agents, however in a difficult horse this may be hard to do. Intramuscular sedation is possible, although rarely required.

Neuropraxis

Neuropraxis is a temporary paralysis. In horses, this can occur in facial or limb nerves and is usually caused by pressure on the nerve during anaesthesia.

In **facial neuropraxis** the muzzle visibly droops on the affected side. In **limb neuropraxis** the limb drops e.g. in radial nerve paralysis the elbow drops and appears lower than the other side. The affected limb is poorly controlled by the horse, and they often put less (if any) weight on it.

There is **no specific treatment for this condition,** which usually resolves spontaneously over a few days, and it is important to avoid neuropraxis where possible. Extreme care should be taken with limb positioning during anaesthesia in horses to ensure there is no pressure on specific nerves.

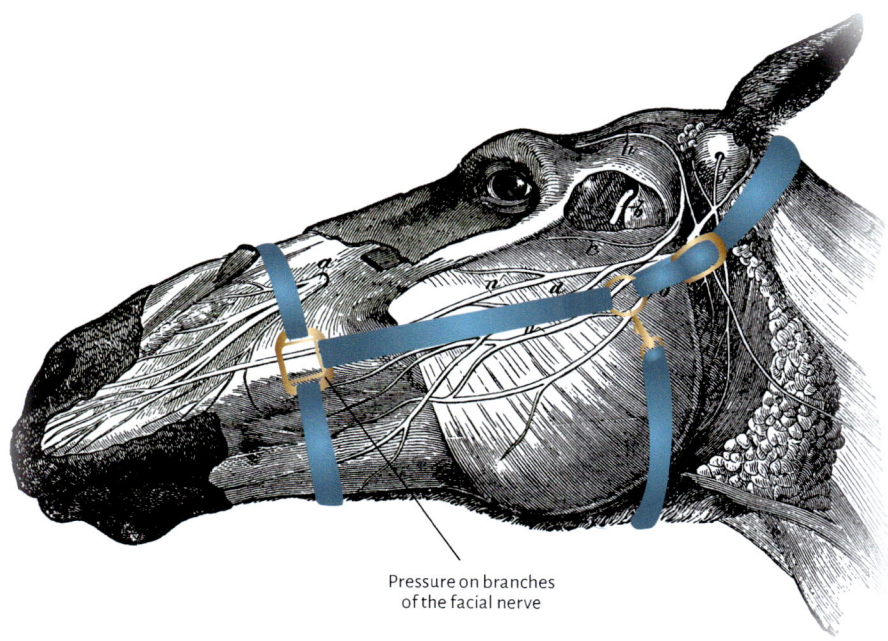

Pressure on branches of the facial nerve

Figure 2. Headcollar with metal pieces.

One common cause of facial nerve neuropraxis is if the horse wears a headcollar during anaesthesia (Figure 2). Most headcollars have metal pieces on each side and possibly buckles for adjustment. These commonly lie across the facial nerve, which is very superficial in horses with little natural covering or protection.

For this reason, most anaesthetists remove headcollars. If this is not practical, for whatever reason, soft padding between the hard metal pieces and the horse's skin reduces the risk of nerve compression.

Gut Motility

Horses are hind gut fermenters. They are herbivores, and grass is not an easy substance to digest. The horse has a simple stomach (similar to a dog or human), but the colon is very large and heavy in the horse and contains lots of bacterial flora which aid digestion.

It is important to keep the guts moving; gut stasis or ileus is a big problem in horses, since they rely on almost constant movement through the gastrointestinal tract. Some horses exhibit colic (abdominal pain) related to gut distension and tympany associated with lack of motility.

Factors that increase the risk of ileus or gut stasis include lengthy starvation, drugs, or pain. There is much discussion about ideal periods of food withdrawal prior to anaesthesia, and the ideal feeding prior to and immediately after anaesthesia.

Horses do not vomit, so this is not a reason to withhold food. Many hospitals try to minimise starvation periods and encourage horses to eat small amounts of easily digestible food soon after recovery, without bingeing on large quantities. Because the largest volume in the abdomen is the hindgut/colon, the bulk of the abdominal contents are not much depleted by starvation either, so many people consider it of little benefit.

Opioids can reduce gut activity, which is more of a problem for long term or infusion use rather than short term perioperative analgesia. Importantly there is some evidence that **antibiotics also affect gut function** and may be a factor in postanaesthetic colic. **Pain** increases sympathetic system activity and decreases parasympathetic activity, hence decreasing gut motility.

Fitness

Some horses are exceptionally fit, and this affects anaesthesia. **Fit horses can be very difficult to manage under anaesthesia** and may swing rapidly from light to deep planes of anaesthesia (or vice versa) and are more prone to hypotension.

Ideally, a fit horse should not be anaesthetised for an elective procedure. If anaesthesia is required, then allowing a period of 7–10 days rest prior to the procedure is useful. This means reducing very high energy feed (which affects the gut flora and gas production, which could produce tympany). Training work should also be reduced, so the horse is not at peak fitness. It should be noted that this refers to the very fit horse, e.g. a racehorse in training, rather than an active everyday riding horse.

Interestingly, the same factors can be present in other species too. Anaesthetists in human hospitals report fit young athletes are difficult to anaesthetise and some veterinary surgeons see similar factors in racing Greyhounds. This may be related to the relative preponderance of parasympathetic activity, i.e. a lower resting heart rate and blood pressure.

Recovery Injuries

FRACTURES
The recovery period is very high risk for all animals, which is especially true for horses which have some particular problems.

Horses are very heavy animals and **may fracture long bones in recovery;** the most common being a fracture of the tibia, as it is used in the push when a horse stands. Although a small animal is less likely to sustain a fracture in the recovery period, if it did occur repair is possible in most cases. However, **in horses, a long bone fracture is almost never repairable** (there may be exceptions, but these are rare). The weight of a horse means that metal plates and implants which are strong enough to resist bending or breaking without being unmanageably heavy have not been developed. This means it is likely the horse would require euthanasia.

Horses may also fracture their spine. For example, if a horse is recovering and stumbles forward towards a wall, the horse's head impacts against the wall, but the body keeps moving forward, breaking the cervical spine. The impact does not need to be forceful, and it is likely to be fatal. However, some injuries in recovery are minor, such as cuts, grazes, and bruises, which are common.

OCULAR INJURIES
Horses may injure their eyes by hitting their head on the wall or floor of an induction area. This can cause bruising, grazes, and inflammation.

In addition, **corneal damage may occur due to desiccation of the cornea,** as seen in small animals. It is also possible that the cornea is scratched or a foreign body (e.g. grit, sand or stone) enters the eye due to the location of most anaesthetic inductions. As in small animals, eyes should be lubricated and protected (e.g. by covering) as much as possible. **Scrub solutions or spirit coming into contact with the eyes should be avoided.**

MYOPATHIES
Horses may suffer from postanaesthetic myopathy (muscle injury). This usually becomes apparent during recovery when the horse develops hot, hard, painful muscles. It may be localised to one muscle group or more widely distributed. The horse may struggle to stand if the myopathy is widespread. If localised, the horse may be able to stand but unwilling to place weight on one limb or stand unevenly.

Damaged muscle fibres release myoglobin into the circulation; myoglobin is related to haemoglobin. As it circulates, it is excreted via the kidneys into the urine, **producing myoglobinuria (causing urine to become a dark reddish brown colour).**

Treatment of myopathies includes administering fluids to flush any myoglobin out via the kidneys (it can cause renal damage). **Analgesia is important** as usually horses are in pain. Many hospitals also use supportive therapies such as bandaging other limbs to provide support, cold/hot therapies (cold to reduce inflammation in the initial phases, warm to encourage good blood supply for healing later), laser/ultrasound, or other physiotherapy type measures.

In most cases the horse recovers within a few days. It may be a significant problem and if the horse is unable to stand or unable to bear weight, severely affected horses may require euthanasia.

Other species can develop myopathies, but it is particular problem in horses as their size/weight causes compression of muscle groups (which reduces blood flow) and the way horses' muscles are compartmentalised means pressure can build up in the muscle and affect blood flow.

Careful management helps reduce the incidence of myopathies. **Good positioning is vital with the horse's weight evenly distributed over a soft surface.** Limbs should not be held in awkward positions. Pulling a limb out/forward can be as bad as compression under the body, as this also affects blood flow.

Other factors affecting the incidence of myopathies are hypotension, duration of anaesthesia, and possibly hypoxaemia. Both the risk of death and the risk of myopathies increase in anaesthetics of greater than two hours duration, so it is wise for anaesthesia time to be reduced as much as is practical.

Factors which are key to reducing the incidence of myopathies are:
- good padding
- positioning
- maintenance of blood pressure
- minimisation of anaesthetic duration.

MYELOPATHIES
Whereas a myopathy is muscle injury, **a myelopathy is where the damage occurs to the spinal cord.**

This is a rare condition, seen mostly in young, male horses and often heavier breeds (although not always) anaesthetised in dorsal recumbency. The anaesthetic period may have been uneventful, with adequate/good blood pressure and no other abnormalities noted. In recovery, all goes well at first. Progressively, the horse becomes more alert and moves the head, and soon afterwards the forelimbs. In myelopathies, there is little movement if any in the hindlimbs which progresses to a complete paralysis of the hind limbs. Testing for skin sensation, the horse is likely to be insensitive to needle pricks caudal to the level of spinal injury.

Unfortunately, this condition is **unlikely to be treatable and often requires euthanasia.** It is difficult to know how to prevent this condition as its development is not fully understood. There is a suggestion that it may be associated with selenium, but this has not been absolutely proven. Research is limited as the condition is so rare.

Hypoxaemia

Horses are prone to developing hypoxaemia during anaesthesia. A normal arterial oxygen tension (PaO_2) in room air in a conscious animal is around 80–100 mmHg. When oxygen is supplemented during anaesthesia, in theory a horse on 100% oxygen would have a PaO_2 five times this, however this is not the case in all animals.

Of course, other species may also become hypoxaemic. What is unusual in the horse is a reduction in PaO_2 is relatively common in healthy animals (not just those with respiratory or other relevant diseases). This is due to changes within the lungs which lead to ventilation perfusion mismatching (Figure 3).

Figure 3 is a diagrammatic representation of the two lungs of a horse, lying in lateral recumbency. **The lower lung (nearer the ground, whichever recumbency) becomes compressed.** This is related to the size of horse and weight of the tissues. The larger and heavier the horse, the more this compression occurs. This compression means the lower parts of lungs may have little or no airflow. Upper areas of the lungs inflate well.

There are also changes within the circulation. **Due to gravity, blood tends to pool in the lower areas of the lung.** Less blood goes to the uppermost areas of lung (whichever part is furthest from the ground, in whichever position the horse is in), this also happens in people and other animals. Humans have greater ventilation of the parts of the lungs nearer the head when standing, but more blood nearer the abdomen. In horses, the sheer size of the thorax means this effect is particularly dramatic, the top parts and lower parts are just further apart compared to in a person.

The haemoglobin in the blood in the upper areas of lung picks up as much oxygen as possible. The blood in the lower areas of lung may only pick up a little (if any) oxygen. These mix as the blood returns to the heart and is then circulated around the body. The circulating blood is not fully oxygenated and if a significant decrease in oxygenation is seen, this causes hypoxaemia. This can happen in other situations too, particularly in various forms of respiratory disease, but the difference here is it can happen in a totally normal healthy horse.

There are reflexes (hypoxic pulmonary vasoconstriction) which shut down blood vessels in poorly ventilated parts of the lung and direct blood to the better ventilated areas of lung in the conscious person/animal, however these are often reduced or abolished during anaesthesia.

Treatment

Treatment for this condition is beyond the scope of this chapter but includes lung recruitment manoeuvres (to reinflate the poorly ventilated parts of lungs), bronchodilators, or treatments to alter perfusion. Normal ventilation of the lungs alone is unlikely to work as the gas just goes to the open areas of lung. Some anaesthetists use an air-oxygen mixture of gases in horses, the aim being to use the nitrogen (which is not absorbed) to keep the lungs more open.

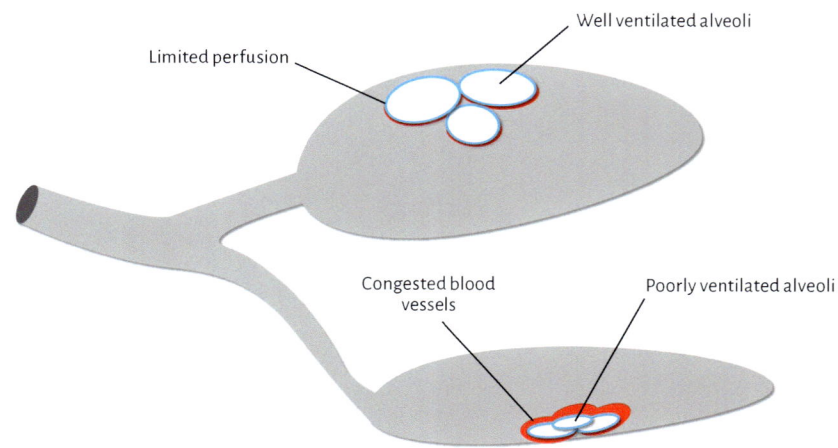

Figure 3. Diagram of lungs with open and closed alveoli.

Positioning the Horse

The position of the horse is relevant; changes happen in whichever position the horse is in, but other factors also come into play (Figure 4).

In the standing horse, this contributes to a large thoracic capacity (along with the 18 ribs of the horse compared to 13 ribs in most species) aiding high performance with both speed and endurance. **Under anaesthesia, however, in the horse the large and heavy loops of colon (due to them being hind gut fermenters), push down on the diaphragm causing even more compression of the lower areas of lung, producing even poorer blood oxygenation.**

If possible, **dorsal recumbency should be avoided in the horse,** although for some types of surgery it is essential.

Legislation

Under EU law, horses are considered food producing animals. It is important to check individual country regulations, as certain drugs preclude the horse from entering the food chain.

In many countries, the equine passport has a section with a declaration stating that the individual horse cannot enter the human food chain. This gives much more flexibility to the veterinary surgeon regarding the drugs they can prescribe. At the time of writing the UK has left the EU and how this will affect future legislation is not yet clear.

Drugs

Many, but not all, of the drugs used for equine anaesthesia are also used in small animals, but with slight differences in usage and effects. In this section, the focus is to highlight specific relevant differences in action in horses which should be used in conjunction with general pharmacology in chapter 2.

Acepromazine

Acepromazine (a phenothiazine tranquiliser) is commonly used in equine anaesthesia. As in small animals, when used alone it does not produce much sedation, but is useful in combination with other drugs. It has a **long duration of action** (up to six hours) and can be given **IM or IV** (oral preparations are also available). It has vasodilatory effects which mean it is not as suitable for dehydrated animals. Acepromazine has some antiarrhythmic effects which can be beneficial.

In the horse preparations of 5 or 10 mg/ml are easier to use than the 2 mg/ml small animal concentration. It is often given as a preparatory premed IM or IV and can calm horses e.g. when entering a strange induction box.

Under sedation with most drugs male horses often develop a flaccid penile protrusion (paraphimosis), but acepromazine is claimed to cause priapism (a persistent erect penis). It is debatable how likely this is to occur. The reports of priapism were almost exclusively with Large Animal Immobilon (a preparation which is no longer in general use containing acepromazine and etorphine), and the combination of drugs may be important. Many anaesthetists avoid acepromazine in breeding stallions, in case of penile injury, but some do use acepromazine on the basis that the risk of priapism is low. If priapism does occur, it should be treated quickly as penile damage can occur which results in amputation being required.

> **Findings from the CEPEF study suggest that using acepromazine may decrease anaesthetic risk in horses, which makes it popular for that reason.**

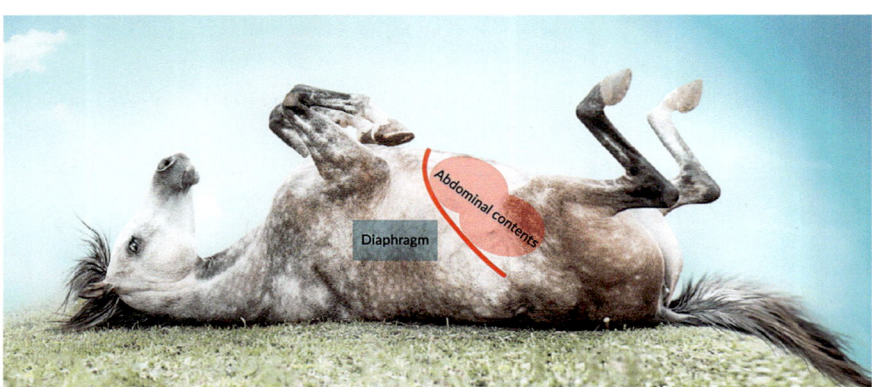

Figure 4. A horse in dorsal recumbency. The diaphragm in a horse is at a much more acute angle than in most other species (the dorsal attachment is more caudal than the ventral attachment). As in other species, the diaphragm is a dome shape but this alteration in position gives a more angled line.

α-2 agonists

General effects of α-2 agonists are similar to those in other species, with common side effects being a reduction in heart rate and an initial increase in blood pressure.

α-2 agonists can produce marked sedation, depending on dosage, and this group of drugs also has analgesic properties. Usually, α-2 agonists are **administered IV in horses,** but they can be **used IM or absorbed across mucous membranes** (there is a gel form of detomidine). Although the transmucosal route is less commonly used, it should be remembered that drugs can be absorbed this way, as accidental splashes into the eyes or mouth of people are very well absorbed and the concentrated equine drug can have dramatic adverse effects.

In the UK three main drugs are used in horses:
- xylazine (Chanazine™, Rompun™)
- romifidine (Sedivet™)
- detomidine (available under many tradenames e.g. Hipnoton™, Domosedan™, Equimidine™ and others).

The properties of these three drugs are summarised in the diagram in Figure 5.

It is useful to think of these drugs together and compare their effects.
- Xylazine:
  - has the shortest onset and shortest duration of action; and
  - produces a lot of muscle relaxation and ataxia.
- Romifidine:
  - has a slow onset of action with a long duration of action;
  - produces very little muscle relaxation and ataxia; and
  - in the author's opinion provides little analgesia compared to the others.
- Detomidine is somewhere between xylazine and romifidine.

Guaiphenesin

Guaiphenesin, also known as glycerol guaicolate ether (GGE or GG), is **a muscle relaxant with no anaesthetic or analgesic properties.** It is therefore never used alone but is useful in combination with other drugs.

Guaiphenesin can come in a 10% commercial form as Myorelax™ from Dechra. Large volumes are needed so it is usually given by infusion, as part of induction or maintenance of anaesthesia.

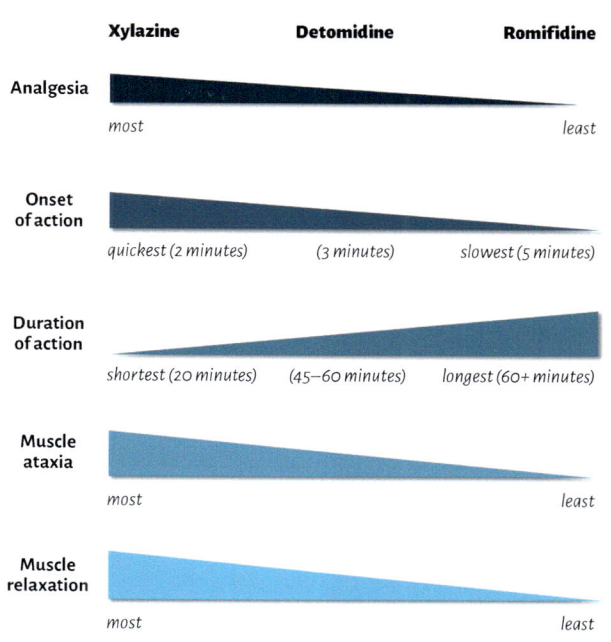

Figure 5. Drug action diagram.

Ketamine

Ketamine is the mainstay of equine anaesthesia for induction and is also commonly used for injectable maintenance of anaesthesia.

Ketamine is classed as a dissociative anaesthetic. In most countries, ketamine use is tightly controlled, for example in the UK it is in the legal category of a Schedule 2 controlled drug and must be stored appropriately, and its use recorded.

Ketamine should never be used alone, and it is important there is reasonable sedation on board before use in horses. Ketamine does not produce good muscle relaxation and so using other agents to improve this is important. It has a **slow onset of action,** so the onset of anaesthesia may only be seen after a couple of minutes and potentially even longer for its full effects.

> Ketamine can allow retention of reflexes, e.g. swallowing and ocular signs.

Thiopental

Although rarely (if ever) used nowadays for anaesthesia induction in horses, many anaesthetists find thiopental a useful product to have in stock. The previously used veterinary preparation is not currently available, so the small vials used in human anaesthesia may be purchased.

Thiopental has a fast onset of action which makes it ideal for use as a top up agent. A 600 kg horse could cause considerable damage to itself, staff, or equipment (e.g. theatre lights) if it started kicking or became light during anaesthesia. A small dose of thiopental, in a small volume, can rapidly regain control. The abolition of swallowing etc. may also be helpful in some types of surgery (e.g. to the palate) if the retention of reflexes with ketamine are problematic.

Benzodiazepines

In the UK the two main benzodiazepine in use are **diazepam and midazolam** (others are available, e.g. climazolam in Switzerland).
- Midazolam is currently licensed for use in horses in several European countries including the UK.
- Diazepam may be used as a human preparation, although under the cascade veterinary surgeons should use a licensed product where it is available.

Benzodiazepines are mainly used at induction, to improve muscle relaxation. They can also be used as part of an injectable maintenance combination of drugs (e.g. with ketamine and an α-2 agonist).

Diazepam is not readily soluble in water, so is either produced in an oily propylene glycol solution or in an emulsion (white) form. This difference is relevant. **It is common practice to mix diazepam or midazolam with ketamine at induction to enable use of a single syringe.** There are anecdotal reports of horses' sudden fatal responses when anaesthesia has been induced with the emulsion preparation of diazepam mixed with ketamine. This has not been reported with the other form of diazepam.

Inhalational Agents

Isoflurane is the main volatile agent in use today. Commonly used in small animals, there are some differences in its' properties when used in horses.

Horses are more likely to suffer **marked respiratory depression during anaesthesia with isoflurane** (compared with dogs), e.g. only breathing four times a minute. This often leads to a **notable hypercapnia.** If using isoflurane, many anaesthetists mechanically ventilate the lungs from the start of anaesthesia, however some wait and evaluate the end tidal/arterial carbon dioxide.

Isoflurane allows for a faster recovery from anaesthesia than older agents such as halothane, but this does not necessarily improve recovery quality with some horses being **uncoordinated and ataxic at recovery. For this reason, it is common to sedate horses with a small dose of α-2 adrenergic agonist for recovery.**

In most countries, sevoflurane is not currently licensed for use in horses. Although time to standing may not be particularly different between isoflurane and sevoflurane, many anaesthetists feel the type and quality of recovery shown is quite different. Horses become more aware sooner and manage themselves, becoming steady on their feet much more quickly with sevoflurane use. This is an important difference, particularly in horses likely to cause themselves injury; for this reason, some anaesthetists use sevoflurane off license.

Sevoflurane may also be useful in foals when a volatile induction is required (due to its rapid onset), as well as enabling the foal to return to the dam sooner.

Non-steroidal Anti-inflammatory Agents (NSAIDs)

Non-steroidal anti-inflammatory agents are used a great deal in horses but are not always the same drugs used in small animals. There is no equine product containing carprofen. In the UK, licensed products containing meloxicam are available for horses however it is less commonly used than in small animals. It is important to always check the drug regulations in the country you practice in.

Phenylbutazone (PBZ) is often used in horses. It is an old drug but has been used successfully for many years. An injectable preparation is available as well as oral sachets of powder which are popular for longer term analgesia.

Importantly phenylbutazone can induce marked bone marrow suppression in people (as well as individual sensitivity reactions e.g. to skin contact) so PBZ should never be used in horses which might enter the human food chain. Many horses are not likely to enter the food chain, however it is relevant considering legislation and the potential export of animals.

Flunixin meglumine is also a popular drug for use in horses and is marketed under several tradenames (e.g. Cronyxin™, Finadyne™, Pyroflam™ and others). It is an effective anti-inflammatory and analgesic, to the point where some veterinarians can worry about the analgesia masking signs of disease progression (e.g. in colic with abdominal pain due to distension or torsion of the guts). In these cases, a smaller dose is preferred (e.g. 20% of the usual dose).

Opioids

For many years opioids were used less commonly in horses than small animals, due to concerns about side effects. **Opioids can reduce gut motility in horses, although this is more likely to be a clinical problem with longer term or continuous use, rather than immediate perioperative use.**

Also, opioids are quoted as producing excitement, albeit in older studies when the doses used were much larger compared to current recommendations. This is perhaps not really excitement, but a marked increase in locomotor activity resulting in horses that persistently box walk round and round in circles. If the horse is prevented from doing so (e.g. in a restricted situation such as stocks) then frequent lifting of the feet may be observed.

There are a few important points to note about locomotor activity associated with opioids in horses. Firstly, side effects are more likely to be seen if the animal is not in pain, as seen in healthy research animals given the drug. If given clinically this may be less likely (though not impossible). The effect may also be dose related; also note that even small amounts of sedation will abolish any box walking.

Opioids used in horses are morphine, methadone, buprenorphine, pethidine, and butorphanol.

PETHIDINE
Pethidine, also used in small animals, is a full mu (µ) agonist opioid. It is licensed for use in horses (in the UK) but **is not practical as it is given by IM injection (to reduce the likelihood of histamine release) and the large volume may be painful to inject.** The duration of action is only around an hour.

METHADONE
Methadone does not have an equine licence in the UK but is popular in some other countries for use in horses.

MORPHINE
Morphine is cheap, effective, and popular for use in horses in the UK, particularly those undergoing more painful surgical procedures. Doses of 0.1–0.2 mg/kg are used with a duration of action of up to 4 hours. **Morphine can be used in an epidural** where it provides long lasting effective analgesia with less risk of systemic side effects, which is particularly good e.g. for seriously painful hindlimb lameness.

BUPRENORPHINE
Buprenorphine has a veterinary license in horses in the UK. **It has a slow onset of action, even after IV injection, but a long duration of action of 6–8 hours and is increasing in popularity for use in horses.**

Anecdotal reports indicate buprenorphine may produce more locomotor or gut motility side effects in horse. This may be partly due to the long duration of action, after any residual sedation has been eliminated, whilst buprenorphine action continues, but may be a dose related effect, whilst some veterinarians report only seeing these problems in larger horses. Decreasing the dose per kilogram in larger horses compared to small horses/ponies may reduce the incidence of side effects. The licensed dose is 6–10 µg/kg.

Others

Other drugs and fluids may be more commonly used in horses than in other species.

TETANUS ANTITOXIN
Although not an anaesthetic drug, it is important to remember tetanus antitoxin. **Horses are usually vaccinated against tetanus,** however if they are not, some hospitals have a policy to provide tetanus cover.

HYPERTONIC SALINE
Another useful agent in horses is hypertonic saline. Usually 7.2 or 7.5% NaCl (compared to the 0.9% of normal isotonic saline) which is a concentrated solution which **must only be given IV.** The concentration of NaCl is such that water is drawn into the circulation from the intracellular fluid and surrounding spaces. **This gives an initial expansion of circulating volume much greater than the volume of fluid administered.** It has a brief effect though, with maximum effect reached at or before 30 minutes after administration, after which the fluid is redistributed, and the volume effect lost.

Hypertonic saline is particularly useful in a sick and dehydrated horses which need urgent surgery. These animals are a very high anaesthetic risk, and it can be difficult to provide adequate fluid volume replacement quickly enough. Hypertonic saline achieves temporary support for the blood volume during the induction and initial maintenance of anaesthesia. It is important that isotonic crystalloid fluids are continued afterwards, as the hypertonic saline exerts its effects by encouraging fluid shifts in the body, not correcting any deficits. These deficits can be replaced during anaesthesia.

DOBUTAMINE
Dobutamine predominantly acts at β-adrenoreceptors in the heart and therefore **administration increases contractility and cardiac output. It is a popular treatment for hypotension in the horse.** Excessive doses can induce an increase in heart rate, however this problem is seen more commonly in foals or very small ponies, when it may be easier to inadvertently overdose if given via gravity (rather than using a volumetric pump). Dobutamine is given by infusion, and it has a rapid onset.

Steps in Equine Anaesthesia

In this section, the different steps used to anaesthetise the horse are discussed, starting with preparation and sedation of the horse, progressing through options for standing sedation, before moving on to induction, maintenance, monitoring and recovery.

Introduction

The first decision to be taken is **whether or not the horse requires a general anaesthetic (GA)**, and if so which broad type. Many horses are anaesthetised in field situations where an ambulatory veterinary surgeon has been called out to see the horse. This can mean limited equipment availability and also limited numbers (if any) support staff. In most cases, **field anaesthetics are limited to short procedures in healthy horses or ponies,** for example castration or sarcoid removal (sarcoids are locally invasive fibrosarcomas (skin tumours) which are common in horses).

Another option is to **anaesthetise the horse for surgery in an operating theatre.** However, many veterinary practices do not have the facilities to anaesthetise horses and they are therefore referred (to a private or teaching hospital) for procedures readily undertaken in first opinion small animal practice.

Given the high risk of equine anaesthesia, no general anaesthetic in horses should be undertaken lightly. In some cases, it may be appropriate to delay the anaesthetic (e.g., in a recently foaled or due to foal mare, or to decrease fitness) a short delay also permits stabilisation (for example, a horse injured in an endurance ride may be dehydrated).

Increasingly, more procedures are performed standing under sedation, e.g. ovariectomies, dentals. and even various orthopaedic procedures. Although there is a lack good evidence of morbidity and mortality associated with this type of standing surgery, it is assumed there is less risk for the horse than general anaesthesia.

Definitions: SCR and SSA

Standing chemical restraint (SCR) is a term often used instead of sedation, and indicates that the horse has received drugs to produce a cooperative and less responsive state (e.g. for imaging), but remains standing.

A newer term is **standing surgical anaesthesia (SSA)** which implies that in addition to the less responsive sedated state, there is desensitisation of an area sufficient to permit surgery. It is useful to differentiate the two states, as it is easy for people to assume the ability to perform surgery when it is not appropriate.

Risks and Problems

Even SCR in horses is not without risk, and there are several factors to consider to ensure a safe and successful procedure.

Head Position
A sedated horse allows their head to droop, depending on the individual and its neck thickness, this may be virtually to ground level. This lowered head relative to the heart allows blood to accumulate in the nasal passages and congestion can affect airflow (horses are obligate nasal breathers, only naturally breathing through the nose, not the mouth). For this reason, **the head should be supported during procedures to prevent too low a head carriage.** There are a few ways this can be done.

Stocks
Stocks are used as a safe place to work on a sedated horse, with side pieces and bars to prevent a horse from falling or staggering sideways (and tread/fall on someone) or moving forward or back (Figure 6). Although useful, care is required with head position when a horse is in stocks. There is a gate or bar across the chest of the horse in most stocks (preventing forward movement), as the sedated horse lowers its head,

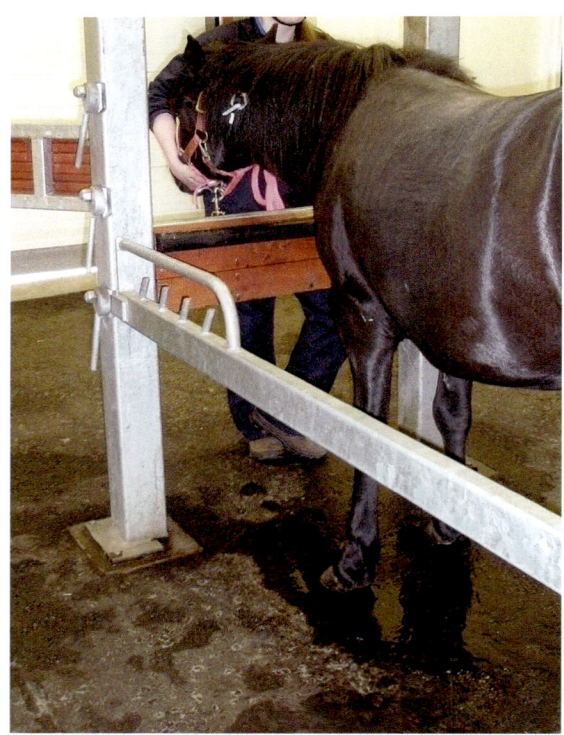

Figure 6. Image of equine stocks.

the horse can lean on this bar causing neck pressure. **If there is significant pressure on the carotid arteries this is reported to cause a fainting episode where the horse suddenly drops to the floor.**

Therefore, it is important to ensure elevation of the head without the neck pressing on a bar or gate. **An assistant can hold the head** in a neutral position, but this is tiring for the handler as horses' heads are heavy. **A headcollar and ropes can be used,** with ropes attached to rings fixed on the stocks, but any metalwork (such as buckles, rings) should be well padded to reduce the risk of pressure causing neuropraxis.

Alternatively, **some hospitals use a head support.** This is an adjustable height stand with a padded bar or plate on the top of which the horse rests their head on. However, close observation is required as the horse's head may slide off the support.

NOISE AND TOUCH
During sedation many horses are touch and/or noise sensitive, so care should always be taken around a sedated horse. Lots of noise may cause reactions, as well as touching the horse unexpectedly may cause it to jump or kick out. It is good practice to run a hand down a leg from the body, rather than suddenly touching a limb, as is usual in the fully conscious animal.

> A horse under sedation is not insensitive to pain, so adequate desensitisation is needed before a painful procedure such as suturing a wound.

Drugs for Standing Chemical Restraint (SCR) and Standing Surgical Anaesthesia (SSA)

A number of drugs are available to sedate horses for SCR and SSA.

ACEPROMAZINE
A small amount of acepromazine, used prior to entering the room or stocks, reduces anxiety and has a synergistic effect with other drugs.

DETOMIDINE
Detomidine is undoubtedly the most popular drug for sedation in horses, often combined with butorphanol. For longer procedures, it is becoming common to use a detomidine infusion to permit titration to effect over time and a consistent level of sedation.

ROMIFIDINE
Romifidine is useful for imaging or other procedures as the horse is less ataxic after receiving this drug.

MORPHINE
Morphine can be used instead of butorphanol for more painful procedures.

General Anaesthesia

Preparation for General Anaesthesia

Long periods of starvation affect gut function and the return of motility. Horses cannot vomit (passive regurgitation is occasionally seen if the stomach is distended, for example in some forms of colic, but this is a different mechanism). **Most veterinarians aim for 6–8 hours starvation without removing water,** but there is little evidence to support a specific time.

SAFETY
Most horses in work wear shoes. **Shoes should always be checked prior to anaesthesia** as a loose shoe wrenched off during induction or recovery can cause considerable damage to the foot. Raised clenches (where the ends of the nails are raised) can be sharp and cause damage to the contralateral limb.

Most hospitals remove shoes before anaesthesia, which prevents shoe associated risk to the horse and protects the expensive surfaces in an induction box from damage. Alternatively, feet can be taped or bandaged, but it is important to ensure the horse has a good grip underfoot.

As grazing herbivores, horses may have grass or food particles in the mouth, especially around the molars. **Washing the horse's mouth out before anaesthesia** helps remove these, to ensure they are not taken into the trachea during intubation. An large syringe with a metal nozzle is used to push water into the caudal areas of the mouth, with the nose lower than the larynx to ensure water falls forward bringing residual food as it does so. It is important to ensure both buccal and lingual aspects of the dental arcades are flushed.

INTRAVENOUS CANNULATION
The jugular vein is the most common site for venous cannulation in the horse. The catheter may be placed upwards (i.e. with the tip pointing towards the head) or downwards (pointing towards the body); each technique carries advantages and disadvantages (Table 3).

Turbulence is important, as jets circulating in the blood vessel may increase the damage to the intima of the blood vessel, increasing the likelihood of thrombophlebitis. **Thrombophlebitis (inflammation of the blood vessel associated with clots and obstruction to blood flow) is a significant problem in horses,** particularly if both jugulars are affected.

Table 3. Advantages and disadvantages of placing a catheter upwards or downwards.

Upwards	Downwards
Technically easier to perform.	Technically more difficult to perform.
Against blood flow.	Aligned with blood flow.
Turbulence.	Less turbulence.
If the cap is dislodged, blood flows via the catheter. This will clot, and flow will cease before significant blood loss occurs.	If the cap is dislodged, air may enter catheter producing an air embolus.

In many other species, if the jugular veins are occluded or have reduced flow, blood drains from the head via vertebral blood vessels. However, horses are almost totally reliant on the jugular veins, so if both jugulars have impaired blood flow, blood cannot drain away causing swelling over the head. This is not treatable. To try to reduce the risk of jugular occlusion, **intravenous cannulae are usually placed in horses with sterile gloves and after full sterile preparation of the site.**

Turbulence in the jugular vein increases the risk of thrombophlebitis, even in the absence of infection. For this reason, downwards facing catheters are recommended for longer stays (anything over a few hours) and if large volumes of fluids are administered, as this increases the turbulence. An upwards facing catheter, however, is useful as a quick and easy placement for short term use such as for field castration in horses.

A risk of downward catheter placement is air embolism, which causes a variety of clinical signs in the horse. Reports suggest neurological signs (e.g. blindness, ataxia, pruritis) are possible, also agitation, tachycardia, tachypnoea, and muscle fasciculations, and may be fatal in a proportion of cases. Due to under-reporting in the literature, it is difficult to be certain of fatality rates, but one study suggests six out of 32 horses with an air embolism died (Parkinson et al, 2018).

Preanaesthetic Medication

If the horse does not tolerate intravenous catheter placement, sedation may be required. Many horses permit a quick off-the-needle injection into the jugular vein when intravenous cannulation (a longer and slower procedure) might not be possible. However, **in difficult to handle animals, intramuscular injection of sedatives can be used.**

Acepromazine is often used as part of premedication. It can be given IM prior to IV catheterisation, or IV. Doses of 0.01–0.03 mg/kg are commonly used, not usually exceeding 0.05 mg/kg. As in small animals, acepromazine alone is unlikely to produce much sedation but can exert a mild calming effect and acts synergistically with other drugs.

Intravenous Sedation

The main sedation or premedication is usually administered IV via a catheter. It usually consists of an α-2 agonist, plus or minus an opioid. Typical doses are up to a maximum of 100 µg/kg romifidine or 20 µg/kg detomidine. Lower doses are often adequate with an opioid such as butorphanol or morphine, as these increase sedation. Some anaesthetists give an opioid after induction, however, in most cases provided there is the start of onset of sedative activity before onset of opioid action (which is likely to be slower than α-2 agonist onset time) there will be no signs of the adverse effects which may occur when opioids are given alone to horses.

Intramuscular Sedation

For IM sedation, using a combination of an α-2 agonist, acepromazine and an opioid produces synergistic effects. When choosing the α-2 agonist, it is important to remember that about three times the IV dose is required IM; detomidine is useful due to the smaller injectable volume. Acepromazine and butorphanol are reasonably well absorbed IM, using similar doses to IV, but most vets give towards the higher end of the dose range.

> **It is important to leave adequate time** to allow the drugs to exert their effect (20–30 minutes) without stimulating the animal.

It is unlikely IM sedation will produce adequate sedation to induce anaesthesia, however it is then possible to place an IV cannula and top up sedation IV as necessary.

Induction of Anaesthesia

In a field situation, induction is performed in a confined place which is large enough so the horse will not fall into walls or objects (such as a menage, riding school, or small paddock). The surface should be soft, reasonably flat, and well drained. In theatre situations, specifically designed induction boxes are used. These usually have padding on the walls and a floor with a rubber surface which both gives a good grip but also is not hard if the horse falls on it.

There are different ways of restraining horses at induction.

Induction Gate

One of the most popular ways of inducing anaesthesia is the use of **an induction gate.**

The horse enters a specifically designed padded box and is sedated. With the horse standing against one (padded) wall, a padded gate is moved out from a door or wall. and held in place to maintain the horse in a restricted position. A rope may cross in front of the horse to help pull the gate towards the wall. One handler is in front of the horse. As anaesthesia is induced, the horse goes down into a sternal position, then the door is opened to allow the animal to fall out into lateral recumbency.

Wall

If an induction gate is not available, it is possible **to use several people to hold the horse against the wall for induction.** This is still done relatively frequently; however, it does pose risks as the horse goes down, as falling on a handler causes significant injury. It is important that handlers are aware of the movement of the horse and move quickly out of the way if they find themselves in a dangerous situation.

These guided inductions are particularly useful for horses with some instability or poor weight bearing, such as chip fractures of the olecranon, but can be used in other horses too.

Freefall

Alternatively, the horse can be guided into a lateral position in a more open way. This is necessary in a field situation but can also be done in an induction box. Two ropes are attached to a head collar on the horse, one on each side, and held by two handlers, each in front of and to the side of the horse, creating a 'V' formation with the horse's head.

In these situations, the induction agent is administered, then as the drugs take effect, the handlers tighten the ropes to prevent the horse raising the head and tipping backwards. After going down into a sternal position, the horse is then guided over into lateral recumbency.

Drugs for Induction of Anaesthesia

Ketamine is used to induce anaesthesia at a dose rate of around 2–2.5 mg/kg IV, although higher doses are reported in some studies. If used with an α-2 agonist such as romifidine where muscle relaxation is poor, it is common for a benzodiazepine to be added. This type of induction combination is given as a bolus (not to effect as is usual in small animals). Muscle relaxation can also be provided with guaiphenesin (also known as GGE).

If using guaiphenesin, the induction method is slightly different. The GGE infusion is started first. As the horse becomes weaker (knuckling of the limbs is observed) then the bolus of induction agent is given, with the infusion of GGE continuing until anaesthesia is induced.

Bolus administration of drugs such as diazepam and ketamine can be used both in a restrained or a free induction technique. However, GGE combinations are best used in a restrained induction such as with an induction gate, due to the slow onset and ataxia produced before induction.

Maintenance of Anaesthesia

PROTOCOLS

In a field situation, anaesthesia is usually be maintained with injectable drugs as other options are unlikely to be available.

For a short anaesthetic, **a bolus top up of ketamine** (with or without more α-2 agonist depending on its duration of action) is appropriate. **If a longer duration of anaesthesia is required, drug infusions should be used. A common choice is GGE combined with an α-2 agonist and ketamine; an example is described below.** Because there are usually three drugs included in this infusion, it is sometimes colloquially termed a triple drip; however it is important to be aware there are many different triple drip combinations in use.

> **Intravenous maintenance of anaesthesia:**
> - 1 x 500 ml container 10% guaiphenesin
> - + 500 mg xylazine
> - + 2.5 g ketamine.
>
> Administration should be at approximately 1 ml/kg/h: a faster rate of administration may be needed initially and the rate slowed later.

Horses maintain their airways well and there is usually no need for intubation for shorter anaesthetics. **As a guide, anaesthesia should not be maintained for more than about 30 minutes in dorsal recumbency or 45 minutes in lateral recumbency unless oxygen is being supplied** (due to the ventilation/perfusion imbalances which may lead to hypoxaemia). In a field anaesthetic, this could be provided from a small cylinder with nasal tubing.

> **If driving with an oxygen cylinder on board a vehicle, most countries require use of a safety sign to indicate pressurised gases are on board.** (Requirements vary depending on the country).

In a theatre situation, injectable anaesthetic infusions can be used to maintain anaesthesia, but care is needed for longer anaesthetics. During an anaesthetic of about two hours of duration, GGE can accumulate, causing weakness and ataxia in recovery with an undesirable effect on the horse's ability to stand.

Inhalational agents, such as isoflurane, are commonly used for maintenance anaesthesia in the horse. Increasingly a combination technique is used with an infusion of one or more drugs given throughout anaesthesia, which reduces the requirement for volatile agents; this is known as **PIVA (partial intravenous anaesthesia)**. Drugs used in this way include ketamine, lidocaine, or α-2 agonists such as romifidine.

Equipment for Maintenance of Anaesthesia

It is important to remember the principles of large animal anaesthetic equipment (despite their intimidating appearance) are the same as the more familiar small animal machines (Figure 7). There are **gas inputs** (usually from pipeline supplies), **flowmeters** to control the flow, a vaporiser, and a **circle system.** Non rebreathing systems are rarely used in horses; the gas flow requirements are impractical in anything other than very small miniatures or foals. The reservoir bag on the circle system should be large enough for the size of animal, usually 30–35 litres for adult horses.

Some newer machines look a little different (for example Tafonius, made by Vetronics/Hallowell). This has the same basic features, but with **built in multiparameter monitoring,** and batteries facilitating use away from a power source. This machine has a piston arrangement which the horse moves during spontaneous ventilation or ventilation provided by moving the piston mechanically.

Tracheal Intubation

Tracheal intubation is standard practice in a theatre based anaesthetic, even when using injectable drugs, so ventilation can be supported if required. Endotracheal intubation is most commonly performed orally, or nasally.

Oral Endotracheal Intubation

Oral endotracheal intubation is performed with the horse in **lateral recumbency.** The horse's head and neck should be positioned in a straight line running from the nostril, poll, withers, and hindquarters to straighten the airway. Pulling the horses head back (dorsally) to straighten the neck is not ideal as nerves in the neck, such as the recurrent laryngeal nerve, are stretched with reports of induced laryngeal paralysis.

A **blind technique** is used (i.e. without visualisation). A gag should be inserted between the upper incisor teeth and lower dental arcade; this can be a specially designed metal gag or a piece of drainpipe connection. The endotracheal tube should be passed through the gag, into the mouth, rolling the endotracheal tube 360 degrees if the tube does not pass easily beyond the teeth. The next obstruction is usually the larynx. Care should be taken as horses can go into laryngospasm, although the use of local anaesthetic is not routine.

Visible condensation in the tube confirms the tube is near the larynx. The tube should enter easily, if it does not, the tube should be withdrawn slightly, rotated about 45 degrees, and then gently moved forward again. Timing, insertion with inspiration may be beneficial, as the glottis may open wider during this phase. A large horse usually takes a **30 mm ETT**

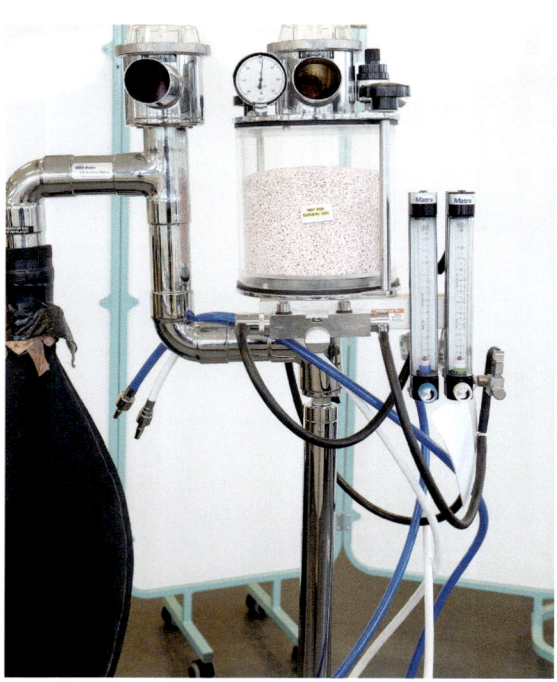

Figure 7. Image of a basic large animal anaesthetic machine.

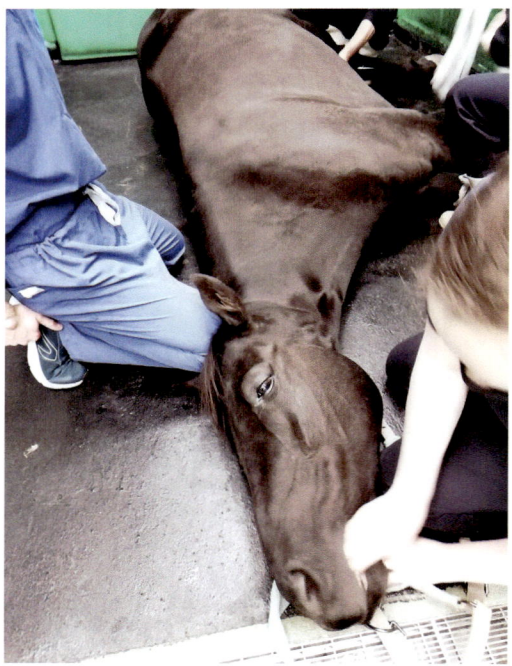

Figure 8. Horse position for intubation.

(endotracheal tube). Rough intubation can cause laryngospasm or trauma and postanaesthetic swelling.

Nasal Endotracheal Intubation
A smaller tube is required for nasal endotracheal intubation (e.g. 20 mm instead of 30 mm). The tube should be generously lubricated. A thumb should be used to press down on the tube as it is inserted into the nostril, pressing ventrally and medially, to ensure it passes into the ventral meatus, which is the largest passage. A crunching sensation may mean the tube is in the middle meatus at which point it should be withdrawn and reinserted.

Nasal endotracheal intubation is not routine but may be helpful for some dental or oral procedures.

Anaesthetic Positioning

In a field situation, the horse usually remains where they fall. In a theatre, hobbles can be placed on the limbs (bags or gloves are usually placed on the horse's feet to prevent mud and other debris from falling into the theatre). The horse is lifted using a mechanical hoist, either straight into the theatre or more commonly into a preparation corridor. Here it is placed on the operating table and the endotracheal tube connected to oxygen and anaesthetic maintenance agents. The table is then moved, often manually, from the preparation area the short distance into the theatre.

Careful positioning on the operating table is vital to reduce risks of myopathies and neuropathies.

Lateral Recumbency
If the horse is in lateral recumbency, a thick mattress with sufficient density such that the horse sinks in, spreading their weight evenly should be used. A mattress which is too hard creates more pressure over small areas of the muscles.

The lower forelimb should be pulled forward to reduce pressure on nerves and blood vessels on the limb's medial aspect, tension on the limb should then be released. Maintaining a position where a limb is drawn significantly forward or backwards should be avoided as the tension causes stretching of blood vessels, which is as deleterious as pressure in its impairment of blood flow and increases the risk of a myopathy.

Most operating tables have areas where leg supports can be attached. Supporting the upper limbs so they are parallel to the floor reduces tension on the muscles. Alternatively, cushions can be used between the limbs, but this is less satisfactory due to a risk of increased pressure on medial nerves.

Dorsal Recumbency
When positioning an equine patient in dorsal recumbency, most equine operating tables have side pieces which are moved upwards to create a trough shape. There is always padding on the table, but extra can be added with foam, an air mattress, or a bean bag. Again, the aim is to **distribute the horse's weight over as large an area as possible and minimise focal pressure points.** Inflatable cushions can be used on either side of the shoulders to support them.

Squeezing hind limbs together (e.g. with cushions or table side pieces) excessively should be avoided. This can produce tension in the muscles and may be a factor in development of gluteal myopathies.

Monitoring Anaesthesia

There are some differences when judging the depth of anaesthesia in horses compared to small animals.

Eye Position
The eye position can be used to help judge depth of anaesthesia; however, the changes are not the same as in small animals. **Horses' eyes rotate less than in small animals** and the movement may be less obvious, as horses often have a pigmented sclera. In horses, the eye tends to rotate forward (i.e. looking towards the nose) rather than ventrally.

> It is important to remember to lubricate the eyes.

Palpebral Reflexes
Assessing the palpebral reflexes is useful in horses. Elicitation of reflexes is more reliable in horses by brushing a finger over the upper eyelashes rather than touching the corner of the eye, as used in a dog.

Nystagmus
Nystagmus is common in a lightly anaesthetised horse. Slow, gentle nystagmus may not be a significant concern, but a sudden, rapid nystagmus could indicate possible imminent movement of the horse. However, if anaesthesia is maintained with ketamine, they retain a central eye and reflexes including swallowing and palpebral reflexes.

Heart Rate
The heart rate tends to remain constant at varying depths of anaesthesia in horses and is therefore not a good indicator of depth. An increasing heart rate may indicate inadequate analgesia but could also be a cardiovascular response to volume status.

Blood Pressure
Blood pressure can be useful in indicating depth with higher

arterial blood pressure relating to lighter anaesthesia. This is particularly relevant if a sudden increase is observed.

Respiratory Rate and Pattern

The respiratory rate and pattern are useful indicators of anaesthetic depth, and indeed in a field situation or with maintenance with ketamine combinations, may be the most reliable signs to use. As depth of anaesthesia lightens, larger tidal volumes and increased respiratory rate are seen. Respiratory signs are not helpful if the horse's lungs are mechanically ventilated (e.g. in an operating theatre).

Anal Reflex

The anal reflex is considered very useful by many anaesthetists. To elicit this reflex, the anal ring should be flicked and speed of a closing response assessed. This is abolished at deeper planes of anaesthesia.

Additional Monitoring Equipment

The Electrocardiogram (ECG)

Normal limb leads (as in small animals) are rarely used in horses, and indeed the cables may not be long enough to allow this. **Most anaesthetists use a triangle of leads around the heart (placed one side of the horse if necessary)** (Figure 9). One configuration used is the base apex; this involves placing the red electrode (RA) on the jugular, LA (left) on the sternum behind the heart and the green LL is placed on the thorax. Note, this produces a negative deflection of the waveform in the normal horse. Other configurations are acceptable, but the electrodes should span the heart.

Arterial Cannulation

Arterial cannulation is commonly performed during theatre anaesthetics.

Arterial cannulation enables direct measurement of blood pressure for accuracy and real time assessment of changes. As hypotension increases the risk of other complications, such as myopathy, accurate measurement allows the anaesthetist to act if required.

Placing an arterial line also allows access for arterial blood sampling. In the case of ventilation perfusion mismatching, non-invasive monitoring tools such as **capnography and pulse oximetry may not truly reflect the situation in arterial blood.** Blood gases give more information about oxygen and carbon dioxide in the case of ventilation perfusion mismatching.

Sites for arterial catheterisation include the facial **artery or the metatarsal artery.** Periosteal inflammation and infection have been reported after insertion of metatarsal arterial lines, so it is important asepsis is maintained and care is taken not to damage the periosteum. Aseptic preparation of the catheterisation site should be performed, although over scrubbing should be avoided as this can cause the vessel to spasm. The facial artery is most commonly used except where the face is hidden e.g. during head surgery.

Non-invasive Blood Pressure Measurements

Non-invasive blood pressure measurements are used in horses with a cuff placed on the tail. Oscillometric machines are reported to give reasonable results, although the Doppler technique is not considered accurate. For short procedures, where arterial cannulation is not considered necessary, oscillometry could be used for blood pressure measurement.

Pulse Oximetry

Pulse oximetry is commonly used. Modern pulse oximeters are better able to cope with tongue thickness in the horse than older devices. It is important to remember that SpO_2 decreasing is a late indicator of falling arterial oxygen partial

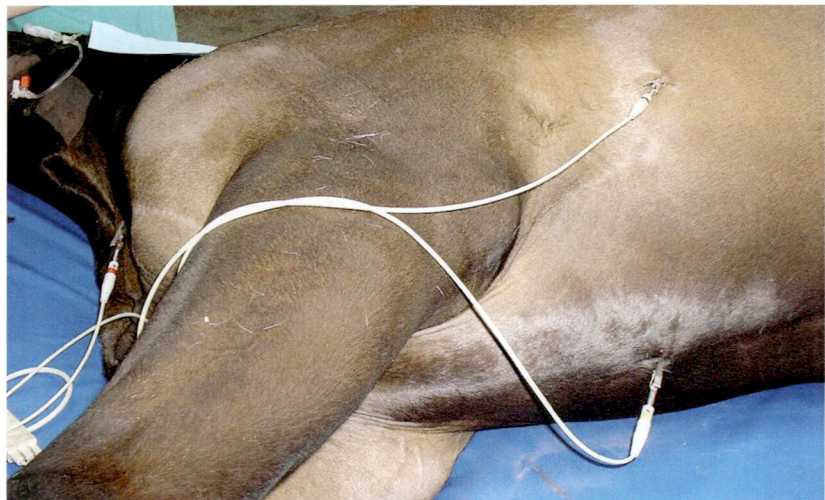

Figure 9. ECG on a horse.

pressure due to the shape of the oxyhaemoglobin dissociation curve.

CAPNOGRAPHY
Capnography is useful but again may not truly reflect the arterial values of carbon dioxide if perfusion with the lung is greatly affected and blood is shunted away from inflated areas of lung.

Recovery from Anaesthesia

For horses that received modern volatile agents as maintenance, it is usual to administer more α-2 agonist for recovery e.g. 20 µg/kg romifidine or 0.1–0.2 mg/kg xylazine. Romifidine appears a sensible choice in most situations as it is long lasting and produces little ataxia (Robinson et al., 2013).

Due to their different onset of action, romifidine (longer onset of action) is given just before the horse is lifted off the table, or if using xylazine (shorter onset of action), it is given once the horse is in the recovery box at the time of or close to extubation.

A recovery box may be the same box as used for anaesthetic induction or a similar (perhaps smaller) padded area. The horse is usually placed in lateral recumbency. After hindimb surgery, it is preferable for the sound leg to be underneath, as this limb is the one which requires most strength to push up into standing. The lower forelimb should be pulled forward as before.

Opinions vary on the risks associated with turning the horse into the other lateral position for recovery. Some anaesthetists are concerned that the atelectic lung is then uppermost and the underneath lung compresses before the upper lung opens. If turning is essential, it is possible to pause with the horse in a dorsal position, give a few large breaths and then place them in the other lateral position to ensure the alveoli are as open as possible. A towel under the lower and over the upper eye is useful to reduce both light and dirt entry.

EXTUBATION
Horses tolerate endotracheal intubation well, meaning that **swallowing is only observed at very light planes of anaesthesia.** Extubation at this point may stimulate the horse to attempt to stand, so many anaesthetists extubate a little earlier.

Congestion can occur in the nasal passages, especially if the horse's head was below the level of the heart during anaesthesia (which is likely if the horse was in dorsal recumbency). Gentle insertion of a finger into the nostril allows for an assessment. A congested nasal passage feels puffy with little space around the finger. Some anaesthetists use **phenylephrine spray into the nose to reduce swelling** (given when the horse is moved into the recovery box). It is helpful to prevent congestion with careful positioning during anaesthesia, meaning phenylephrine is rarely required.

Watching for an increase in respiratory rate, with a more forceful expiration and possibly seeing the return of the active component of expiration may indicate time to extubate. The horse has a normal active component of expiration (this would be abnormal in other animals such as the dog). The horse is seen to breathe in, then out (passive), then an active part (a visible squeeze of the abdomen). There is a brisk palpebral reflex at this time.

The tube with deflated cuff should gently be removed. It should be ensured that the airway is patent (i.e. airflow through nose), and a nasopharyngeal tube inserted if there is doubt. This is a short tube passing from the nostril to the pharynx (i.e. it does not pass through the larynx). If this is necessary, it is important to bear in mind that passage into congested nasal passages can cause epistaxis, but on the other hand as large a tube as possible is beneficial as horses can panic when their airway is small.

It is not essential to remove the endotracheal tube prior to recovery in horses. If there are concerns about the airway, a nasotracheal or even orotracheal tube may be left in situ for recovery. An oral tube should pull slightly through the diastema to ensure it is not bitten during recovery, as the gag is removed. Many anaesthetists deflate the cuff of this tube to make it easier to remove in recovery, but also to reduce the risk of occlusion of the total airway if the tube kinks or is blocked e.g. by the head pressing against the wall. Some airflow can hopefully pass around the tube. The endotracheal tube should be carefully secured with tape.

In recovery, oxygen is initially supplied via the ETT and after extubation into the nostril. At least 15 l/min should be used for a large horse, less is not effective. The tube falls away from the nose as the horse lifts its head.

ASSISTING RECOVERY
There are various ways the anaesthetist attempts to support and assist in recovery, to reduce the incidence of potentially fatal complications.

With very small individuals, an assistant can guide the head and another guide the tail. Alternatively, a hand firmly gripping the mane at the withers can be a good steadying influence, but this should only be tried in small ponies or foals.

For larger horses many practices use ropes with pulley systems. One rope is attached to a headcollar (which must be firmly attached to ensure it does not pull off during recovery). Specially designed headcollars are usually used which are stitched flat without metal pieces which could press on facial nerves. Another rope is attached to the tail, with a secure, quick release knot. These ropes pass through rings at the top of the box and then through a mechanism to allow the tension to be held. It is important to note these ropes are not intended to lift the horse, but they are used to guide the horse and ensure once standing it stands still, not walking around the box or falling over.

As yet there is no convincing evidence that using ropes reduces mortality; horses can still fracture limbs and indeed there are other complicating factors (such as the risk of tail damage) but many people feel they tried to reduce injury. A young, unhandled horse could panic with ropes and may be better without.

Other methods to support recovery can include slings, inflatable supports and even swimming pool recoveries; but none of these aids are perfect.

Foals

Young foals may require anaesthesia for correction of angular limb deformities or other conditions, and very young foals for injuries sustained during birth, such as a ruptured bladder.

Foals have a much larger surface area than adult horses and need temperature support much more than adults, e.g. insulation, heat pads and/or warm air blowers. They can become **hypoglycaemic,** so a young foal which is not yet on solid food should not be starved.

The mare should also be considered; in most situations, both the mare and foal are brought to the induction box. The dam is sedated, then the foal anaesthetised, and the mare led away to a nearby box.

Benzodiazepines produce good sedation in the very young and/or very sick foal. Inhalation induction of anaesthesia can be performed, (using a mask or nasotracheal intubation), but is usually reserved for the very young.

Foals are better developed than a pup or kitten of an equivalent age, so aspects such biotransformation of drugs are not too much of a problem especially after about one month of age, though many anaesthetists select shorter acting agents (e.g. xylazine instead of romifidine).

The body composition of foals varies from adults in that they have a higher water content and less fat; and as a result, have higher fluid requirements. This may alter the distribution of drugs, but this is not necessarily observed clinically.

The ductus arteriosus is a blood vessel which (in the foetus) links the pulmonary and systemic circulation, decreasing the amount of blood directed to the lungs. The ductus closes after birth and permits blood to go to the pulmonary circulation, however it may be patent for up to seven days in the foal. As the pressure on the systemic side of the heart is higher than that on the pulmonary circulation, this means blood flow tends to divert towards the pulmonary circulation.

When stressed, foals are prone to ulceration of the gastrointestinal tract and stomach. Hospitalisation (even without anaesthesia) can induce these gastric ulcers and therefore many practices use preventative ulcer medication for hospitalised foals.

A rapid recovery is desirable to return to the dam, particularly in the very young foal.

More information on anaesthesia of paediatric and neonatal animals is found in chapter 8.

SMALL MAMMALS ANAESTHESIA

Small mammals pose specific difficulties for anaesthesia, and it is worth considering general problems before considering individual species.

General Considerations

Although many practices deal with a fair number of small mammals, it is likely these numbers are fewer than dogs and cats. Unfamiliarity is relevant for mortality as there is a tendency to be less attuned to detecting changes or complications in unfamiliar situations. However, it is important to remember the principles of anaesthesia are the same for whichever species, i.e. pink mucous membranes, heart beats, circulation, and breathing.

Handling

Small mammals can be tricky to handle and may have specific issues such as tail slip in gerbils and degus. Specific concerns for individual species are dealt with later in this chapter.

Allometric Scaling

The drug doses given to small mammals may appear high compared to those used in cats and dogs; this is an effect known as **allometric scaling with small mammals usually requiring a higher dose per kilogram than larger animals.** Care should be taken when extrapolating doses from different species and a resource such as the BSAVA Formulary is useful for checking doses.

Accuracy

Although the dose per kilogram may be higher, a very small mammal still requires a tiny volume of some drugs. **For accuracy, insulin syringes (U-100) are useful and in some cases, making a dilution of a drug also helps.** Care should be taken as the amount of drug remaining in the hub of the syringe can make a dramatic difference to the volume, so drawing saline into a syringe which contains drug already produces inaccuracy.

> ### Making a 1 in 10 drug dilution.
>
> This produces a tenth of the concentration, e.g. when using medetomidine (1000 μg/ml) a concentration of 100 μg/ml is produced.
>
> - 0.45 ml of sterile water for injections or saline should be drawn up.
> - 0.05 ml of drug should be drawn up in a separate syringe.
> - The volumes of saline and drug should be injected into a sterile, empty container (e.g. a third syringe). Mixing is often easier if there is a little more space, so a 2 ml syringe may help. Residual drug in the hub of the syringe should **not be ejected.**
> - The solutions should be mixed well, and this dilution used by drawing the amount required for the animal from this solution.
>
> To accurately draw up required amounts it is important to know the animal's weight; the scales used for dogs and cats are not suitable for very small mammals.

Equipment

Anaesthetising small mammals requires some specific equipment requirements. For example, drawing up the required drug amounts requires an accurate knowledge of the patient's weight, whilst the scales used for dogs and cats are not sensitive enough for small mammals.

Inhalation inductions are frequently used for small mammals, for which **a chamber is useful.** These range from basic devices to Perspex type containers. The size should be appropriate for the animal; too large a chamber is as difficult as too small as it will require high oxygen flows to make a change within the chamber and also the animal may move around more during induction. A good seal is essential to ensure a lack of environmental contamination with volatile agent. The chamber should have two ports; one for the tubing or breathing system to supply gases, the other to connect to the scavenging.

Face masks are needed in a range of sizes and suitable for different anatomy such as long or short noses. There are specifically designed snout masks for rats available. A double mask delivery system is used e.g. in laboratory settings, with a mask inside another mask; the inner tube delivers the anaesthetic and oxygen, whilst a larger tube outside is connected to a fan system drawing gas away.

Low resistance breathing systems (e.g. T-piece) are useful as small mammals may not be able to overcome resistance easily.

Small animals have a smaller tidal volume and therefore consideration of the dead space in the breathing system is important. The dead space is the gas which does not participate in gas exchange, so equipment dead space is that area between the animal and the parts of breathing system where fresh gas flushes through. The smaller the animal, the more important it is to minimise dead space. Specially designed low dead space connectors for endotracheal tubes are useful. Note that if using side stream capnography with a relatively high gas flow e.g. with the T-piece breathing system, there can be some dilution of the measured end tidal carbon dioxide (i.e. it reads a little lower than the actual value). The use of uncuffed ETT in small mammals may also result in a small leak, also reducing the value of carbon dioxide obtained.

Maintaining Respiratory Function

The smaller the animal the smaller the airway, and the easier it is for **secretions to create an obstruction.**

The animal is also less able to overcome other restrictions to breathing; it is important to consider instruments or hands which could press on the thorax during surgery as these can significantly reduce or stop ventilation.

Ocular Damage

Corneal damage is a particular problem in small mammals. In addition to the same contributory factors as in other species (reduced tear production and inability to distribute the tear film over the cornea during anaesthesia) in small animals there are risks such as the mask causing physical damage. The gas flow during an inhalation induction can also promote drying of the cornea and possibly irritation caused by inhalational anaesthetic agents.

Lubricating the eyes is important and, if tolerated by the animal, helpful before induction in a chamber. Care should be taken with the mask positions and where the edge of the diaphragm is. If eye position is not required to indicate the depth of anaesthesia, then taping the eyelids shut should be considered.

Heat Loss

Small mammals are prone to heat loss, leading to hypothermia as they have a large surface area to volume ratio. Attempts to maintain the room and environmental temperature higher than the usual temperature should be made where possible. Much heat loss happens at the start of anaesthesia, so keeping the animal warm just prior to and during induction is as important as heat retention mechanisms afterwards. Using insulation and warming methods (e.g. bubble wrap, heat pads, warm air blowers etc.) is important.

Glucose and Oxygen

Small mammals have a higher metabolic rate than cats and dogs, which means **they use more glucose and more oxygen. Hypoglycaemia or hypoxaemia** can develop readily if glucose or oxygen use exceeds supply, and a very small animal in particular has minimal energy reserves.

Minimal starvation periods help ensure reserves remain as high as possible. Oxygen is usually supplied e.g. with a volatile agent, but care should be taken if there is something else which could increase glucose or oxygen consumption further, for example shivering in recovery. If this happens supplying supplementary oxygen for the initial recovery period is recommended.

Preanaesthetic Examination

It can be difficult to obtain full examination information, such as detecting a heart murmur, in very small animals. Depending on the owners and situation, the history may also be limited.

It is certainly possible for disease processes to be undetected in these animals, and this is probably one factor promoting their increased anaesthetic risk of death. It may be difficult to take preanaesthetic blood samples for further investigation, and although pet insurance for rabbits is common, there may be financial constraints for some small pets.

Normal values quoted (e.g. for heart rates and respiratory rates) vary considerably between sources, which shows how difficult it may be to obtain reliable resting rates. Guide indications for heart and respiratory rates are provided under the section for each species.

Fluids and Drug Administration

Intravenous Access

Small mammals have small vessels which are fragile, therefore care is needed so as not to cause damage. It may be impractical to gain intravenous access in some very small mammals and so other options are needed for fluid administration and drug administration.

Very small cannulas are necessary for intravenous access e.g. 24 or 26G. In addition to those sites commonly used for cats and dogs (e.g. cephalic, saphenous) other options to consider are the **ear vein** (particularly useful in the rabbit), the jugular vein, or other large vessels not usually used for routine venous access e.g. the femoral. Which vein to choose is highly species dependent, and not all are appropriate in all cases.

The **weight and drag of a giving set** or attached tubing are not well tolerated by some small animals. One option is giving frequent **bolus administration,** for example giving fluids once an hour in recovery.

EMLA

EMLA cream (a eutectic mixture of local anaesthetics) is very useful for use in small mammals. It can be used to provide local topical anaesthesia e.g. prior to cannulation of a vein.

Gloves should be worn and EMLA applied to the area after clipping, then covered with a non-absorbent material (e.g. a trimmed part of a vinyl glove held in place with tape or self-adherent bandage, or even cling film can be used). This prevents the animal from rubbing off the EMLA, prevents it drying out, and improves the results. As well as desensitisation of the skin, EMLA produces some local vasodilation which is very beneficial with small vessels.

EMLA requires time to work, with this time being dependent on the thickness of the skin it needs to penetrate. About 15–20 minutes is adequate for most small mammals as they often have thin skin.

Ethyl Chloride

Ethyl chloride spray is marketed to provide a localised freezing effect on the skin. It can be slightly unpleasant for the animal, but rather than spraying directly on the skin, **a small amount can be sprayed onto a swab which is then dabbed onto the area.** There is good evidence for efficacy in larger animals. In very small animals, there may be concerns about not freezing a large area (which can be difficult to minimise) as it may affect body temperature. It is also worth noting that vasoconstriction may be produced in response to the cold effect.

Intraperitoneal Injection (IP)

Intraperitoneal injections are rarely used in larger species; however, this route can be useful for drug or fluid administration in small mammals. (Figure 10).

There is a risk of hitting internal organs (the liver if the injection is given too far cranial). A reasonable volume can be

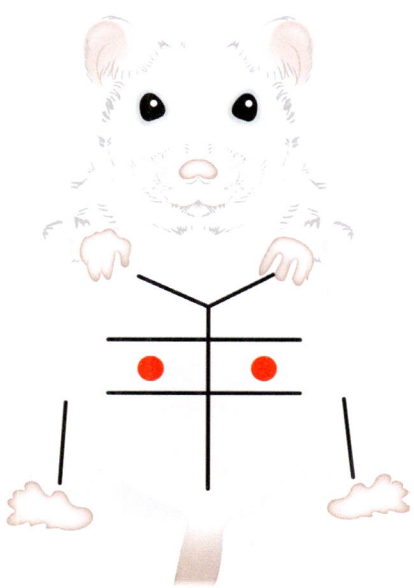

Figure 10. Intraperitoneal injection. The location used is off midline and in a caudal quadrant. Some authors recommend tilting the animal, either on its back (almost head down) or vertically.

given by this route (unlike some other routes of administration), but a very large volume of fluid at one time could impair diaphragmatic movement. (At the time of writing, in the UK it is inappropriate for veterinary nurses to perform a procedure entering a body cavity.)

Drugs and fluids administered intraperitoneally are relatively well absorbed. However, some drugs are irritant (e.g. chloral hydrate which is an older drug and not currently recommended, in part due to the irritant effect when given IP). Also, fluids administered directly into the abdomen, during abdominal surgery, are absorbed during recovery from anaesthesia and can be beneficial.

Intramuscular Injection (IM)

Intramuscular injections can be used in small animals, with **the main limitation being the small volume that can be administered.** A guideline is not to use more than 0.2 ml/kg per site. Although this volume is reasonable for a 2 kg rabbit (0.4 ml), for a 500 g rat this volume is lower, and for a small gerbil or hamster may not be practical. More than one site of injection can be used if required.

These limitations are why intramuscular injections are useful for animals over 1 kg, but rarely used for very small animals.

The selection of muscle group to use depends on the species and the individual animal, and a well developed muscle group to inject into. The quadriceps muscles can be used, but the lumbar muscles are also a good option in many animals. Care should be taken with very small animals not to go through the muscle group and hit the transverse processes of the spine or miss the muscle to give an unintentional intraperitoneal injection.

Gluteal muscles should be avoided as well as the musculature at the caudal side of the hind leg due to risks of nerve damage.

Some people recommend rubbing the area afterwards to reduce the pain, but this assumes the animal permits this. With larger volume injections, it may be wise to displace the skin over the site (i.e. so the skin puncture does not align with the muscle injection hole when released) as this reduces losses emerging from the skin.

Subcutaneous Injection (SC)

Subcutaneous drug administration may be easier to administer than intramuscular injection and is reasonably well absorbed in various small animals. This route often requires a higher dose and/or a longer time to exert effect.

Fairly large volumes of fluids can be given subcutaneously. It is not absorbed as quickly as some alternatives but is useful e.g. to give fluids after a routine castration. Large volumes are more painful in species which have tight skin. For example, in guinea pigs, which are relatively tight skinned, it can be uncomfortable (less so in the lumbar area rather than the scruff). Hamsters, however, tend to have loose skin so subcutaneous injection may be well tolerated and effective. **As a rough guide it is acceptable to use 1 ml/kg per site in rabbits, 5 ml/kg in rats and 10 ml/kg in mice.**

The environmental temperature affects absorption; at cooler temperatures, absorption of fluids is slower if the animal is vasoconstricted to retain body temperature. Similarly, in a dehydrated and hypovolaemic animal, vasoconstriction reduces and slows uptake. Other routes of fluid administration may be appropriate in these circumstances.

Hyaluronidase is a substance which breaks down the intercellular material to increase uptake and can be used to speed up absorption of drugs or fluids e.g. from a subcutaneous site. There are known drug interactions, so it should only be used with drugs where it has been shown to be safe and effective. **Local reactions are common,** which is unsurprising given the effects on the tissue. People who have had this type of injection report it to be painful. Using hyaluronidase is not common, however it is a possibility. It is probably best reserved for when subcutaneous injection is the best option to administer fluids, but dehydration or other matters reduce the uptake.

Intraosseous Injection

Intraosseous injections of fluids or drugs are as well absorbed as intravenous administration. Care should be taken with the volume administered as the receiving tissue is a no distensible bone and a rapid bolus can be uncomfortable. Therefore, it is best to use an infusion with a syringe driver.

The most frequently used sites of administration are the tibia, and to a lesser extent the femur. (Figure 11). This is a good option for administration when intravenous access is difficult or impossible to perform (e.g. in very small, dehydrated animals).

Intraosseous needle insertion is quite painful so local anaesthesia should be provided in the area or the needle placed under general anaesthetic. The needle provides a route for infection to enter the bone marrow cavity, so it is important to maintain sterility when placing and subsequent dressing/cleanliness. A spinal needle is good to use as the central stylet prevents a plug forming within the needle.

Fluid Administration

Fluids can be administered via a variety of routes; subcutaneous, intraperitoneal, intravenous, or intraosseous. The oral route of administration is not usually appropriate during or immediately after anaesthesia, but is, of course, important for longer term care.

Fluids should be warmed before injection; a cold bolus of fluids could decrease core temperature significantly.

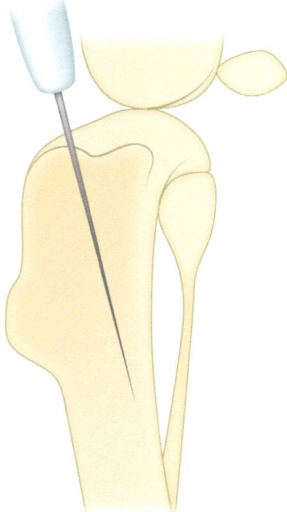

Figure 11. Intraosseous needle insertion in small mammals. The aim is to align the needle with the length of the bone and imagine where the bone cavity is running down inside.

Warming is easily achieved by placing the syringe in a jug of warm water or running under a hot tap, using an incubator, warming oven, or a warmer designed for babies' bottles. However, care should be taken to ensure the fluid is well mixed, especially microwave warmed fluid as hot spots can be generated. Sterility should be maintained during warming.

Fluids should be warmed to around 40 °C, but it is important not to overheat as hot fluids cause tissue damage.

Small Animal Anaesthesia

Inhalation Inductions

Inhalation inductions using a chamber are commonly used in small mammals. Although there are slight variations of technique, this is one effective technique which may reduce apnoea. Sevoflurane may produce a more rapid induction and recovery than isoflurane and is possibly less irritating.

The animal should be placed in a chamber, which should preferably not be too large as this makes it difficult to change the concentration of anaesthetic agent. Oxygen flow alone should be used initially so the animal becomes accustomed to the flow of entering gas. The volatile agent should be introduced with the vaporiser set at 1%, and the animal observed for three or four breaths to ensure there is no breath holding, the percentage should then be increased by 1%. This should be repeated until the vaporiser is set as high as it will go: 5% isoflurane or 8% sevoflurane.

The vaporiser flowmeter should be set to match the size of chamber. A flow which fills the chamber in a minute should be used (e.g. minimum of 1 l flow for a 1 l chamber). Higher flows make changes occur more rapidly; however, they are less pleasant for the animal, more likely to dry the eyes, and/or more irritant.

Once the highest vaporiser setting has been achieved, the animal should be watched for the loss of righting reflex which indicates when to remove the animal from the chamber. This is not an exact reflex. The chamber can be tipped e.g. to 45 degrees sideways; observing whether the animal corrects its position, or moves with the chamber.

When the **righting reflex has been lost,** the animal should be removed and connected to a close fitting mask to complete induction. Immediate opening of the chamber would result in considerable quantities of volatile agent entering the atmosphere (and probably being inhaled by staff) so as much as possible should be removed from the chamber before opening by pressing the oxygen flush button on the machine after the vaporiser is turned off. This stage needs to be done quickly, especially with sevoflurane, so the animal does not recover before attaching a mask; an extra pair of hands makes for a slick exchange. If done well, there should be minimal personnel exposure to volatile agents, however it is wise to try to perform this in a well ventilated area and not allow pregnant staff to participate.

Monitoring Small Animals

A variety of means can be used to aid clinical monitoring in small mammals, e.g. ECG, pulse oximetry, capnography, and blood pressure monitoring. The smaller the animal the more difficult it is to monitor.

CLINICAL MONITORING

Clinical monitoring of depth can include **righting reflex and withdrawal reflexes** (where the toes are pinched firmly, and limb withdrawal is observed). Jaw tone is useful to determine depth but is less easy to evaluate if using a mask for maintenance delivery of anaesthetic vapour. Eye position is difficult to assess in very small animals and may not rotate as expected. Care should be taken with palpebral reflexes as some sources indicate that the palpebral reflex may be retained at surgical planes of anaesthesia in rabbits, and only lost when markedly deep. Some other reflexes may be useful, e.g. an ear pinch reflex in rabbits.

Respiratory rate and heart rate may be used to aid assessment of depth of anaesthesia.

Counting pulses is tricky when the rate is very fast, it can be easier to count over six seconds instead of 15 seconds, (perhaps even three if the rate is very fast). This gives a better indicator than losing some beats. Femoral vessels or apex beats may be the only palpable areas in the very small animal, but peripheral pulses are easy to monitor in larger species such as the rabbit. An **oesophageal stethoscope** can be used in larger animals e.g. rabbits, or a Doppler probe applied to the thorax of very small mammals to give an audible indicator of the heartbeat.

PULSE OXIMETRY

Pulse oximetry can be used in many small mammals, but it is important to bear in mind that much monitoring equipment (whether or not labelled for veterinary use) originates from technology from human monitors. These tend only to count a rate between 30–220 or 250 bpm in most cases. This may be acceptable for use in a rabbit but is an insufficient range for smaller mammals. Some specifically designed veterinary devices count higher rates. The Nonin veterinary designed pulse oximeter counts up to 450 bpm. Some equipment is specifically designed for laboratory or exotic animals (e.g. monitors made by Vetronics).

The desired values for oxygen saturation are the same as for other species (i.e. expected >95%, very concerned <90%).

ECG

Electrode pads for ECG monitoring can be cut down to size and wrapped around limbs to make contact. **Needle electrodes** can be used in very small animals. Although this sounds harsh, they can be less traumatic than crocodile clips. Fine hypodermic needles are placed just under the skin and crocodile clip ECG electrodes are attached to them.

Remember that human designed ECGs may not be able to count the rate, but the waveform will be displayed.

CAPNOGRAPHY

Capnography is useful but there is a need to consider **mainstream versus sidestream capnography,** particularly relating to the dead space and gas withdrawal from the system.

In sidestream capnography, a gas sample is drawn constantly for analysis in the capnograph device. This rate of withdrawal can be a significant amount for a very small animal. Compensatory higher flows mean the capnography sample reads lower than the true reading of CO_2 as fresh gas is also withdrawn (this effect is also seen in cats with small tidal volumes and higher flows). The reading may also be a lower value if there is a leak, e.g. around an uncuffed ETT.

Monitoring is more difficult if the patient does not have an ETT, but there are ways to overcome this such as the use a small cannula in a mask or at the nose. For example, a dog urinary catheter, trimmed to a suitable length, attached to the capnography sampling line then eased under the diaphragm of a close-fitting mask with the tip near the nose; or a small cannula (e.g. such as used for IV) placed at or just inside the nose e.g. in recovery from anaesthesia.

The expected values for end tidal CO_2 are the same as in other species, but artefacts causing lower results as mentioned above should be considered.

BLOOD PRESSURE

Direct blood pressure measurement is possible, particularly in rabbits where arterial cannulation is not difficult, however it is rarely performed in the clinical situation.

Non-invasive methods may be preferable. Cardell (oscillometric) blood pressure monitors, which are popular in veterinary practice, are able to read rabbit blood pressure.

Doppler devices are versatile and useful in a variety of species e.g. rabbits, ferrets, and guinea pigs. A study comparing Doppler blood pressure in rabbits with direct arterial pressures found Doppler to be accurate (Harvey et al., 2012). In very small species it can be used as an audible heart rate monitor.

Blood pressure should be within the ranges expected for other species, e.g. Doppler >80 mmHg approximately.

Temperature

Small mammals are prone to heat loss, and therefore monitoring temperature is very helpful. Care should be taken with the size of thermometers, although most electronic thermometers have quite small tips. Oesophageal or rectal thermistor probes can be used during anaesthesia for a continuous assessment.

Recovery

A warm place for recovery is essential. Temperatures of 26–30 °C are not unreasonable for small rodents. Small incubators can be obtained which are ideal for this purpose, but the animal should be observed at all times. The animal may value some nesting materials.

Anaesthesia of Specific Species

Ferrets

Introduction and Handling

Ferrets are carnivorous, simple stomached animals; this means some of the concerns for other small animals are less relevant. For example, they are used to intermittent feeding, so periods of withholding food are less of a problem. In many ways their physiology is not that different to a cat and in some respects, they can be treated similarly.

Ferrets may nip, so a secure hold is helpful. One method is to put a hand around the chest, with the head between first and second fingers, forelimbs between thumb and index on one side and middle/ring finger on the other to give a safe and secure hold. It is preferable to ensure support to the hind end rather than letting it dangle or swing. Scruffing can be used for aggressive ferrets or for restraint for procedures.

Physiology and Pathology

Ferrets are induced ovulators, requiring copulation to terminate oestrus. If they do not have a mate, female ferrets can have very prolonged oestrus periods. The continuous presence of oestrogen (hyperoestrogenism) can lead to bone marrow suppression and anaemia, with a reduction in platelets which can lead to increased bleeding. Nowadays, chemical contraceptive implants are often used, but a rescued animal may not have been treated appropriately.

Ferrets are prone to adrenal disease which can manifest in a variety of forms depending on which hormones are overproduced.

A normal heart rate is around 120 beats per minute, however this may be higher in an excitable animal when conscious. Respiratory rates are around 20–30 breaths per minute.

Intravenous Access

Intravenous (IV) access is obtained via the cephalic vessels (which are small) or saphenous veins.

If the animal is dehydrated, a larger vessel is preferable, e.g. the jugular. If the veins are very collapsed, then it is worth considering an intraosseous approach. In a wriggly, bright ferret, prior sedation will help.

Drug Combinations

The drug combinations used when anaesthetising a ferret in part depend on their temperament.

Acepromazine/opioid combinations provide mild sedation and may be effective to allow inhalational induction of a cooperative ferret (if a dark mask is available, the ferret may even helpfully insert its own head into the required place).

For more wriggly or difficult to handle animals, ketamine combinations, similar to those used in cats, work well. There are many possible drug combinations which can be used successfully in ferrets, here are a few examples:

- acepromazine 0.05–0.1 mg/kg + buprenorphine 0.02–0.03 mg/kg IM, inhalation induction;
- ketamine 5 mg/kg + medetomidine 40–50 µg/kg + butorphanol 0.1–0.2 mg/kg IM; or
- ketamine 5 mg/kg + midazolam 0.5 mg/kg IM, inhalation induction.

Endotracheal Intubation

The trachea is relatively large in ferrets and the mouth opens wide to permit good visualisation (provided there is adequate muscle relaxation). For these reasons, intubation is not usually difficult. Uncuffed endotracheal tubes maximise the airway; 3–3.5 mm is suitable for most ferrets.

A small laryngoscope helps with visualisation. The assistant holding for intubation should ensure the neck is straight which is not always easy due to the extreme flexibility of the ferret's body. It is not usually necessary to use topical local anaesthetics, however some veterinarians may opt to do so.

Securing the ETT is not easy, as bandage tends to pull off easily. Narrow adhesive tape can be passed under the ETT and then crossed over the upper muzzle, but other techniques are also acceptable.

Maintenance and Monitoring

As endotracheal intubation is so easy, maintenance with inhalational agents is usually employed. For monitoring the depth of anaesthesia, withdrawal reflexes, palpebral reflexes, and jaw tone are appropriate.

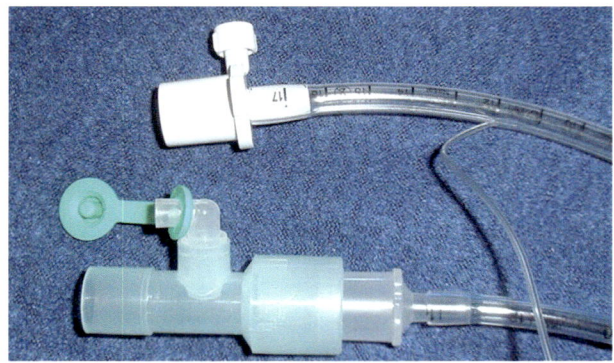

Figure 12. Using a low dead space connector (upper) is advisable for small animals.

A low dead space ETT connector facilitates capnography (Figure 12). Even in darker haired ferrets, the pads are often unpigmented, so if the pulse oximeter clip does not work well on the tongue, the paw is a good alternative.

An ECG can be used with pads cut to size and then secured to the paws or around the limbs. Doppler blood pressure measurements can sometimes be taken by placing the cuff above the elbow with the probe on the medial side of the forelimb, between carpus and elbow. Temperature monitoring is important as heat loss is a big problem in all small mammals.

Rabbits

General Considerations and Handling
Rabbits are the third most common pet in the UK and commonly presented for anaesthesia in veterinary practice.

Care should be taken when handling, as a rabbit can kick out forcefully. The rabbit may be more comfortable with a hold which permits the head to be hidden, and it is important to **ensure the hindquarters are always supported.**

Check for Preexisting Disease
Although owner and veterinary awareness of respiratory disease in rabbits (often termed *Pasteurella*) has improved, however, it is still possible to encounter animals with poorly controlled respiratory conditions. Sometimes it is unclear how relevant the diagnosis of *Pasteurella* may be.

Normal heart rates are around 220 beats per minute, with respiratory rates around 50 breaths per minute. It is important to bear in mind that stress causes these values to increase, whilst the use of α-2 agonists (in particular) decreases them.

Ileus
Rabbits are prone to poor gastrointestinal motility (ileus). Ileus is a multifactorial condition, with stress, pain, and drugs all contributing to a decrease in gastrointestinal motility in rabbits.

In rabbits the aim is to **avoid starvation** and ensure they eat again soon after anaesthesia to maintain gastrointestinal function. Many veterinarians use metoclopramide to encourage motility around anaesthesia. A fast recovery and eating soon after an anaesthetic reduce the problems with ileus, but of course a comfortable rabbit eats better, so pain relief is important.

Positioning
Rabbits have a large volume of guts (not dissimilar to the horse) and this pressure on the diaphragm limits ventilation. If possible, a tilted table should be used for anaesthesia to maintain a head up posture. A rolled pad under the thorax of the rabbit is not ideal, as the rabbit may develop a curved spine which compresses the thorax. If a tilting table is not available, a board which is elevated at one end can be used.

Intravenous Access
It is usually possible to obtain IV access in rabbits, but when this is not possible then the intraosseous route should be considered.

The most common site for intravenous access is the **marginal ear vein,** with most anaesthetists using the caudal edge of the ear. However, care should be taken not to enter the artery, unless this is the desired vessel. The cephalic vein can also be used, which is a reasonable option in a very small Netherlands Dwarf with petite ears.

EMLA is very useful and is particularly effective on the ear where the skin is very thin in the rabbit, and also produces some vasodilation. Further local vasodilation can be encouraged by warming the ear (e.g. holding a glove filled with warm water on the ear for a few minutes).

Everyone has their own preferred methods for taping catheters into the ears. A few swabs on the inside of the ear can be useful, however excessive weight e.g. rolls of bandage should be avoided, as this is unpleasant for the animal and counterproductive.

Arterial Access
The auricular artery in the ear is readily accessible and suitable for sampling blood gases or direct blood pressure measurement if desired. Although not likely to be used in day to day practice, arterial access is useful when dealing with very sick rabbits e.g. liver torsions.

Premedication and Induction
Premedication in rabbits consists of a variety of drugs, including α-2 agonists, midazolam and/or opioids.

Examples of premedication drugs include:

- medetomidine 0.1–0.3 mg/kg + buprenorphine 0.01–0.3 mg/kg IM;
- buprenorphine 0.03 mg/kg IV followed by midazolam 0.5–1 mg/kg IV five minutes later; or
- ketamine may be added to medetomidine/opioid combinations and to produce anaesthesia with high doses.

Subcutaneous injection of drugs is popular in rabbits but requires a longer onset time and slightly higher doses than needed for IM.

Some rabbits possess an atropinase enzyme which rapidly inactivates atropine should it be required.

INDUCTION

In the UK, alfaxalone is now licensed for use in the rabbit and is a popular induction agent. It is usually used intravenously but can be given intramuscularly for sedation; the disadvantage of intramuscular use being the large volume required.

Propofol is adequate, however has a short duration of action in rabbits.

Inhalational inductions should be avoided except if the patient is heavily sedated. Inhalation inductions are useful for many small mammals, but not the rabbit, as rabbits find inhalation inductions very stressful. The only times this may be reasonable are in the profoundly sedated animal or the very sick and unresponsive.

ENDOTRACHEAL INTUBATION

Endotracheal intubation is not easy in rabbits, with many variations of the techniques used.

Many anaesthetists use visual techniques. The larynx is not easy to visualise, due to the narrow gape and preponderance of soft tissue in the mouth and pharynx. A small laryngoscope can be used or often an otoscope. Once visualised, some practitioners drop some local anaesthetic on the larynx, but many do not.

The ETT may be inserted directly or a guide (e.g. dog urinary catheter) inserted first and then the ETT guided over the top. Noncuffed ETT's are usually used in rabbits, with sizes 2.5–3.5 mm being suitable for most rabbits. It may be helpful to ensure a straight airway by lifting the head (Figure 13).

Blind techniques are also used. For this it is easier for the operator to hold the head themselves in one hand, lift the head, straighten the neck, and place the ETT just in front of the larynx; airflow is then heard or felt against the side of the face. As the ETT is advanced, loss of airflow means the tube has entered the oesophagus, so it may be withdrawn slightly

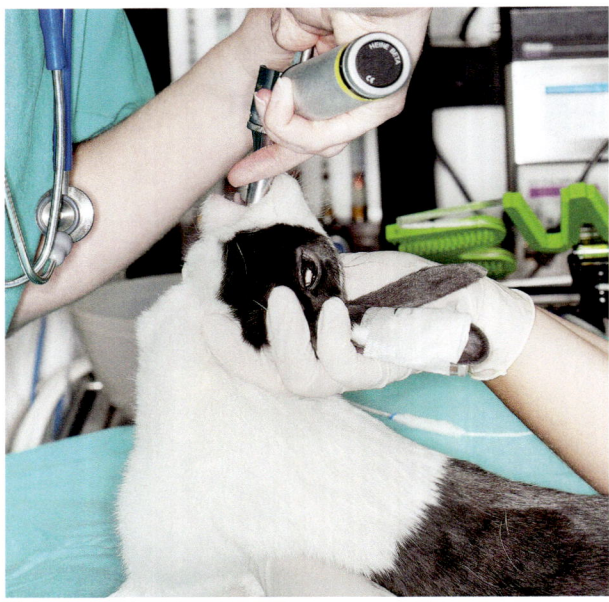

Figure 13. Head lifted for intubation.

and the procedure reattempted. Nasal intubation is possible in larger rabbits, again, the neck should be straightened upwards and the ventral meatus targeted.

PROBLEMS WITH ENDOTRACHEAL TUBES IN RABBITS

It is important to recognise laryngospasm; subsequently apnoea will occur, followed by cyanosis. It is possible to give some ventilatory support to the nonintubated rabbit by rocking it gently backwards and forwards, this pushes some air in and out of the lungs, or alternatively air can be forced in via a mask (although this also causes some stomach distension).

An excessively long ETT may enter one bronchus and produce one lung ventilation. In this case, the tidal volume is small, and cyanosis may occur. To recognise this has occurred, thoracic movement should be observed as there may be a visible asymmetry, and air movements not heard on one side of the thorax. To avoid this, ETTs should be measured carefully against the rabbit and passing tubes past the thoracic inlet should be avoided. However, an ETT which is too short is readily dislodged.

Kinking of the tube which occurs especially at the junction of the connector should be checked for. Other occlusions of endotracheal tubes can occur, e.g. if food particles are wedged in the lumen.

It is also possible the ETT may become disconnected from the connector and aspirated.

Trauma to the larynx during intubation leads to mucosal inflammation and swelling, and possible airway obstruction after extubation. There are also reports of airway inflammation after chemical irritation (e.g. from a cleaning solution not fully removed) (Grint et al., 2006).

ALTERNATIVES TO INTUBATION

It is not essential to intubate the trachea in most cases for rabbits, however, it is preferable and does permit ready support of ventilation if required. Alternatively, a close fitting mask can be used, the corner of the mandible should be pushed forward and into the mask to ensure a clear airway.

Laryngeal mask airways are devices which sit on top of the glottis without entering the trachea per se, hence they are also known as supraglottic devices. Devices designed for people may be used in rabbits, but the size and shape are not necessarily perfect, as they are not designed for this species. The inflatable cushion can be adjusted to seal the pharynx.

The V-gel (Docsinnovent™) is a specially designed laryngeal mask airway device for rabbits. There is also a cat version, so it is important to ensure the correct species' device is selected as the shapes are different. This laryngeal mask airway has a gel surround which sits in the pharynx. A piece enters the top of the oesophagus and has a series of baffles to block it off. The epiglottis is pushed down by the epiglottic rest. Correct positioning of the tube should be confirmed using capnography.

During long procedures (particularly in larger rabbits) discolouration of the tongue may be observed, which is related to pressure by the epiglottic rest. It may be advisable to move the position of the device slightly to permit blood flow.

The epiglottis can be pushed back into the larynx during placement of the device and the seal for ventilation is not as effective as when using an endotracheal tube. Although many veterinarians would use an ETT as a first choice, V gel airways are useful as a backup should intubation not be possible or for ease of placement for short procedures.

Chinchillas

Great care should be taken when handling a chinchilla to **avoid fur slip.** This is a condition whereby the animal sheds a lump of hair in response to being trapped or held in a stressful situation, and is a risk when restrained for injections etc.

Small blood samples (e.g. a single drop to check blood glucose) are readily taken from the ear in chinchillas. Larger samples are better taken from the jugular vein. For IV access, the saphenous vein is accessible or intraosseous (tibial) techniques can be used.

Heart rates can be between 150–250 beats per minute with respiratory rates of 40–80 breaths per minute.

Ketamine/midazolam (5–10 mg/kg plus 0.5 mg/kg IM) provides good sedation, with anaesthetic induction completed with volatile agent as required. Medetomidine can be substituted for midazolam (e.g. 0.06 mg/kg) but it is best that this is only used in healthy chinchillas. An opioid such as buprenorphine 0.05 mg/kg SC can be added for a painful procedure.

Maintenance may be with a mask and volatile agent. It is possible to intubate the trachea in chinchillas with a 1 or 1.5 mm ETT (e.g. made by Cook). A blind technique similar to that used in rabbits is used or a rigid endoscope (if available) to guide insertion.

Guinea Pigs

Guinea pigs do not vomit but do have pharyngeal pouches. Green liquid material may emerge from these pouches which looks similar to regurgitant material. Although a long starvation is not advisable, withholding food for two to three hours prior to anaesthesia may help to reduce the contents of the pharyngeal pouches.

Guinea pigs do not ventilate well under anaesthesia, and it is common for paradoxical ventilation to be seen.

A normal heart rate is around 280 beats per minute.

ANAESTHETIC DRUG COMBINATIONS

For a well-handled guinea pig, acepromazine and buprenorphine are often adequate sedation for an inhalation induction. Atropine can be added to this combination to reduce respiratory secretions and dilate airways.

For more lively or difficult to handle guinea pigs, ketamine combinations (e.g. with medetomidine and buprenorphine) are used. Some published doses are high, and these can cause slow recoveries, a smaller amount could be used with induction completed with a mask and volatile agent if required.

For example, some texts recommend 250–500 µg/kg medetomidine and 40 mg/kg ketamine for sedation, but in the author's experience medetomidine at 50–100 µg/kg with 2–5 mg/kg ketamine is more than adequate for sedation; higher doses of ketamine will induce anaesthesia if desired.

INTUBATION

It is possible to intubate the trachea of a guinea pig, but this is best performed with endoscopic guidance.

MONITORING ANAESTHESIA

Doppler can be used for anaesthetic monitoring. Placing a cuff above the elbow with a probe on the medial aspect of the limb produces credible results.

Hamsters

Hamsters are not the easiest animals to handle and it is best to gently cup them in the hands. It is possible to restrain hamsters using the scruff but care should be taken as the protuberant eyes proptose if the skin is pulled excessively.

Normal heart rates are around 350 beats per minute with respiratory rates of around 80 breaths per minute.

There are reports of hamsters self-mutilating after intramuscular injections of ketamine and xylazine. This may be from irritation; ketamine appears to sting on IM injection in various species. Intraperitoneal drugs can be used, but many people rely on inhalational techniques.

Care should be taken with hamsters' eyes. The protuberant eyes in this nocturnal species mean they can be easily damaged accidentally, for example with the edge of a mask.

It is possible to access the cephalic or saphenous veins if the hamster is still enough, although small, "off-the-needle" injection may be feasible. The vessels are small but readily visible. The skin is very thin so care should be taken to ensure a superficial approach.

Gerbils and Degus

Handling of gerbils and degus should be gentle, but it is important to hold them firmly around the body. **It is important to be aware of tail slip,** where improperly handled gerbils or degus (e.g. if the tail is grabbed) lose hair or even skin over the tip of the tail.

Gerbils have normal heart rates of around 260–300 beats per minute with respiratory rates of around 90 breaths per minute. For degus, the heart rate is lower (100–150 bpm) and the respiratory rate is around 75 breaths per minute.

There are reports of gerbils receiving Saffan® (an older preparation of alfaxalone) IP, however the newer formulation of alfaxalone (Alfaxan®) has not been reported as being used in this way. Ketamine combinations or inhalation inductions are the main techniques used.

Rats and Mice

Rats and mice are generally not too difficult to handle. Mice can be held securely by holding the skin along the back. Rats respond well to being handled along an arm or hand but do not like being scruffed at all, so this is not recommended. It is acceptable to hold a tail if required in these species.

Normal heart rates are around 350 beats per minute for a rat and can be over 500 for a mouse. Respiratory rates are around 70–100 breaths per minute for rats and 100–200 for a mouse.

DRUGS

There is a lot of information on rats and mice, from laboratory animal work. It is useful as a reference, but laboratory animals are usually young and healthy animals so care should be taken when extrapolating results to sick pets.

Ketamine combinations and inhalation anaesthesia are often used.

INTUBATION

It is possible to intubate the trachea of larger rats, using a small laryngoscope to aid vision, as the mouth opens wide enough to allow visibility. Size wise, a 1–1.5 mm ETT can be used or an IV cannula in smaller animals (it is important to ensure it is a soft material which does not kink easily, this can be tested by bending one in the hand).

INTRAVENOUS ACCESS

Intravenous access in rats is obtained via the tail vein or cephalic in larger specimens.

MONITORING

Blood pressure monitoring using Doppler may be obtainable in a bigger rat. In a mouse, Doppler can be used to obtain an audible heart rate if placed over the heart. A pulse oximeter probe can be used on a paw as they usually have unpigmented pads. This works well in rats, but probes may be rather large for mice.

Pain and Analgesia in Small Animals

Introduction

It is not always easy to evaluate pain in small mammals. There are many similarities in evaluating pain across species, but also some differences. More information on pain scoring is found in Chapter 6, but it is worth thinking about how pain can be recognised in small mammals.

General Signs of Pain in Small Mammals

There are a variety of **general (nonspecific) signs of pain in small animals.** It is important o bear in mind some of these signs are indicative of general malaise, of which pain plays a part.
1. Unkempt coat due to a decrease in self grooming.
2. Respiratory changes, e.g. faster respiratory rate or irregular patterns.

3. Reduced appetite.
4. Teeth grinding, in rabbits in particular and other herbivores.
5. Inactivity, interspersed with bouts of marked (not particularly controlled) activity.

Specific Pain Behaviours

The University of Newcastle have studied small mammals for years, as part of their work to improve laboratory animal care and welfare. They identified specific pain behaviours and signs in small mammals, which they describe as arch, writhe, twitch, stagger, and press. These behaviours have specifically been studied in rabbits, rats, and mice, but due to the similarity between species it is fair to assume that gerbils, hamsters and other rodents also show similar movements.

RABBITS
- Arch: an upward movement of the spine into a curve.
- Flinch: a sudden unusual movement of the body.
- Wince: a sudden grimace.
- Twitch: a sudden movement of the skin, e.g. over the back.
- Press: the spine is moved ventrally, pressing into the floor.
- Stagger: when moving about, the animal appears unsteady.

Unfortunately, rabbits often do not demonstrate these behaviours when watched, and they are more clearly seen when there is a camera used to take video footage without an in person observer. It is often wise to treat pain based on knowledge of a procedure in other species rather than respond to visible pain signs.

RATS
Rats are more demonstrative than rabbits. The arching and pressing signs can be dramatic, large movements. They can also show a writhing movement of the body.

MICE
Mice show some similar movements to rats, with flinching, pressing staggering, and twitching readily observed. Other small rodents are likely to show similar behaviours.

Facial Indicators of Pain

Over the last 10 years there has been growing interest in so called pain faces or grimace scales where characteristic changes in facial expression are used as a guide to pain assessment.

Some years ago, an interesting research project used video observation and eye tracking to follow people's eye movements when watching a video of rabbits to evaluate pain (Leach et al., 2011). The key finding was most people focus on the face of an animal for a considerable proportion of time. The suggestion at the time was that perhaps people do not look to see pain, however there is more evidence now that facial expressions can be used to assess pain. Facial expressions have also been used in nonverbal children and in cats.

There are a variety of signs to look for, with many broad similarities and some differences, between species.

ORBITAL OPENING
Orbital tightening is a clear sign of pain, where the eyes become narrowed and are held closed more tightly. This is seen in cats and other species.

EARS
In rabbits, the ears close more tightly or fold and pull back over the back (with lop eared animals this sign is not as clear). In rats and mice, the space between the ears appears wider, as the ears pull downwards and to the side.

WHISKERS
In comfortable animals the whiskers droop slightly, the muscles at the base of the follicles are relaxed. As the animal becomes painful, there is more tension in these muscles and whiskers look as if they are standing out on end.

NOSE
In rabbits, increased muscle tension pulls the tip of the nose towards the mouth and the shape becomes more angular, more V shaped. In mice, the area above the nostrils bulges as the muscles become tenser, but in rats it flattens out more. In all cases the area looks different to the normal relaxed animal.

CHEEKS
In rabbits and rats, the cheeks flatten and from the front this gives a sunken appearance, or the face looks longer and narrower. In mice, however, there is bulging of the cheeks.

The main things to look out for are changes from a normal appearance, as all these changes are related to increased muscle activity, the face being tense rather than relaxed.

The National Centre for the Replacement Refinement and Reduction of Animals in Research's website has excellent visual resources available on the grimace scales in rats, rabbits and mice: https://nc3rs.org.uk/grimacescales.

Scoring systems generally include an intervention level when the animal is considered to be in pain and analgesia is required. However, these have generally not been well defined in grimace scales, although there is a suggestion for an intervention level in rabbits (Varga, 2016) These signs are very useful however in helping assist clinical judgement in management.

Analgesia in Small Mammals

Analgesia is well researched in common laboratory species.

Most is known about **buprenorphine and NSAIDs** which are generally the first choice for postoperative analgesia. However, it is important to remember laboratory research is conducted in animals which are usually young and healthy, and dose alteration is required in sicker and older clinical cases.

Local anaesthetic can be used but with extreme care when dosing for small animals. Up to 4 mg/kg lidocaine or 1.5 mg/kg bupivacaine is appropriate. When this volume is very small, it can be diluted (in normal saline) to make a reasonable volume if required. Local anaesthetics may be used to infiltrate around a surgical site, as specific nerve blocks (e.g. the femoral or sciatic nerve), or for regional techniques (such as in epidurals which are useful techniques in rabbits and ferrets).

Other opioids such as methadone may be used, but less is known about their effects in these species. That said, fentanyl was available in a product known as Hypnorm™ for many years (which is no longer available), so this has been widely used and would appear to be a good choice for additional analgesia if required.

Ketamine is commonly thought of as an induction agent, however it may be used for analgesia as a supplement to first line therapies.

ANAESTHESIA IN BIRDS

Introduction

It is important to note that birds are in a different class compared to mammals and there is a **huge difference in both anatomy and physiology.** Differences in the respiratory tract, in particular, are highly relevant for anaesthesia. This chapter is an introduction to the major points regarding birds and avian anaesthesia, rather than a comprehensive review.

It is not appropriate to try to treat all birds in the same manner; this is a little like trying to treat a mouse like a dog or an elephant. **Extrapolation between species** is necessary, however, and perhaps even more so than in mammals as there is often less research information available on which to base decisions.

There are many variations of anaesthetic drug combinations, and it is impossible to give absolutes for every situation. Included here are some guidelines and suggestions, but it is important to work as a veterinary team to ensure the selection is appropriate for the individual animal.

Anatomy

Avian Respiratory System

The respiratory system in birds has many important differences to more familiar mammalian anatomy and physiology. These differences include anatomy of the upper and lower respiratory tracts, and functional differences.

LARYNX

The larynx in birds is a much simpler structure than in mammals; it not the organ responsible for vocalisation, so precise muscular control is not required. There is no epiglottis and therefore it is usually easy to intubate (subject to the beak shape permitting access).

TRACHEA

The trachea in birds has **complete tracheal rings,** rather than the incomplete (C-shape) rings seen in mammals. This is an important difference, as it means there is no distensibility of the trachea. For this reason, cuffed endotracheal tubes are best avoided.

Some species of bird have a tracheal sac or extra long loops of trachea (these features aid increased resonance). The names of bird species with these features may give a clue to their presence such as the whooper swan (Figure 14). **Extra long tracheas with loops increase dead space considerably.** However, birds can overcome this being as much of a problem as expected by their altered respiratory pattern, and their efficiency of ventilation.

Figure 14 shows a diagram of the respiratory tract of a whooper swan. From the larynx, the trachea descends the neck in an S-shape, but before entering the thorax it passes backwards under the keel bone (the equivalent of the sternum in mammals) and over the outside of the body cavity in a large loop before returning and entering the thorax.

In other species of birds the trachea may divide into two, as if the two mainstem bronchi are joined together, with only a short trachea above them (Figure 15).

In some species, there is a shorter septum dividing the trachea which may only be a short piece above the bifurcation of the trachea or may extend further towards the larynx. There is therefore a risk of entering one lung or hitting the septum if long tubes are used in these species.

LOWER RESPIRATORY SYSTEM

It is important to note that **birds do not have a diaphragm.**

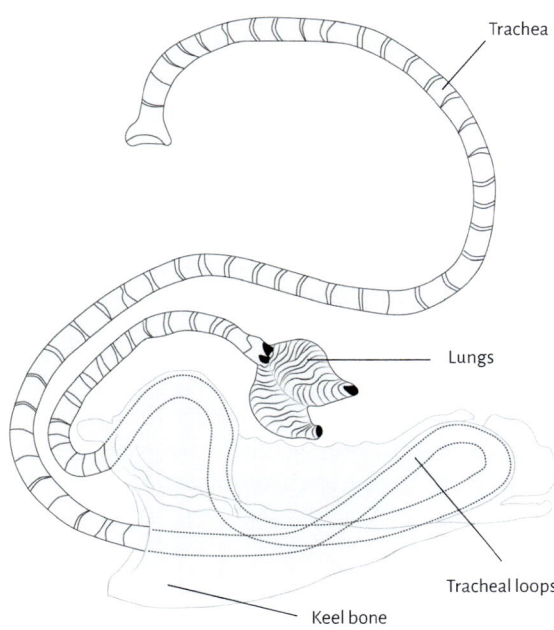

Figure 14. Diagram showing whooper swan respiratory tract.

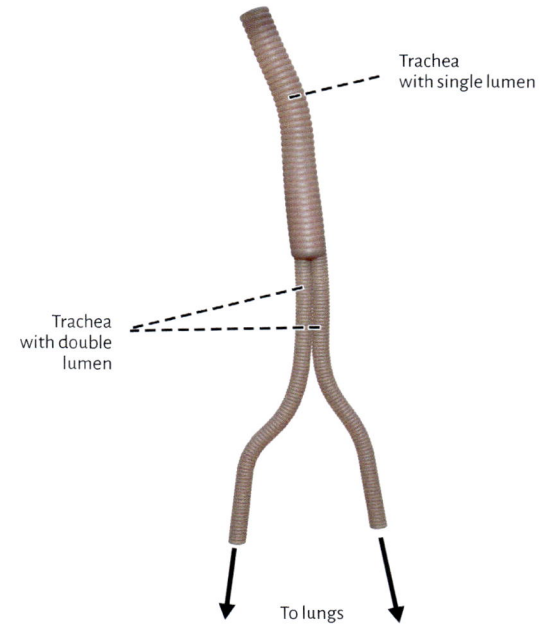

Figure 15. A divided trachea can be seen in some penguin species e.g. the yellow eyed penguin from New Zealand.

The body cavity (coelom) is one chamber. **This means birds are reliant on movement of the keel bone/ribs to inhale.** In a mammal if the thorax is restricted, the diaphragm can still move caudally and permit air entry, but this does not happen in birds.

The organ for vocalisation in birds is the syrinx, which is located around the bifurcation of the trachea. This location means some noises may be heard e.g. when providing ventilation to an anaesthetised bird.

The bronchi divide and divide again into parabronchi. These are rigid tubules which are the main area of gas exchange, equivalent to the alveoli in mammals, and are known as paleopulmonic lung tissue. Birds may have a variable proportion (depending on species) of what is known as **neopulmonic lung tissue,** the construction of which is more like mammalian lung, but this is generally not so important.

The parabronchi tubules are rigid and nondistensible, so there needs to be other means of allowing expansion in the coelom to allow gas passage through the lung tissue. This is a one way system in birds. As the thorax increases in volume, this generates a subatmospheric pressure and gas is drawn in from the larynx and stored in the air sacs. These are literally **storage sacs, which do not participate in gas exchange** (Figure 16). Gas passes from the air sacs and then through the tubules of lung tissue via a complicated sequence of

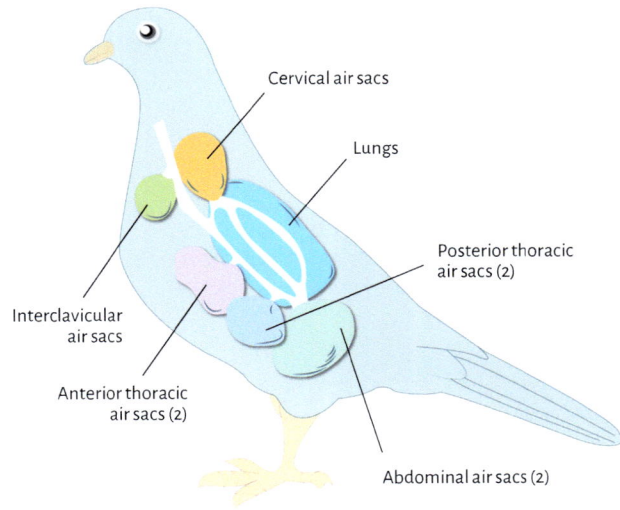

Figure 16. Diagram showing the orientation of the airsacs in a bird.

movements, which contribute to the efficiency of the respiratory system in birds.

Both the inhalation and exhalation phases are active in birds, meaning they require muscle activity to pull gas in and to push gas out again (unlike in mammals where inspiration is active, but expiration is passive). Respiration may therefore be affected by excessive muscle relaxation during anaesthesia.

The exact numbers/locations of air sacs or air flow through them are perhaps less important to remember, but a note should be taken particularly of the abdominal airsacs which are large and easily compressed by accident.

As the lungs are not distensible, the air sacs must be allowed to distend to produce inhalation and movement of gas through the oxygen absorbing parabronchi. It is important to note that **the air sacs connect with the wing skeleton;** these pneumatic bones contribute to the lightness of a bird's skeleton (helpful in flight). Other pneumatic bones commonly found in domestic bird species include the vertebrae and the skull. This is relevant for anaesthesia, especially if the intraosseous route is used for fluid administration, making it vital to check the relevant species to ensure fluids are administered in appropriate nonpneumatised bone.

The gas flow through the parabronchi is unidirectional and there is what is known as a cross current mechanism (blood flows in the opposite direction to the airflow) which permits efficient absorption of oxygen from inspired gas (Figure 17).

Avian Cardiovascular System

Blood
The red blood cells in birds are an ovoid shape and nucleated. This is relevant for anaesthesia, for example when monitoring with pulse oximetry; if light absorption is affected by the nuclei in the cells, this could affect results. This factor probably explains the variability in response of pulse oximetry in birds.

Heart
In birds the heart has four chambers, as in mammals, with a similar function but there are some differences. Within the valves of the heart are myocardial fibres and electrical connections (which mean they close tightly). The different electrical configuration means the **ECG looks different, with a predominant negative S wave** (Figure 18).

Renal Portal System

Birds have a renal portal system, which means blood from the hindlimbs preferentially perfuses the kidney before entering the systemic circulation. Although the importance of the renal portal system is debatable, it may be relevant to drug uptake for an injection given in the hindlimbs.

The amount of blood passing through the portal system varies and is controlled by the sympathetic/parasympathetic systems. However, it is perhaps less important for anaesthetics, as the effect of the drugs is visible and additional drug can be given if required.

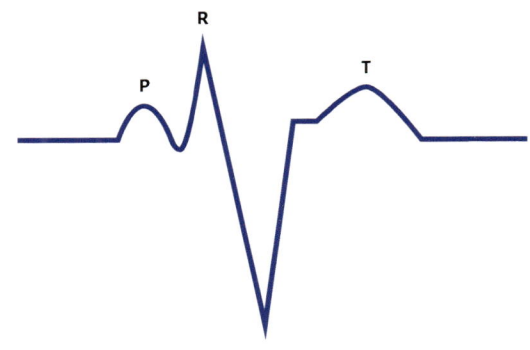

Figure 18. Avian ECG.

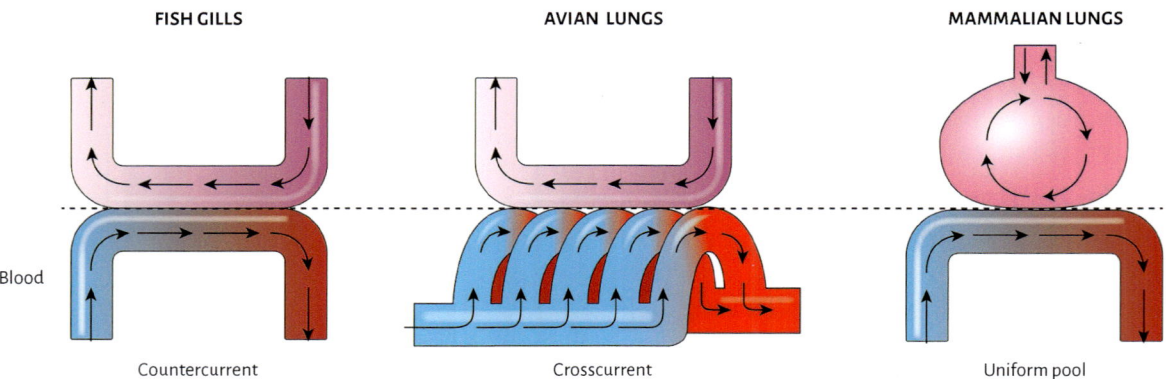

Figure 17. Crosscurrent mechanism which permits very efficient absorption of oxygen from inspired gas.

Techniques in Avian Anaesthesia

Intravenous Access

In most birds the **right jugular** is more developed and used for intravenous access. Wing veins are useful in medium sized birds. Waterfowl that have sturdier legs than some birds also have good vessels e.g. the dorsal metatarsal vein which is a good access point for swans. The intraosseous route is another option (but the wing should not be used) with the tibia a useful route in small, debilitated birds.

Drug Combinations

Examples of the drugs appropriate for use in birds are given below, but the veterinary team must determine the best option in an individual case:
- ketamine combinations (with diazepam or medetomidine or dexmedetomidine): e.g. 25–75 µg/kg dexmedetomidine with 2–5 mg/kg ketamine;
- inhalation techniques (+/- midazolam premedication);
- isoflurane/sevoflurane requirement is similar to mammals;
- intravenous alfaxalone (3–5 mg/kg) or propofol can be used to induce anaesthesia e.g. in waterfowl;
- atropine/glycopyrrolate may be used to reduce respiratory secretions.

Inhalational Induction

Inhalation induction is often used in birds. One reason for this is their efficient respiratory system means inhalation inductions/recoveries are much faster than in mammals, with the drugs taken up or eliminated more quickly.
- It should be ensured that the keel bone can move freely when the bird is restrained for induction.
- It is important to ensure that there is no air sac compression, especially of the abdominal sacs as this impairs ventilation.

> **Due to the variability of facial shape, some creativity with masks may be required in birds.**

Intubation

Intubation is generally quite easy in birds, subject to beak anatomy allowing access to the oral cavity. The simple larynx means it is usually quite easy to enter the glottis. However, there are risks and problems associated with avian tracheal anatomy (e.g. the complete tracheal rings and possible presence of a septum). For this reason, a different type of tube is recommended for birds. These are called Cole pattern tubes. Although normal uncuffed endotracheal tubes are acceptable, acquiring a set of Cole pattern tubes is recommended for any practice that anaesthetises a significant number of birds. The Cole tube is short and uncuffed. The narrow tip sits within the glottis and the wider shoulder creates a seal against the larynx.

An alternative to traditional endotracheal intubation is to **place a tube into an air sac.** This requires a cut-down endotracheal tube, which is surgically placed in an air sac. Ventilation is provided through this tube (there may be some leak from the larynx) but requires a veterinary surgeon to perform the surgical procedure. This is a technique used in specialist practices.

Monitoring Anaesthesia

To monitor the depth of anaesthesia, **useful tools are heart rate and respiratory rate, but also jaw tone and the corneal reflex.**

The eye position stays constant in birds, as the globe does not rotate. Pinching the toe may produce a withdrawal reflex during lighter anaesthesia, and the wing muscle tone (where it is practical to stretch the wing out) can also be evaluated.

Some authors use the palpebral reflex (somewhat like in mammals), if the response is unclear an alternative is the corneal reflex (Figure 19). To test the latter, a moistened cotton bud can be used to gently touch the corneal surface. The normal reflex is a withdrawal of the globe into the head and the movement of the third eyelid across the cornea (or a blink in some species).

MONITORING EQUIPMENT: ECG
An ECG can be used, but it is important to remember the ECG appears different to that of mammals. In smaller birds, crocodile clips can traumatise the skin and pads are unlikely to stick, in which case **needle electrodes are used.** These are fine hypodermic needles, passed just under the skin and the clip of the ECG is then attached to the needle; this might appear rough but is less traumatic than harsh clips. Heart rates are fast for most small birds (around 350–450 bpm) so it is worth checking the maximum rate the monitor can display, as not all can cope with such a fast rate.

DOPPLER
In larger birds Doppler evaluation of blood pressure is possible, with a cuff above the elbow on the wing and the probe on the medial aspect of the wing. A minimum blood pressure of 90 mmHg should be aimed for.

CAPNOGRAPHY
Capnography is useful in birds as respiratory rates tend to be high at any time.

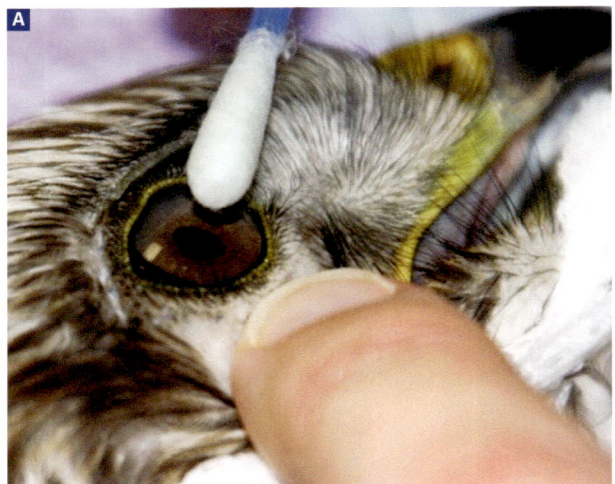

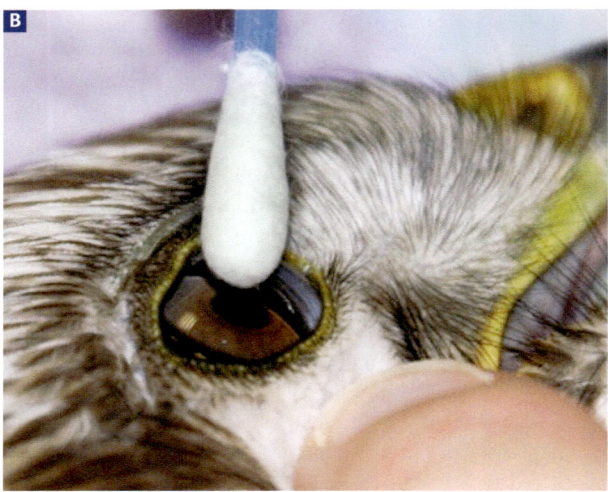

Figure 19. A. Shows the eye before it has been touched with the cotton bud; particular attention should be paid to the medial edge of the eye which is towards the right hand side of the picture; **B.** Shows the eye after the cornea has been touched; note the medial aspect of the eye, to see how the globe is withdrawn. Images courtesy of Emma Love.

PULSE OXIMETRY
Pulse oximetry may be used but may be inaccurate due to avian nucleated red blood cells.

THERMOMETER
Most of these animals are small and liable to heat loss, so monitoring temperature is important.

General Anaesthetic Considerations

Due to anatomical differences, a number of considerations must be taken into account when anaesthetising birds.

- It is important to **avoid air sac compression.** Hands should be positioned carefully when holding a bird to ensure the keel bone is able to move (for example one hand cranially and one hand caudally behind the legs).
- **Most birds do not ventilate well in dorsal recumbency** as this position can compress the air sacs.
- As with all species, it is important to ensure the airway is patent. The airway can get blocked with secretions and some veterinarians reduce this risk of this by the use of atropine or glycopyrrolate.
- A risk at induction and recovery is that the bird may flap its wings and cause itself trauma. Wrapping the bird in a towel loosely to prevent it from being able to extend its wings and flap can be helpful. It is of course vital that the bird's ventilation is not constricted.
- Birds should be extubated at the last minute but jaw tone should be monitored to ensure a sharp beak does not cut or constrict the tube.

Avian Pain Assessment and Analgesia

Pain Assessment

Many signs of pain in birds are **nonspecific.**

In the postoperative period, it can be useful to look for signs of irritation/attention to the operative site and monitor the bird for signs of general malaise such as appetite.

In more chronic pain, signs include:
- anxiety
- apprehension
- restlessness
- decreased appetite
- dullness
- elevated respiratory rate
- inactivity
- increased aggression
- escape attempts
- immobility
- fluffed up appearance
- salivation
- scratching painful area
- social isolation
- vocalisation
- refusal to allow grooming.

Some of these signs are only visible when observed in the interaction of a group (e.g. in an aviary or flock of hens) but the owner may report indications. Some signs also appear contradictory such as escape attempts or inactivity, restlessness, or immobility, therefore looking for **behavioural changes from the norm is important.**

Analgesia

Butorphanol is the most popular opioid for use in birds.

One often quoted fact is that there is a greater density of kappa opioid receptors found in birds (and therefore a kappa agonist such as butorphanol may be superior). The original study which sparked this statement regarding kappa receptors was in pigeons (specifically referring to the forebrain, there are differences in different parts of the CNS) (Reiner et al., 1989), and it is unclear how valid this assumption is in other species.

Morphine, pethidine and other agents have been used in a variety of species; however, many reports are contradictory and may reflect species and dosing differences. Tramadol has been used in ducks and parrots.
- butorphanol: 0.05–2 mg/kg IM
- pethidine: 1–4 mg/kg IM
- oral tramadol: 30 mg/kg reported in ducks
- NSAIDs can be useful and have anti-inflammatory effects as well as providing analgesia (for example meloxicam: 0.5 mg/kg IM).

LOCAL ANAESTHETICS

There are reports of birds being more sensitive to local anaesthetics than mammals, however this is unlikely to be true. However, many birds, especially pets such as budgerigars, are much lighter than estimated, as the feathers are deceptive. Birds have a pneumatic skeleton, so it is important to remember the bones are lighter than those of an equivalent sized mammal.

Unless experienced in doing so, estimating bird weights is not recommended and accurate scales should always be used. If using an accurate weight, up to 3 mg/kg lidocaine can be used in birds, diluted to make a reasonable volume if required. There is an increasing tendency for exotics veterinarians to use sedation and local anaesthetics in some birds.

ANAESTHESIA IN REPTILES

Introduction

Reptiles pose different challenges for anaesthesia. One thing which is very different to mammals (and birds) is that **these animals are poikilothermic (cold blooded)**, which is relevant as it affects their physiology and response to drugs.

The respiratory and cardiovascular systems in reptiles are also quite different in anatomy and physiology from other more common species, whilst their anatomy also presents challenges for intravenous access.

Additionally, there is little good quality evidence of anaesthesia and analgesia in these species. Reptiles vary hugely, so although it may not be ideal, extrapolation between species may be necessary.

Reptilian Biology

Thermoregulation

Being poikilothermic means the animal is totally dependent on its surroundings for its body heat (unlike a mammal or bird which can maintain a body temperature above that of the surroundings).

Metabolism affects everything. **The temperature of the environment therefore affects heart rate and drug biotransformation in reptiles.** It is an important differentiation meaning that reptiles are much slower regarding everything related to anaesthesia and metabolism compared to mammals (note the intervals of analgesic administration presented later in this section). It is important these animals are kept at the correct surrounding temperature for the species (e.g. an appropriate vivarium). **Cold decreases drug elimination** even further.

Some **common species preferred temperature ranges** are shown below (Table 4). These values are taken from Veterinary Nursing of Exotic Pets by Simon Girling (2003), published by Blackwell, but checking the preferred temperature range of the specific species being dealt with is recommended.

Table 4. Some common species preferred temperature ranges.

Species	Temperature
Mediterranean tortoise	20–27 °C
Green iguana	25–32 °C
Bearded dragon	25–32 °C
Corn snake	23–30 °C

The practice of placing a tortoise in the fridge before performing a procedure, with the aim of making handling easier is not recommended. It is very important to recognise that although this reduces movement by slowing down the animal, it does not provide analgesia and all procedures will be felt.

Respiratory System

The reptilian respiratory system varies considerably between species, so the points below are intended as examples of aspects important for anaesthesia.

SNAKES

In snakes, the left lung is absent or vestigial. There is no diaphragm, which is important if surgery enters the body cavity. Snakes often show episodic breathing; this is where a few breaths are seen close together and then there is quite a long pause before more breathing is seen and is likely to be related to the slow circulation times in reptiles. In snakes, the tracheal rings are usually incomplete, but there is a tubular structure passing through the mouth which is more rigid.

CHELONIANS

Chelonians (e.g. tortoises) have a short trachea which quickly divides into the two main bronchi. The trachea has complete tracheal rings. The primary bronchus does not divide down in the same way seen in mammals, indeed the whole lung structure is much simpler.

The bronchi enter ediculi, which are simple flattened chambers or crypts, and there is little if any distensibility in the lungs of chelonians, as they are bound by the shell. Although the upper and lower parts of the coelomic cavity are separated by a membrane, this is not muscular and does not function as a diaphragm. Chelonians are reliant on muscle movement for ventilation and their legs move in and out when they breathe. Excessive muscle relaxation seriously affects ventilation and so mechanical ventilation is usually provided for chelonians.

LIZARDS

Lizards have incomplete tracheal rings, and their lungs can vary, being either simple or multichambered structures (but no reptile has the lung complexity of mammals or birds).

Like in birds, lizards perform active inspiration and expiration. Although not likely to be relevant for the species encountered in most practices, it is interesting to note that some species of reptiles have other forms of respiration e.g. sea snakes can absorb oxygen through their skin, other species through the cloaca (the common outlet for gastrointestinal and urinary systems) or through the pharynx.

Cardiovascular System

Differences in the cardiovascular system are highly relevant to anaesthesia.

Like birds, reptiles have **nucleated red cells** which look different to the shapes seen in mammals, being more oval in appearance. The heart in reptiles is different from mammals and varies between species. Generally, **the reptilian heart has three chambers: two atria and a single ventricle** (Figure 20). Muscular divisions come into force as the heart contracts, but there is no full wall creating a division into a right and left ventricle.

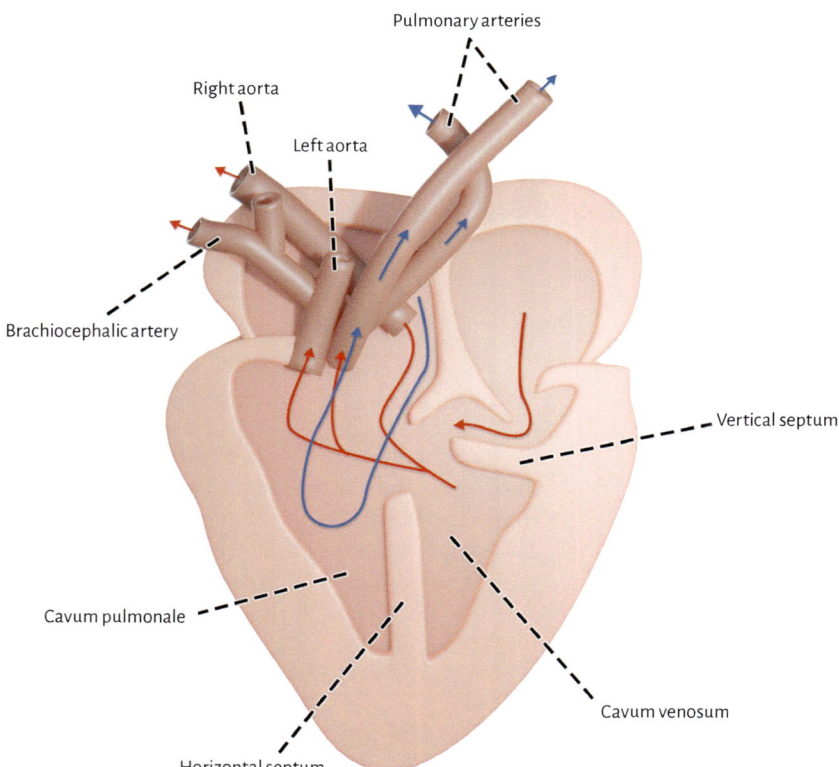

Figure 20. Illustration of a reptile heart.

This means as the heart contracts, blood which has come from the lungs could go back to the lungs again and some blood from the body may go back around the systemic circulation and bypass the lungs completely. How much this happens is related to the balance of sympathetic and parasympathetic nervous input. Capnography does not reflect the arterial tension of carbon dioxide, as some blood containing carbon dioxide is likely to bypass the lungs.

Reptiles also have a renal portal system, as in birds, meaning a variable proportion of blood from the rear of the animal circulates directly through the kidneys before circulating throughout the body.

Handling

Reptiles come in different shapes and sizes. Species specific handling requirements should be employed as some species are dangerous to the handler, or other species may be injured inadvertently.

SNAKES

Snakes can be restrained by **controlling their head.** The thumb should be placed over the back of the head and the fingers curled under the chin, ensuring their weight is supported, and moving slowly.

For large, aggressive, or venomous species, **professional advice should be sought.** Specifically designed snake hooks are used to pick up snakes or restrain the head, but a trained handler for dangerous animals is recommended.

CHELONIANS

Most chelonians are held with fingers on the carapace and the plastron (upper and lower parts of shell). It is important to beware of the beaks and claws of more aggressive species, and keep hands towards the back legs to reduce the risk of being bitten. A rubber speculum can be placed in the beak of snappier animals.

A significant problem when handling tortoises is their tendency to withdraw their heads. There are a few things which can be tried to coax them out. Some authors recommend gently tipping the head downwards, which can persuade a shy animal to protrude, whilst touching the hindlimbs can encourage their head to move forward.

LIZARDS

Certain types of lizards, such as geckos, are fragile and their skin easily damaged, so they should be handled with nitrile gloves and soft cloths. Other lizards such as iguanas, are aggressive and care should be taken as their tails can lash out in a whip like fashion.

Lizards should never be restrained by their tails as many species shed their tails in response to stress, but not all species will regrow them so they could be left tailless.

Many species of reptile have *Salmonella* bacteria as a normal part of the bacterial flora in their digestive systems and the bacterium can be found all over their body. To prevent zoonotic disease, hygiene is therefore very important when handling these patients.

Anaesthesia

Intravenous Access

Venous access is difficult in reptiles. The **jugular vein is used in tortoises** and is the preferred site of blood sampling, but an alternative is the dorsal tail vein or the subcarapacial sinus for injection of substances (not recommended for sampling). The ventral tail vein can be used in lizards and snakes.

For collapsed tortoises or lizards, the intraosseous route of administration of fluids is easiest and just as effective as intravenous administration. Some authors suggest abscessation can be a problem at injection sites, so ensuring cleanliness is important.

Preparation for Anaesthesia and Drugs

In snakes, no prey should be offered for at least 48 hours prior to anaesthesia and in larger species the fasting period may need to be up to one week. Chelonia and lizards rarely regurgitate, but live prey should not be fed to insectivorous reptiles within 24 hours of anaesthesia.

Drugs

Ketamine is a useful sedative/anaesthetic in reptiles, sometimes used with diazepam or midazolam. Ketamine alone may show effects for one to three days after anaesthesia in snakes.

Alfaxalone has been used in some species, as has propofol. For both of these drugs, there is a slower onset of action than that for mammals and a longer duration of action.

Inhalation induction using isoflurane (or sevoflurane) is commonly employed in reptiles. It may be slow, due to the shunting of blood reducing uptake from the lungs. However, inhalation induction is not advised in diving species, as it may induce a diving response where ventilation ceases and the heart rate slows.

Isoflurane requirements for maintenance of anaesthesia are often considered to be somewhat higher than those in dogs.

Intubation and Ventilation

Intubation in snakes is quite easy, due to the simple larynx which is situated rostrally.

In lizards and chelonians, the tongue is fleshier and the larynx more caudal and intubation obtained with relative ease.

An IV cannula may be used as an endotracheal tube in small animals, but it is important to ensure it is soft and does not kink.

Mechanical ventilation is useful during procedures involving entering the body cavity, for longer anaesthetics, and where muscle relaxation affects the ability to ventilate (e.g. chelonians). Many ventilators used in small animal practice are not suitable for these types of animals. The mechanical thumb type of ventilator is appropriate for many of these small species; for example the SAV04 ventilator produced by Vetronics, but other makes are also suitable.

Monitoring Anaesthesia

It is a challenge to judge the depth of anaesthesia in reptiles.

It is important to remember that many physiological functions are temperature dependent. So, for example, the heart rate slows if the animal becomes cooler; a heart rate of 30–40 beats per minute is not unusual during anaesthesia. Respiration often slows and many animals become apnoeic requiring ventilation.

Use of some of the usual reflexes used for mammalian anaesthesia are not possible in reptiles.

THE RIGHTING REFLEX
Loss of a righting reflex may be an early indicator of the onset of anaesthesia but is more reliable in snakes and lizards than in chelonians.

MUSCLE RELAXATION
Muscle relaxation is a key feature of anaesthesia, for example noting limp limbs in chelonians.

JAW TONE
Jaw tone can be used to assess muscle relaxation and can be used as in other species.

EYE POSITION
In most reptiles, the globe cannot rotate in the orbit, so eye position is not helpful.

THE CORNEAL REFLEX
The corneal reflex may be used (as in birds) in tortoises but is not useful in snakes and some lizards where there is a spectacle (a clear scale which covers the eye). The spectacle protects the cornea, and as it is not touched directly there is a lack of response.

TONGUE WITHDRAWAL
In snakes, tongue withdrawal can be assessed by gently pulling the tongue out with atraumatic plastic forceps. This reflex is retained until quite deep levels of anaesthesia so helps judge excessively deep anaesthesia.

OTHER METHODS
An ECG may be used in reptiles, using needle electrodes, where fine needles are inserted subcutaneously and then ECG crocodile clips are attached to the metal. A doppler probe may be used as an audible indicator of a heartbeat, e.g. in snakes. It is important to bear in mind that in some lizards the heart is more cranial heart than expected.

Capnography may be used in reptiles, but importantly the expired end tidal carbon dioxide is likely to underestimate the arterial carbon dioxide, due to the variable amount of blood recirculating in the heart from the systemic circulation. However, it may be useful for monitoring trends.

There are varying opinions on the reliability of pulse oximetry in reptiles, but some people use a reflectance probe inserted into the cloaca or orally.

Monitoring temperature is useful, however most clinical rectal thermometers do not read temperatures as low as necessary. Thermistor probes from multiparameter monitors may be suitable and may be inserted into the cloaca (the common outlet for the intestinal/urinary tracts).

Anaesthetic Recovery

A suitable temperature should be ensured during the recovery period, and it is important to be aware recovery can be slow after injectable agents.

With IPPV, endotracheal intubation should be maintained and the rate of ventilation slowed to one breath per minute (some people recommend even slower), until effective ventilation returns. Some veterinarians recommend changing from oxygen to air when ventilating the lungs during recovery from anaesthesia.

Fluid therapy should not be forgotten. Maintenance requirements are considered to be 20–25 ml/kg day. Subcutaneous fluids may be administered in snakes and lizards in the lateral body wall. Intravenous or intraosseous techniques may be used in some species when more rapid absorption required.

Some veterinarians use doxapram to stimulate recovery, but this is a drug which is no longer easily obtained in the UK. It may be available in some other countries.

Pain and Analgesia

In acute pain, reptiles may adopt an abnormal posture, as in other species. Locomotion may be altered, and with chronic pain signs are likely such as anorexia, immobility, or behavioural changes such as increased aggression.

There is a lack of reliable evidence regarding analgesia in reptiles. Many of the research studies available use thermal nociceptive responses to assess analgesia in reptiles (where a heated probe is applied to the skin). It is controversial how useful this system is to replicate clinical pain, or indeed whether a reptile's response to heat is the same as mammals.

NSAIDs

Ketoprofen has been investigated in iguanas, with a dose of 2 mg/kg given IM or IV suggested to last 36 hours (Tuttle et al., 2006). Meloxicam has a slow onset in iguanas, with a dose of 0.2 mg/kg suggested to be effective after 48 hours (Divers et al., 2010), dosing can be continued orally daily for five days and then changed to every other day dosing for longer term treatment.

Opioids

Some suggested opioid doses for reptiles are presented in the Table 5. Butorphanol or morphine have been suggested in different species. The choices should be discussed with the veterinary team and might also depend on availability.

In the table below, note the long interval between doses in reptiles, which is related to their much slower biotransformation and elimination of drugs.

Table 5. Opioid doses for reptiles.

Drug	Dose	Route	Frequency
Butorphanol	0.5–2 mg/kg	Intramuscular injection	Twice daily
Buprenorphine	0.02–0.2 mg/kg	Intramuscular injection	Once daily
Morphine	0.4 mg/kg	Intramuscular injection	Twice daily
Tramadol	10 mg/kg	Oral	Every 4 days

Local Anaesthetics

Local anaesthetics are a useful adjunct in reptiles for surgical interventions. A dose of 3 mg/kg lidocaine or 2 mg/kg bupivacaine should not be exceeded. For very small reptiles, this can be diluted in saline for ease of use.

References

- Brodbelt, D. C., Blissitt, K. J., Hammond, R. A., Neath, P. J., Young, L. E, Pfeiffer, D. U., & Wood, J. L. (2008) The risk of death: the confidential enquiry into perioperative small animal fatalities. *Veterinary anaesthesia and analgesia.* 35(5), 365–373.
- Brodbelt, D. C., Pfeiffer, D. U., Young, L. E., & Wood, J. L. N. (2007) Risk factors for anaesthetic-related death in cats: results from the confidential enquiry into perioperative small animal fatalities (CEPSAF). *British Journal of Anaesthesia.* 99(5), 617–623.
- Divers, S. J., Papich, M., McBride, M., Stedman, N. L., Perpinan, D., Koch, T. F., Hernandez, S. M., Barron, G. H., Pethel, M., & Budsberg, S. C. (2010) Pharmacokinetics of meloxicam following intravenous and oral administration in green iguanas (*Iguana iguana*). *American journal of veterinary research.* 71(11), 1277–1283.
- Grint, N. J., Sayers, I. R., Cecchi, R., Harley, R., & Day, M. J. (2006) Postanaesthetic tracheal strictures in three rabbits. *Laboratory Animals (London).* 40(3), 301–308.
- Harvey, L., Knowles, T., & Murison, P. J. (2012) Comparison of direct and Doppler arterial blood pressure measurements in rabbits during isoflurane anaesthesia. *Veterinary anaesthesia and analgesia.* 39(2), 174–184.
- Johnston, G. M., Eastment, J. K., Wood, J. L. N., & Taylor, P. M. (2002) The confidential enquiry into perioperative equine fatalities (CEPEF): mortality results of Phases 1 and 2. *Veterinary Anaesthesia and Analgesia.* 29(4), 159–170
- Leach, M. C., Coulter, C. A., Richardson, C. A., & Flecknell, P. A. (2011) Are we looking in the wrong place? implications for behavioural-based pain assessment in rabbits (*oryctolagus cuniculi*) and beyond? *PloS One.* 6(3), e13347-e13347.
- Parkinson, NJ, McKenzie, HC, Barton, MH, et al. (2018) Catheter-associated venous air embolism in hospitalized horses: 32 cases. *J Vet Intern Med.* 2018; 32: 805–814.
- Reiner, A., Brauth, S. E., Kitt, C. A., & Quirion, R. (1989) Distribution of mu, delta, and kappa opiate receptor types in the forebrain and midbrain of pigeons. *The Journal of comparative neurology.* 280(3), 359–382.
- Tuttle, A. D., Papich, M., Lewbart, G. A., Christian, S., Gunkel, C., & Harms, C. A. (2006) Pharmacokinetics of ketoprofen in the green iguana (*Iguana iguana*) following single intravenous and intramuscular injections. *Journal of zoo and wildlife medicine: official publication of the American Association of Zoo Veterinarians.* 37(4), 567–570.
- Varga, M. (2016) Analgesia and pain management in rabbits. *Veterinary Nursing Journal.* 31:5, 149–153.
- Woodhouse, K. J. Brosnan, R. J., Nguyen, K. Q., Moniz, G. W., & Galuppo, L. D. (2013) Effects of postanaesthetic sedation with romifidine or xylazine on quality of recovery from isoflurane anaesthesia in horses. *Journal of the American Veterinary Medical Association.* 242(4), 533–539.

Test

Answers on page 140

1. In a rodent, where should an intraperitoneal injection be given?
    a. Caudal quadrant of abdomen, midline.
    b. Caudal quadrant of abdomen, off midline.
    c. Cranial quadrant of abdomen, midline.
    d. Cranial quadrant of abdomen, off midline.

2. Which bone is most commonly used for intraosseous injection in small mammals?
    a. Humerus.
    b. Radius.
    c. Tibia.
    d. Ulna.

3. Which species of birds may have a divided trachea/septum?
    a. Ducks.
    b. Hawks.
    c. Penguins.
    d. Swans.

4. Which artery might be used for catheterisation if horse is undergoing surgery on the head (e.g. for molar removal)?
    a. Auricular artery.
    b. Facial artery.
    c. Metatarsal artery.
    d. Radial artery.

5. Which body position will produce the most ventilation-perfusion mismatching in horses?
    a. Dorsal recumbency.
    b. Left lateral recumbency.
    c. Right lateral recumbency.
    d. Sternal recumbency.

6. Which sympathomimetic agent is most commonly used to treat hypotension in horses?
    a. Adrenaline.
    b. Dobutamine.
    c. Dopamine.
    d. Noradrenaline.

7. At which stage of anaesthesia will a snake stop tongue withdrawal?
    a. During induction of anaesthesia.
    b. Very light anaesthesia.
    c. Very deep anaesthesia.
    d. It will not be lost during anaesthesia.

8. How does end-tidal carbon dioxide relate to arterial carbon dioxide in reptiles?
    a. Likely to be lower due to shunting of blood in the lungs.
    b. Closely related due to the rapid equilibration of carbon dioxide across the lung membranes.
    c. Likely to be lower due to some systemic blood bypassing lungs.
    d. Likely to be lower due to the slow metabolism in reptiles.

9. Which is the largest wave of the ECG in birds?
    a. P.
    b. R.
    c. S.
    d. T.

10. Which species may shed skin on the tail if it is used for restraint (so-called "tail slip")?
    a. Chinchilla.
    b. Gerbil.
    c. Mouse.
    d. Rat.

Clinical Case 1

The owner of a 6-month-old Netherlands Dwarf rabbit weighing 0.8 kg wishes to book an appointment for neutering (ovariohysterectomy).

1. What instructions do you give regarding withholding food and water prior to the appointment tomorrow morning?

2. Premedication.
   A premedication of medetomidine 50 µg/kg and buprenorphine 0.03 mg/kg IM has been selected (along with a NSAID for analgesia). Calculate the volume of medetomidine required (the rabbit weighs 0.8 kg, and the concentration of medetomidine is 1 mg/ml) and the volume of buprenorphine required (the concentration of buprenorphine is 0.3 mg/ml).

3. Which muscle should be used for this injection?

4. After premedication, which vein would you choose to cannulate for IV access?

Self-assessment

5. How could intravenous cannulation be eased in this animal?

6. After induction of anaesthesia with IV alfaxalone, what are the options for maintaining anaesthesia and supplying oxygen?

7. How would you position the rabbit for endotracheal intubation?

8. During the intubation process, it is noticed that the mucous membranes are becoming cyanotic. What may be happening and what action should be taken?

9. As intubation was not successful, you maintain anaesthesia using a mask. Where can you apply the pulse oximeter?

10. How should the rabbit be positioned during surgery?

11. During surgery, the vet notices some blood loss. You retrieve the swab and weigh it to determine how much blood has been lost. If the bloody swab weighs 12 g and a dry swab weighs 4 g, how much blood is present?

12. If this 0.8 kg rabbit is estimated to have 70 ml/kg blood volume, what percentage of blood volume does this haemorrhage represent?

13. Is this amount of blood loss significant?

14. What are particular priorities for monitoring recovery for this case?

Clinical Case 2

A budgerigar is presented for surgical removal of a small mass from its pectoral region. It weighs 30 g.

1. How does the risk of anaesthetising a budgerigar compare to the anaesthetic risk in dogs?

2. The budgie is well handled. After a premedication of butorphanol has been administered, the budgie undergoes a mask induction. Which breathing system and gas flow should be used?

3. Why is it important not to hold the bird too tightly?

4. Induction of anaesthesia is very rapid in this bird. Why?

5. What factors should be taken into account when positioning this animal for surgery?

6. How can anaesthesia be monitored in this bird?

7. If local anaesthetic is to be infiltrated around the site of the mass removal, calculate a safe volume to administer. The budgie weighs 30 g and you have 1% lidocaine.

8. How could fluids be administered to this bird before recovery and how much would be an appropriate amount? The anaesthetic duration was 30 minutes.

9. What might be an appropriate analgesic for recovery in this bird?

Notes

Self-assessment

Correct Answers:

Test

1. b
2. c
3. c
4. c
5. a
6. b
7. c
8. c
9. c
10. b

Clinical Case 1

1. **What instructions do you give regarding withholding food and water prior to the appointment tomorrow morning?** Do not withhold food or water.

2. **Calculate the volume of medetomidine required (the rabbit weighs 0.8 kg, and the concentration of medetomidine is 1 mg/ml) and the volume of buprenorphine required (the concentration of buprenorphine is 0.3 mg/ml).**
   - Medetomidine
     - 0.8 kg x 50 µg/kg = 40 µg
     - 40 µg/1000 µg/ml = **0.04 ml**
   - Buprenorphine
     - 0.8 kg x 0.03 mg/ml = 0.024 mg required
     - 0.024 mg/0.3 mg/ml = **0.08 ml**

3. **Which muscle should be used for this injection?** Rabbits have good lumbar muscles, and this would be a good choice for IM injection.

4. **After premedication, which vein would you choose to cannulate for IV access?** The marginal ear vein is most used in rabbits. It can be very small in small rabbits and those with small ears such as this Netherland Dwarf however, so an alternative would be the cephalic vein if the ear is difficult.

5. **How could intravenous cannulation be eased in this animal?** Using EMLA will desensitise the area and may cause some vasodilation. Local warming e.g. with a warm water filled glove may also enlarge the vessel.

6. **After induction of anaesthesia with IV alfaxalone, what are the options for maintaining anaesthesia and supplying oxygen?** A facemask can be used (push the mandibles forward to maintain the airway), an endotracheal tube, or a supraglottic airway (e.g. V-gel). Anaesthesia can be maintained using isoflurane or sevoflurane.

7. **How would you position the rabbit for endotracheal intubation?** Although not performed by everyone, there are benefits to holding the rabbit with the neck straight and head lifted.

8. **During the intubation process, it is noticed that the mucous membranes are becoming cyanotic. What may be happening and what action should be taken?** This may be laryngospasm caused by the intubation attempts. Intubation attempts should be stopped. A mask can be used to supply oxygen and even give a breath if needed. Air movement in and out of the lungs can be encouraged by using the weight of the rabbits guts against the diaphragm – tilt the hind end of the rabbit up and down alternately.

9. **As intubation was not successful, you maintain anaesthesia using a mask. Where can you apply the pulse oximeter?** The paws are often very suitable for pulse oximeters.

10. **How should the rabbit be positioned during surgery?** The rabbit will need to in dorsal recumbency. Using a tilted table with the head elevated will help reduce pressure on the diaphragm and aid ventilation.

11. **During surgery, the vet notices some blood loss. You retrieve the swab and weigh it to determine how much blood has been lost. If the bloody swab weighs 12 g and a dry swab weighs 4 g, how much blood is present?**
    - 12 g - 4 g = 8 g.
    - Blood weighs approximately 1.1 g per ml. 8 g divided by 1.1 = 7.27, so 7.27 ml has been lost.
    - For ease of calculation, many people will just use an estimate of 1 g of blood = 1 ml of blood loss.

12. **If this 0.8 kg rabbit is estimated to have 70 ml/kg blood volume, what percentage of blood volume does this haemorrhage represent?** Total blood volume for this rabbit:
    - 0.8 kg x 70 ml/kg = 56 ml blood volume
    - 7.27 ml/56 ml = 0.1298
    - 0.1298 x 100 = **approximately 13% blood volume has been lost.**

13. **Is this amount of blood loss significant?** This is a relevant blood loss, and the volume should be replaced. Crystalloids may be adequate, although more blood loss might require replacement e.g. with colloids.

14. **What are particular priorities for monitoring recovery for this case?**
    - Pain.
    - Gut movement (eating, faeces production).
    - Cardiovascular status related to the haemorrhage:
      a. Mucous membrane colour.
      b. Pulses quality and rate.

Clinical Case 2

1. **How does the risk of anaesthetising a budgerigar compare to the anaesthetic risk in dogs?** Anaesthesia in the budgerigar was reported to be very high risk in the CEPSAF study (1 in 6). It is important that owners are aware that it is a high risk, although of course they should be reassured that all care will be taken of their animal. Data from an individual practice e.g. mortalities could be less than that reported in CEPSAF.

2. **The budgie is well handled. After a premedication of butorphanol has been administered, the budgie undergoes a mask induction. Which breathing system and gas flow should be used?** A low resistance breathing system should be used for this very small animal – an Ayre's T-piece would be ideal. The gas flow as 2–3 x minute ventilation (minute ventilation is the amount of air breathed per minute).

    In birds, the tidal volume tends to be greater than that of a mammal, but the respiratory rate is usually less. Data varies on what minute ventilation is seen in birds and there is little data on the very small animals. A minute volume of 760 ml has been reported for a chicken – but a budgerigar is smaller with a higher metabolic rate. A good estimate of minute ventilation might be 500 ml per kg. For a very small bird, calculating this would give a flow requirement of 150 ml/min for the 30 g budgerigar.

    Realistically, calculating the minute ventilation is not vital. In most cases it would not be advisable to administer less than about 0.5 l/min as the vaporisers are unlikely to be accurate at lower flows. There may also be some leakage from the mask. Practically, a flow of 0.5–1 l would be used for this bird.

3. **Why is it important not to hold the bird too tightly?** There are a couple of reasons for this. Firstly, the bird has no diaphragm, so it is dependent on expansion of the ribcage to inspire. Too tight a hold can restrict the movement of the "keel bone" (the sternum of the bird). Also, the lungs of the bird are very rigid. Birds rely on gas moving in and out of simple air sacs which do not participate in gas exchange, in order to create flow through the unidirectional parabronchi. Excessive restriction may inhibit air sac expansion.

    A tight hold may also be very stressful for the bird. This increase of catecholamine may increase the chances of arrhythmias.

4. **Induction of anaesthesia is very rapid in this bird. Why?** Due to the efficiency of the avian respiratory system, the bird will take up and eliminate volatile agents faster than a mammal.

5. **What factors should be taken into account when positioning this animal for surgery?** The airsacs should not be compressed and the positioning must allow for keel bone movement.

6. **How can anaesthesia be monitored in this bird?**
    - A pulse oximeter can be attached above the hock.
    - In such a small bird, it is unlikely to have an endotracheal tube. It can be more difficult to use capnography, but it is possible to insert a narrow tube (such as an IV cannula attached to the sampling tube) alongside the beak via the diaphragm of the mask.
    - An ECG with needle electrodes could be used, pads or clips are quite aggressive in such a small animal.
    - This bird is probably too small to be using blood pressure measurement.
    - It may be possible to measure cloacal body temperature if your probe is small enough – do be gentle.
    - To judge depth of anaesthesia, the corneal reflex could be used with a moistened cotton bud (very gently) touched on the surface of the eye. Respiratory rate and heart rate can be used too.

7. **If local anaesthetic is to be infiltrated around the site of the mass removal, calculate a safe volume to administer. The budgie weighs 30 g and you have 1% lidocaine.** The budgie weighs 30 g = 0.03 kg. A suggested maximum dose would be 3 mg/kg lidocaine:
    - 0.03 kg x 3 mg/kg = 0.09 mg maximum safe amount

Self-assessment

- 1% lidocaine has 10 mg/ml:
  0.09 mg/10 mg/ml = 0.009 ml

As this is too small a volume to draw up, a dilution of 0.1 mg/ml lidocaine is made. Recalculate the maximum safe volume of lidocaine which can be used.

The maximum dosage of lidocaine for this budgie was 0.09 mg: 0.09 mg/0.1 mg/ml = 0.9 ml.

8. How could fluids be administered to this bird before recovery and how much would be an appropriate amount? The anaesthetic duration was 30 minutes.
A suitable route of administration would be SC. An appropriate amount would be around 10 ml/kg/h allowing for respiratory losses to be quite high.
- 0.5 h x 0.03 kg x 10 ml/kg/h = 0.15 ml.

9. What might be an appropriate analgesic for recovery in this bird? A NSAID such as meloxicam could be used.

Notes

Fluid Therapy and Critical Care Nutrition

Nicki Grint

Chapter Summary:

- Types and uses of different fluids, including colloids.
- A fluid therapy plan and patients monitorization.
- The principles of transfusion medicine.
- The importance of nutrition in the critical patient.

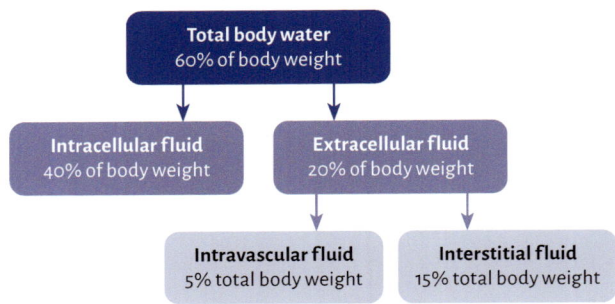

Figure 1. Fluid balance.

This chapter aims to help the reader understand the **different types of fluids and their uses,** how to devise a **fluid therapy plan,** and then **monitor** the patient effectively. It also explains the principles of **transfusion medicine** and the importance of **nutrition in critical care patients.**

THE PRINCIPLES OF FLUID THERAPY

Fluid Compartments

Understanding fluid therapy requires an appreciation of the distribution of water and electrolytes within the body. When these reservoirs become depleted, they requirement replacement, which is where fluid therapy comes in. Crucial to deciding the best replacement fluid to use is to recognize the nature of the loss and then replace it appropriately.

Water makes up 60% of the total weight of an adult's body. Total body water is divided into:
- **extracellular fluid (ECF)**: further subdivided into:
  - **plasma** (intravascular volume)
  - **interstitial fluid** (which bathes the body's cells)
- **intracellular fluid** (Figure 1).

There is a separate category called **transcellular fluid** (e.g. synovial and CSF fluid) which only comprises a small percentage of the total body water and is not further considered in this text.

Types of Fluid Loss

Different losses of fluid, due to different clinical conditions, come from one or more of the fluid compartments listed above.

WHOLE BLOOD LOSS
- **possible causes:** severed superficial arteries or large veins
- **compartment lost from:** intravascular compartment (plasma)
- **components of fluid lost:** water, colloidal particles, red cells and electrolytes, platelets, clotting factors etc.

EXTRACELLULAR FLUID LOSS
- **possible causes:** vomiting, diarrhoea, diuresis
- **compartment lost from:** interstitial compartment and intravascular compartment
- **components in fluid lost:** Na^+, Cl^-, and water.

PROTEIN RICH EXTRACELLULAR FLUID LOSS
- **possible causes:** some pleural/peritoneal effusions, protein losing enteropathies, burns
- **compartment lost from:** interstitial compartment and intravascular compartment
- **components in fluid lost:** Na^+, Cl^-, water and proteins.

PURE WATER LOSS
- **possible causes:** e.g. high respiratory rate or primary water deprivation
- **compartments lost from:** as pure water loss as water moves freely across all compartments, water is lost from all compartments.

Making a Fluid Therapy Plan

The following should be considered:
- the type of fluid that has been lost
- how much of this fluid has been lost
- over how long a timeframe the fluid has been lost.

Knowing the compartment from which the fluid has been lost and what the components of the fluid are, helps answer the first point (what type of fluid has been lost) For example:
- **Pure water losses** are best replaced with crystalloids (hypotonic crystalloids may be indicated but infused slowly so to avoid rapid changes in plasma sodium concentrations).
- **Extracellular fluid losses** from conditions such as vomiting and diarrhoea where water, sodium, and chloride are lost; these are best replaced by isotonic crystalloids (containing water and electrolytes including sodium and chloride).

Hypotonic, Isotonic, and Hypertonic Solutions

The tonicity of a solution refers to the concentration of solutes (such as sodium and other electrolytes) in a solution, compared to another solution.

For intravenous fluid therapy **the fluid is termed hypertonic, isotonic, or hypotonic based on higher, equal, or lower concentrations of electrolytes compared to normal plasma.** Sodium is usually the main electrolyte considered as it is the major extracellular cation (positive ion) and commonly called the osmotic skeleton of the ECF.
- **Hypotonic:** Na^+ concentration is lower than plasma e.g. 0.18% NaCl with 4% glucose.
- **Isotonic:** Na^+ concentration is similar to plasma e.g. Hartmann's solution or 0.9% NaCl.
- **Hypertonic:** Na^+ concentration is higher than plasma e.g. 7.2% NaCl.

These solutes or electrolytes cannot pass through semipermeable membranes whereas water can. Therefore, water tries to follow solutes to even out the concentrations. For example, infusing hypertonic (7.2%) saline intravenously pulls water from the interstitial space into the intravascular space, which then increases the blood volume and blood pressure. This is because the water from the interstitial space follows the solute to try and even out the concentrations between the intravascular and interstitial fluid compartments.

Types of Fluids

Crystalloids are any solution of crystalline solids (the solute) dissolved in water (the solvent). The crystalline substance can be sodium based or dextrose based. If the electrolyte composition of the solution is similar to extra cellular fluid, then the fluid is known as a **balanced electrolyte solution.**

Crystalloids are divided into extracellular fluid volume replacers and maintenance solutions.

EXTRACELLULAR FLUID VOLUME REPLACERS

When the sodium concentration is similar to the ECF sodium concentration, these fluids stay in the extracellular compartment. Therefore, these fluids are good at replacing extracellular fluid loss.

These fluids can be infused rapidly as they do not induce changes in electrolyte composition, especially sodium ions. It is important not to change serum sodium concentrations too quickly, with the rate of change being no faster than 1 mmol/hr.

After IV administration the fluid redistributes between the intravascular and interstitial compartments; thus, for every 1 litre of fluid administered IV, only about 250–300 ml remains in the intravascular space after one to two hours.

Two examples of ECF volume replacers are Hartmann's solution (also known as lactated Ringers) and normal saline. (Box 1).

> **Box 1. Composition of ECF Volume Replacers (lactated Ringers):**
>
> - **Hartmann's** (Figure 2):
>   - 131 mmol Na^+
>   - 5 mmol K^+
>   - 111 mmol Cl^-
>   - 1.4 mmol Ca^{2+}
>   - 29 mmol Lactate.
>
> - **Normal saline** (0.9% NaCl):
>   - 150 mmol Na^+
>   - 150 mmol Cl^-.

- The lactate in **Hartmann's solution** is a precursor to bicarbonate and therefore this fluid is an alkalinising solution.
- **Normal saline** is an acidifying solution.

MAINTENANCE SOLUTIONS

In addition to supplying water, **maintenance fluid should replace electrolytes.** In order to meet specific daily requirements, maintenance solutions have lower sodium and chloride concentrations when compared with the ECF. A **potassium supplement** is often required, because animals treated with maintenance solutions are often inappetant and all potassium is diet derived. The maximum rate of potassium supplementation is 0.5 mmol/kg/hr.

These solutions work because they are isotonic; due to dextrose +/- the small amount of sodium. The dextrose is metabolised and no longer osmotically active, only water remains, which then distributes freely throughout the three fluid compartments. Note that the amount of dextrose present in the solutions described provides negligible energy at the concentrations used.

Hypotonic solutions are not suitable for maintenance, because the sodium concentration is very different to that of the ECF. These fluids should not be given at fast rates, but slowly infused over 24-hours or red blood cell lysis may result. These fluids are of no use for restoring circulating volume but are ideal for **treating primary water loss.**

Examples of maintenance fluids:
- 4% glucose with 0.18% sodium chloride (supplemented with 20–30 mEq/l of potassium for maintenance)
- 5% dextrose (supplemented with 20–30 mEq/l of potassium for maintenance).

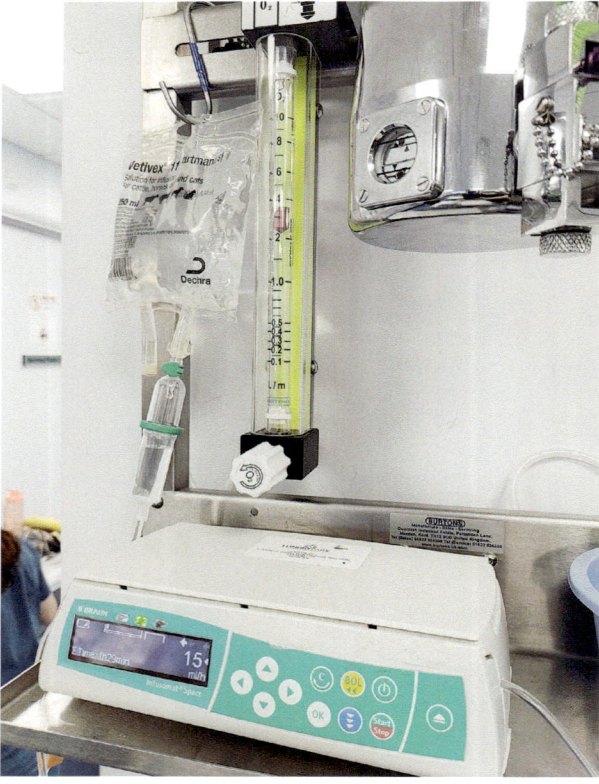

Figure 2. Bag of Hartmann's solution being infused via a drip pump.

Hypertonic Saline

Hypertonic saline is used in **cases of shock.** It causes an increase in blood pressure by several mechanisms, the main one being it draws water from the interstitial space. The effect of hypertonic saline is **transient** and should be followed by the administration of isotonic crystalloids to replace borrowed water. The use of hypertonic saline also carries some potential side effects; hypernatraemia/hypokalaemia, haemolysis, ventricular arrhythmias, and potential for rehaemorrhage

Colloids

Colloids are fluids in which large molecular weight particles are suspended but not visible. **Colloids contain large molecules that cannot pass through the vascular endothelium.** They increase the colloid osmotic pressure of the plasma and in addition to each litre of fluid staying in the intra vascular compartment, they also pull water from the interstitial space into the intra vascular space. To avoid dehydrating the interstitium, **crystalloids should be used concurrently** or just after colloids, to pay back the fluid borrowed from the interstitial space.

Colloids remain in the intravascular space for several hours compared to the hour that crystalloids remain in the intravascular space. Therefore, colloids are also called **plasma volume expanders** and used when **rapid improvement of circulating volume is necessary.** As a general rule **no more than 25%** (usually 20 ml/kg in the dog) **of circulating volume** of an animal should be given as a colloid at any one time (usually within a 24-hour time frame), otherwise haemodilution dilutes out clotting factors etc. Colloids can be used intraoperatively to help maintain blood pressure, or if an animal has a total protein of less than 35 g/litre in order to prevent extravasation of fluid.

There are several types of artificial colloids, such as starches, gelatins, and dextrans (Table 1 and Figure 3).

Table 1. Characteristics of different artificial colloids.

Gelatin based	Gelofusin® Haemaccel®	· Last for maximum 6–8 hours. · May cause hypersensitivity reaction ranging from mild urticarial lesions to anaphylaxis dilutional coagulopathy.
Dextran based	Dextran 40 Dextran 70	· Last approximately 12 hours (D-70). · Hypersensitivity reactions rare (dilutional coagulopathy).
Starch based	Hetastarch	· Last approximately 24–36 hours. · Hypersensitivity reactions rare (dilutional coagulopathy).

Disadvantages of colloid use include volume overload, anaphylactic reactions, and clotting problems. In 2013, meta-analyses showing increased risks related to kidney dysfunction and mortality in septic and critically ill human patients if starches

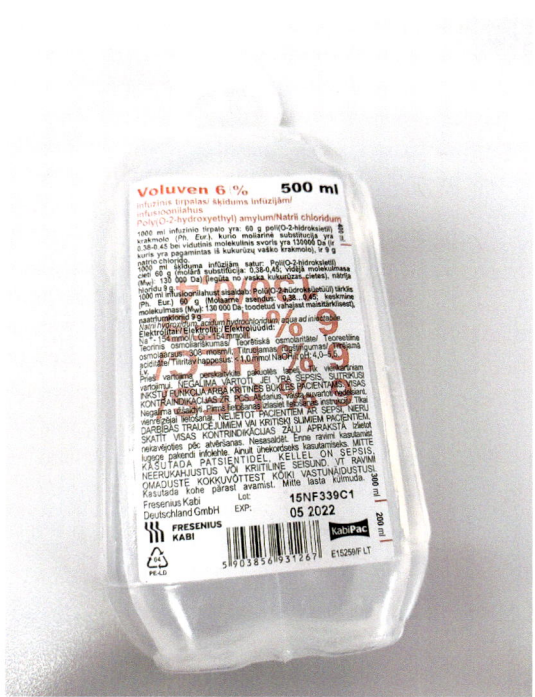

Figure 3. Hetastarch is an example of an artificial colloid.

had been administered. This led to restrictions of starch use in these patient populations by European regulatory authorities, and although the initial ban on the use of starches in Europe has been eased, it can sometimes be difficult to obtain starches for use in veterinary patients. There is no evidence in veterinary patients that there are similar risks with starch use, and large scale randomized studies are needed before any consensus statements are made.

Calculations in Intravenous Fluid Therapy

Maintenance Fluid Therapy

An animal's maintenance requirement is defined as the amount of water and electrolytes required to replace those lost through normal physiological processes, i.e. through respiration, perspiration, and excretion via the alimentary and urinary tracts.

Maintenance fluid therapy rates were calculated as 2 ml/kg/hr, but newer thinking suggests maintenance rates differ between species and sizes of animal. To calculate an individual's fluid therapy rate (total volume over 24 hours) the following formulae should be used (Box 2):

Box 2. Formulae for Calculation of Maintenance Fluid Therapy Rate

- **Cats:** $80 \times$ body weight $(kg)^{0.75}$
  Rule of thumb = 2–3 ml/kg/hr

- **Dogs:** $132 \times$ body weight $(kg)^{0.75}$
  Rule of thumb = 2–6 ml/kg/hr

Clinical Signs of Dehydration

If an animal is admitted with a preexisting degree of dehydration, this deficit needs to be factored in and compensated for in the fluid therapy plan.

First, a combination of clinical signs and laboratory data should be used to decide how dehydrated the animal is. Clinical signs to check include:
- moistness of mucous membranes (when patients become dehydrated their mucous membranes can become tacky)
- skin turgor (i.e. what happens when the skin on the back of the neck is tented)
- sunkenness of eyes (the fat pad behind the orbit can shrink when dehydrated and the eyes appear to 'sink back' in the skull).

These signs should be combined to estimate the degree of dehydration by using the table in Table 2.

Table 2. Clinical signs of dehydration.

Percentage dehydration	Clinical signs
4%	· No clinical signs
5%	· Semi dry oral mucous membranes · Skin turgor normal · Eyes moist
6–7%	· Dry oral mucous membranes · Eyes moist · Mild loss of skin turgor
8–10%	· Dry oral mucous membranes · Eyes retracted · Considerable loss of skin turgor · Signs of hypoperfusion
10%	· Very dry mucous membranes · Severe eyeball retraction · Eyes dull · Complete loss of skin turgor · Altered consciousness · Greater signs of hypoperfusion
12%	· As 10% but moribund
12–15%	· As 10% but dying

Fluid Deficits

The percentage dehydration value from the table in Table 2 indicates the amount of water lost as a percentage of body weight. So if the percentage is multiplied by the animal's body weight, the amount of fluid owing to the animal's fluid deficit can be calculated.

Depending on the severity of the dehydration, the fluid required to restore this deficit is given over 12–24 hours. In more acute situations, deficits are addressed in a shorter time frame, with 30% of the fluid deficit front loaded in the first few hours and the rest administered over the rest of the 24-hour period. If the animal is shocked, the full fluid deficit is administered in a shorter time frame e.g.one to four hours. Another consideration is how long the patient took to lose the fluid; with rapid loss replaced more quickly, than slow, chronic losses.

In addition to restoring the fluid deficit, if the animal is not eating or drinking, then maintenance needs must also be provided over the same time frame that the fluid deficit is being corrected.

If a patient is dehydrated due to vomiting or diarrhoea, it is common for these losses to continue whilst the patient is hospitalised. To correct for these additional losses, additional boluses of fluids for each episode of vomiting or diarrhoea should be given. Volumes equalling those lost should be administered, but measurements this accurate are often difficult (and unpleasant!) so some texts suggest 4 ml/kg per episode.

In a dehydrated patient, water is lost from all compartments and therefore using a crystalloid (where water is the solvent) distributes water freely across all compartments to restore the fluid deficits. If rapid restoration of the fluid deficit is necessary, a balanced ECF volume replacer such as Hartmann's solution should be used, as this fluid has a more similar sodium composition to plasma than a maintenance crystalloid, and therefore is safer to infuse at faster rates. Maintenance crystalloids could be considered for primary water deprivation cases when the fluid deficit is repaid over a longer period of time, e.g. 24 hours.

Anaesthetic Fluid Therapy Rates

Correcting dehydration, as above, helps stabilise a patient before anaesthesia but they also need fluid therapy during anaesthesia. Even a fit and healthy animal, such as a bitch spay, requires fluid therapy in excess of maintenance rates once under anaesthesia. This is required because the anaesthetic agents used tend to produce hypotension via vasodilation or decreasing myocardial contractility. To support blood pressure, on top of the maintenance rates, additional fluids are given to the patient. Also, in the case of the bitch spay, the losses are increased by evaporative fluid losses from the open abdomen and possibly by haemorrhage. Current recommendations from the American Animal Hospital Association (AAHA) suggest **normal healthy dogs start with a crystalloid fluid therapy rate of 5ml/kg/hr and cats with 3 ml/kg/hr and then every hour the rate should be reduced by 25% until maintenance is reached.**

If hypotension (mean blood pressure <60 mmHg) occurs under anaesthesia, the AAHA advise that euvolaemic animals are unlikely to respond to fluid boluses and even though initial crystalloid and colloid boluses can be used, moving on to positive ionotropic or sympathomimetic treatment at an early stage is warranted. An algorithm showing the suggested course of action to treat hypotension is shown in Figure 4.

Intraoperative Blood Loss

The calculations discussed above are to correct dehydration, however there are other types of fluid losses including haemorrhage which need compensating for. If haemorrhage occurs, **it is important to assess how much blood is lost,** in order to decide on the type of replacement fluid and the volume to administer. To estimate blood loss, blood-soaked swabs should be counted and weighed (1 g of weight is approximately 1 ml of blood), and the volume in the suction bottle, on the floor, and drapes estimated. (Figure 5).

From the volume of blood lost, then it should be decided if this volume is significant to the animal e.g. 50 ml blood loss

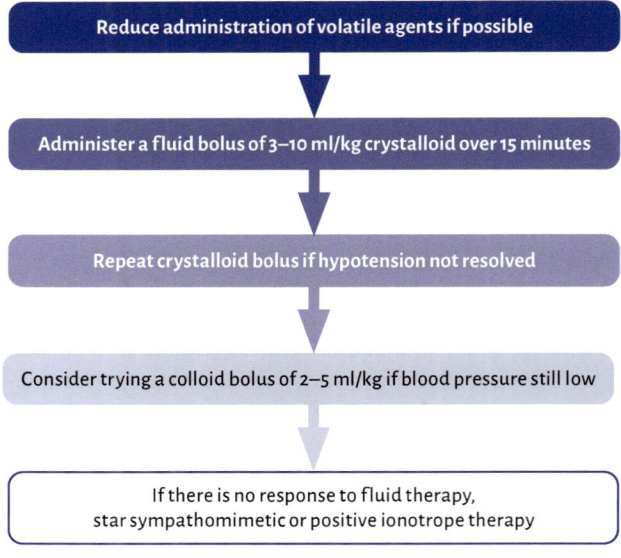

Figure 4. Hypotension flow chart.

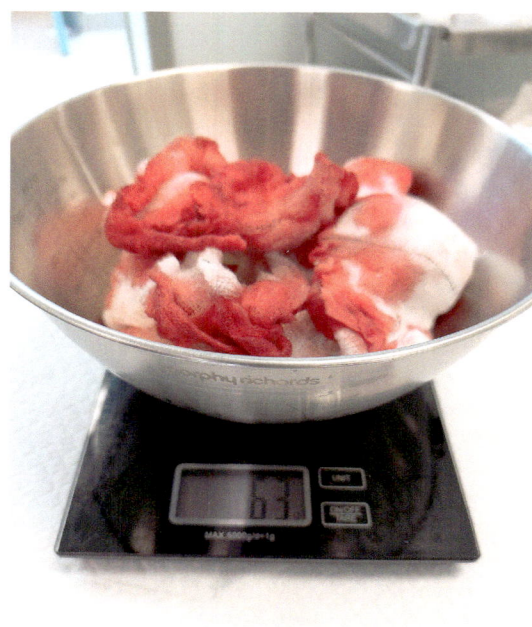

Figure 5. Bloody swabs can be weighed, and the dry weight of the swabs subtracted to estimate surgical blood loss.

has more effect on a 4 kg cat than a 70 kg Bull Mastiff. The first step is to **calculate the animal's blood volume,** which is generally estimated as 90 ml/kg in the dog and 56 ml/kg in the cat (there are other values cited in the literature, the ones specified here represent some of the most commonly cited values for the two species). From these figures (blood lost and the patient's total blood volume) **the percentage blood loss should be calculated.**

$$\text{Percentage blood volume lost} = \frac{\text{volume of blood lost}}{\text{animal's blood volume}} \times 100$$

If an animal loses between 10–15% blood volume and is not already on fluids, then crystalloid fluid therapy should be started. If the amount lost is 15–20% then colloid therapy is more appropriate. Once 20% blood has been lost then the animals oxygen carrying capacity is affected and blood products should be considered.

Only one third of crystalloid fluid remains in the intravascular space after an hour, with the rest passing into the other fluid compartments. So, when using crystalloids to replace small volumes of blood loss, three times the volume of blood loss should be administered in order to replace the intravascular volume. However, when using blood or colloids these remain in the intravascular space and only the equivalent fluid volume to the blood lost is required.

Monitoring Fluid Therapy

Once a fluid therapy plan is made, the patient should be checked regularly to ensure appropriate corrections are made and to monitor for side effects e.g. volume overload. The reason for the initial fluid therapy plan should be reassessed, including the clinical signs or clinical pathology abnormalities; e.g. PCV for anaemic patients having a blood transfusion, hydration status for dehydrated patients whose fluid deficits are being corrected. The minimum frequency of observations is twice daily (including weighing the patient), although more critical patients require more frequent observations.

Arterial blood pressure measurement can be used, especially if hypovolaemia or hypotension is suspected. However, arterial blood pressure is influenced by other factors, not just blood volume (e.g. how vasodilated or vasoconstricted a patient's vasculature is). One blood pressure monitoring technique that gives an indication of blood volume is central venous pressure.

Central venous pressure measurements represent the pressure in the intrathoracic vena cava. It is a measure of the relative ability of the heart to pump the blood returning to it and is a useful tool if a degree of heart failure is suspected. Central venous pressure is also an estimate of the relationship between blood volume and blood volume capacity and can be used to tailor fluid therapy in hypovolaemic animals. Normal CVP in small animals is between 0–10 cm H_2O. Generally, low value ranges indicate relative hypovolaemia, and if the value is increased, it indicates relative hypervolaemia, and the heart's inability to cope with venous return.

A catheter should be placed in the jugular vein heading towards the heart. The tip must lie within the thorax (usually in the anterior vena cava); if overlong it can contact the endocardium of the right atrium or ventricle and stimulate arrhythmias. This catheter should be attached to an electrical transducer (as used in arterial blood pressure monitoring) or to a U-manometer. An electrical transducer displays CVP in mmHg, and a U-manometer reading reads as cm H_2O. The following conversion should be used: mmHg x 1.36 = cm H_2O.

These U-manometers are available in commercial sets, but easily made in-practice with a bag of normal saline, a drip set, a three-way tap, an extension set, a drip stand, a ruler, and a cut down length of drip set. Once flushed through with saline, the three-way tap should be turned to connect the jugular catheter and the column of fluid open to the air.

A zero level should be drawn on the ruler at the level of the animal's heart, and measurements taken in relation to this (see Figure 6).

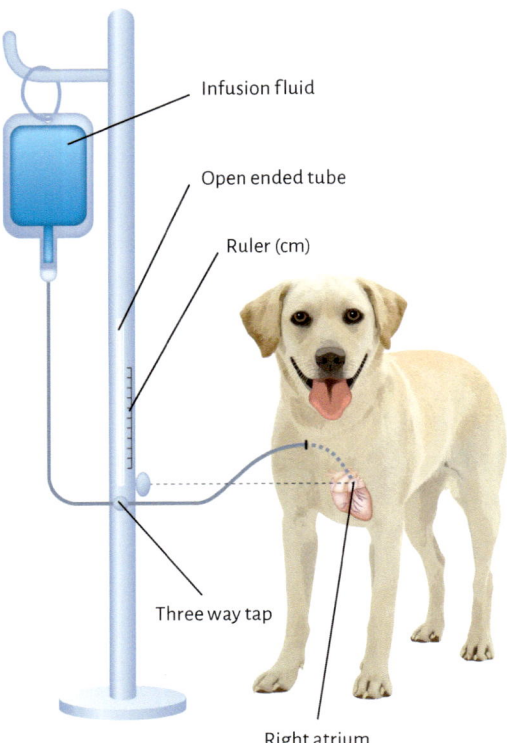

Figure 6. A U-manometer can be used to monitor central venous pressure.

Blood Products

Currently in the UK there are several different blood products stored for use in canine patients in a Pet Blood Bank, but there are no stored blood products available for cats, although this situation may change in the future. Another option in practice, is to collect whole blood canine and feline donations. Depending on the clinical presentation, different blood products are suited to different patients.

Types of Blood Products

Whole Blood
Whole blood contains:
- red blood cells
- white blood cells
- clotting factors
- platelets
- plasma proteins.

One unit is approximately 450 ml in volume for dogs and 45 ml in cats. Whole blood is the best way of transfusing platelets, although the number of active platelets is not significant as they lose viability over the first one to three days.

Blood can be stored for up to three weeks at between 1 and 4 °C (refrigerator), as long as it is collected in a closed system. Whole blood should be transfused as soon as possible after collection. The risk of transfusion reaction increases the older the blood.

Packed Red Cells
Canine whole blood is separated out into packed red cells and plasma. The packed red cells are usually washed with saline and resuspended in minimal saline and SAG-M nutrient solution. The packed cell volume (PCV) of packed red cells is significantly higher than whole blood, between 60–80%. If the PCV is very high, the packed red cells can be resuspended in sterile normal saline to facilitate administration. A sample should be taken aseptically from the packed red cells to ascertain the actual PCV.

A typical canine unit of packed red cells is approximately 200–250 ml in volume. The unit must be stored in the fridge between 2 and 6 °C and used within 42 days of production. (Figure 7).

Fresh Plasma
If the plasma separated from the packed red cells (by centrifugation) is transfused within six hours after harvesting, this is termed fresh plasma. It is rich in clotting factors and platelets, however in most situations the plasma is frozen to create fresh frozen plasma.

Fresh Frozen Plasma
If whole blood is centrifuged and plasma harvested and frozen to -18 °C within six hours this is fresh frozen plasma (FFP). It is rich in clotting factors and also contains immunoglobulins, lipids, albumin, and electrolytes. This product can be stored for up to one year below -18 °C; but after thawing, should be given within six hours.

> A unit of canine FFP is approximately 200 ml in volume.

If FFP is stored at -18 °C for between one and five years, this is classed as frozen plasma. The product still contains non-labile clotting factors (such as II, VII, IX and X), immunoglobulins, albumin, lipids, and electrolytes.

Cryoprecipitate and Cryosupernatent
If fresh frozen plasma is partially thawed and centrifuged, cryoprecipitate is a plasma fraction which is separated from fresh frozen plasma. It is a concentrated product containing

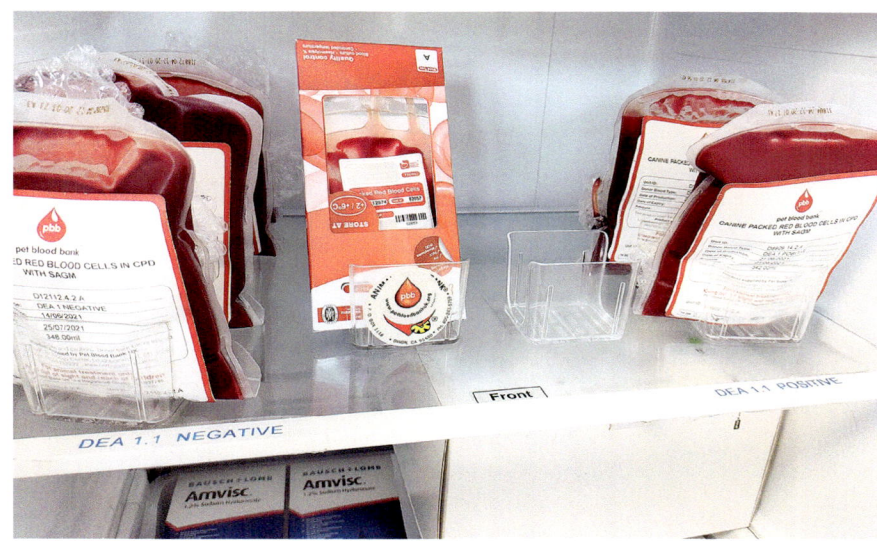

Figure 7. Whole blood and packed red cells must be stored in the fridge.

the labile clotting factors fibrinogen (factor I), factor VIII and Von Willebrand's factor. The remaining fraction is cryosupernatant, containing plasma proteins including albumin, and vitamin K dependant clotting factors II, VII, IX and X. It is stored at -18 °C or below for up to one year.

Canine Blood Transfusion

Canine Blood Donation

When collecting a whole blood donation in a dog, the following are positive attributes in a canine donor:
- friendly and clinically normal
- aged between 1 and 8 years
- large breed dogs (at least 25 kg lean weight)
- easily accessible veins
- a universal donor blood type.

Negative attributes:
- recent bite wounds
- acute vomiting or diarrhoea
- fever
- currently pregnant
- vaccinated within the last 10–14 days
- a history of foreign travel
- a parasite burden
- dogs on any medication
- dogs that have previously received a blood transfusion.

In addition to a preclinical exam, predonation bloods should be taken to include a routine complete blood count and biochemistry or PCV/total protein (as a bare minimum). The results should be checked to ensure there is no underlying pathology, including anaemia, which would make the dog unsuitable as a donor. A portion of the blood sample is also used to ascertain the blood group of the dog.

As well as submitting anticoagulated blood to a commercial laboratory for typing there are commercial blood typing kits available for in-house use.

CANINE BLOOD GROUPS

Blood groups are defined by inherited antigens on the surface of the red blood cell. The presence of an antibody directed against a blood group antigen results in haemolysis.

Canine blood groups are defined by **dog erythrocyte antigens (DEA).** Of the DEAs, DEA 1, and 7 are the most important. Previously, DEA 1 was considered to have three subgroups (DEA 1.1, 1.2 and 1.3) but recent monoclonal antibody and immunofluorescence testing have demonstrated that DEA 1.2 and 1.3 are red cell populations with a lower density of the DEA 1 antigen on them. Therefore, **blood products are described as DEA 1 positive or negative,** where previously the term DEA 1.1 positive or negative was used.

Dogs rarely have naturally occurring alloantibodies, **so the first transfusion is unlikely to cause problems** even if the blood was not of the same blood group. However, it is still advisable to blood type both recipient and donor to check for incompatibility as the life span of the red blood cells may be shortened once transfused into the donor. In addition, if antibodies are generated from an incompatible transfusion, future transfusion potential is limited. **Dogs must be crossmatched for second and subsequent transfusions.**

The process of taking a whole blood donation in the dog is outlined in Box 3.

Box 3. How to Take a Whole Blood Donation in the Dog.

- It is important to wash hands and put on clean examination gloves.
- An assistant should restrain the dog in lateral recumbency. The chin should be tilted up and the forelimbs gently drawn caudally to improve visualisation of the jugular vein.
- A square of hair (5 cm × 5 cm) over the jugular vein should be clipped and this site prepared aseptically (with a final surgical spirit application). The use of a fenestrated sterile drape improves sterility.
- An assistant with a clean pair of examination gloves should remove the collection bag from its plastic storage bag and place it on the scales.
- The scales should be positioned at a level lower than the dog and with the bag in place the weight on the scales should be set to zero.
- If an in-line clamp is provided on the kit, it should be closed off. Alternatively, the haemostat can be clamped approximately 5cm from needle on collection tubing.
- A sterile pair of gloves should be worn.
- The jugular vein should be raised with the non-dominant hand.
- Using a clean stick (preferably) venepuncture should be performed with the bevel of the needle facing upwards.
- The haemostat or clamp should be released.
- Blood should flow from the collection line to the bag easily.
- As soon as the blood starts to enter the collection bag, the bag should be gently rocked to mix the blood with the anticoagulant. This should be repeated regularly (approximately four times a minute) during the collection process.
- The weight of the bag should be checked intermittently. One full unit is 450 ml.
- Once the unit has been collected, the vein should no longer be raised and the collection line clamped again.
- The needle should be removed and firm pressure applied over the venepuncture site with several swabs for two minutes. If required, a neck bandage should be applied.
- If a tube stripper is available, the blood should be stripped from the line into the bag. It should be stopped 5 cm from bag, and the empty tubing should be folded and a knot tied behind the fold. The tubing should be cut on the needle-side of the knot and the needle with tubing discarded into the sharps.
- The donor's demeanour, heart rate, mucous membrane colour and pulse quality should be checked. If the donor is showing any signs of hypovolaemia, such as tachycardia or pale mucous membrane colour, intravenous crystalloid fluid therapy (at three times the volume removed) should be administered.

CROSS-MATCHING

Cross-matching is an in vitro test which investigates potential reactions between the donor's blood and the recipient's blood, which may appear as haemolysis or agglutination. It is the gold standard laboratory procedure used to determine the serological compatibility between the donor and recipient. However, this is not always practical and is restricted to patients receiving more than one blood transfusion.

Cross-matching should be performed in conjunction with blood typing if:
- the recipient received a prior transfusion <5 days earlier.
- there is any suspicion of blood group incompatibility.

There are two types of cross-matching:
- **Major cross-match:** the compatibility between the erythrocytes of the donor and the recipient's plasma/serum should be assessed.
- **Minor cross-match:** assesses the compatibility between the donor's plasma/serum and the recipient's red blood cells.

Cross matching is performed via:
- manual in-house
- in-house gel cross-matching test kit
- external commercial laboratory.

Note: Emergency cross-matches can also be performed (see Box 4).

MANUAL IN-HOUSE CROSS-MATCH PROCEDURE

1. 1 ml of plain and 1 ml of EDTA blood samples should be obtained from both the donor and recipient; ensuring all samples are labelled correctly.
2. Both serum and plasma should be separated at 3000 rpm for 5 minutes. The plasma should be separated and the serum decanted into separate individual tubes. All tubes should be labelled accordingly (i.e. donor serum, recipient serum).
3. 2–3 ml of 0.9% NaCl should be added to the RBC's inverting gently, then centrifuging at 3400 rpm for one minute. The supernatant should be removed. This process should be repeated twice.

Box 4. How to Perform an Emergency Cross-match.

1. On a clean microscope glass slide, 2 drops of recipient serum should be mixed with one drop of the donor's red blood cells.

2. The sample should be examined microscopically for agglutination after 5 minutes.

   Saline agglutination test should be performed prior for both recipient and donor and used as a control. It is important to differentiate from rouleaux formation.

4. The supernatant should be removed from the third above process and resuspend RBCs with saline (i.e. 4.8 ml of NaCl to 0.2 ml RBC's).
5. All tubes should be labelled with one of the following:
   a. major cross-match
   b. minor cross-match
   c. recipient control
   d. donor control.

To perform the test:
1. One drop of recipient serum and one drop of donor RBC suspension should be added to the major crossmatch tube.
2. One drop of donor serum and one drop of recipient RBC suspension should be added to the minor crossmatch tube.
3. One drop of recipient serum and one drop of recipient RBC suspension should be added to the recipient control tube.
4. One drop of donor serum and one drop of recipient RBC suspension should be added to the donor control tube.
5. All four tubes should be incubated at 37 °C for 15 minutes, prior to centrifuging all four tubes at 3400 rpm for 15 seconds.

Manual cross-match procedure interpretation:
- **Macroscopic interpretation:** the tubes should be rotated. With compatible blood there is no agglutination/clumping and the supernatant should not be a haemolysed colour. RBC's should easily float off from the pellet of centrifuged RBC's.
- **Microscopic interpretation:** a drop of serum/RBC mixture should be placed onto a microscope slide with a cover slip. The sample should be checked for agglutination. If compatible there should be no agglutination. Care should be taken to differentiate between agglutination and rouleaux formation.

Feline Blood Transfusion

Blood Donation

The following are positive attributes to look for when choosing a feline donor:
- friendly temperament: although sedation is usually still required
- clinically normal: a predonation exam should be conducted to ensure they are healthy. The Pet Blood Bank also recommends all donors have an echocardiographic examination to check for occult heart disease
- aged between 1–8 years old
- a large cat, of ideally at least 5 kg lean weight
- a high donor PCV (>30%) is preferred
- not pregnant: but previous pregnancy does not exclude a queen from donating
- ideally an indoor cat
- test negative for FeLV, FIV, and FIP
- free from for *Haemobartonella felis*, *Bartonella*, *Dirofilaria*, and *Babesia*.

Feline Blood Groups

- **Group A:** dominant to AB, and most common in the UK, although this may be different in other countries.
- **Group B:** thought to be common in some breeds, e.g. Persian, British Shorthair.
- **Group AB:** recessive to A; codominant with B.

Cats are born with naturally occurring alloantibodies to other cats' blood groups and there is no universal donor in cats, so cross-matching is mandatory, even a check has been performed for compatible blood types between donor and recipient. The potential reactions that may be observed if the incorrect blood type is given to a recipient cat, are shown in Table 3. A more recently identified red blood cell antigen (Mik) is a potential cause for such non-AB incompatibilities.

Table 3. Feline blood groups.

Donor \ Recipient	A	B	AB
A	Ok	Fatal	Reaction
B	Reaction	Ok	Reaction
AB	Reaction	Fatal	Ok

A step-by-step guide on taking a whole blood donation in the cat is shown in Box 5.

> ### Box 5. How to Take a Whole Blood Donation in the Cat.
>
> - Sedation is usually required. The sedation protocol should be based on the temperament and health status of the cat. The author has used alfaxalone intramuscularly or sevoflurane by mask. Others suggest α-2 adrenergic agonist-based protocols although this class of drugs prevents compensatory tachycardia as a response to a loss of blood volume.
> - Flow by oxygen by mask and anaesthetic monitoring should be used for all sedated cats. Their eyes should be lubricated.
> - A typical unit of cat blood is 45 ml; but it should be ensured that no more than 12 ml/kg donation is taken.
> - A ratio of 1 ml of anticoagulant (drawn in a sterile manner from the bag of anticoagulant) to 7 ml of whole blood should be prepared.
> - The area over the jugular vein should be clipped and prepared aseptically.
> - Sterile gloves should be worn.
> - The butterfly catheter and three-way tap should be attached to the 60 ml syringe (containing the anticoagulant amount described above) and anticoagulant injected through the three-way tap into the butterfly needle.
> - The jugular vein should be raised and the butterfly catheter inserted into the vessel, bevel upper most and the blood gently aspirated into the syringe at a rate of 5 ml/min or greater.
> - Once the desired volume is collected into the syringe, the three-way tap should be turned off, and the butterfly needle removed from the vessel.
> - Pressure should be applied to the venepuncture site.
> - The donor's demeanour, heart rate, mucous membrane colour and pulse quality should be checked. If the donor is showing signs of hypovolaemia, such as tachycardia or pale mucous membrane colour, then intravenous crystalloid fluid therapy should be administered (at three times the volume removed).

Transfusion Protocols

Blood Donation Storage

Usually, whole blood is used immediately, but if storage is required, assuming sterile collection then donations can be stored in a fridge (1–4 °C) for up to three weeks. **If sterility was compromised, the blood should be used immediately** (and certainly within 24 hours). When stored in the fridge, the bag should be agitated every two to three days to ensure mixing of contents.

Red cell products should be allowed to warm up gradually, either by allowing them to acclimatise to ambient temperature or by placing them in a warm water bath <37 °C.

A giving set with **an in-line filter must be used** with all blood products (to filter out any debris and microthrombi). Smaller volume whole blood donations (e.g. for cats and small dogs) may be delivered via a syringe driver, and therefore an in-line filter should be used between the syringe and intravenous catheter.

Blood should not be administered through lines with Hartmann's, or other calcium-containing solutions in them. Citrate (part of the anticoagulant in the blood collection bag) binds to calcium in the blood and calcium is required for the coagulation cascade, therefore the citrate stops the blood clotting. Hartmann's contains calcium, and so adding extra calcium to the mix allows blood clots to form where the two fluids mix.

Monitoring the Transfusion

- **The recipient's baseline temperature, pulse, and respiration** (TPR) should be recorded before the start of the transfusion: this makes it easier to note reactions whilst continuing observations during transfusions.
- If the patient is stable, **the initial transfusion rate is 0.5 ml/kg/hr for the first 15 minutes** to check for acute reactions. During this first 15 minutes, the patient must be continuously monitored and further TPR recordings taken every five minutes.
- After the initial 15 minutes, if there are no signs of a transfusion reaction, **the infusion rate should be increased to 5–20 ml/kg/hr.**
- The author suggests further **recordings of TPR continuing every 15 minutes** for the first hour, then half hourly observations for the next hour, and after that hourly observations until the end of the transfusion.
- Ideally, **the transfusion should be completed within four hours.**
- In the dog, the transfusion should be followed with a small (100 ml) bag of 0.9% saline to ensure that blood product is not lost in the drip tubing. Alternatively, in the cat, **sufficient saline should be flushed through the administration line to flush all remaining whole blood into the catheter.**
- For a patient with acute hypovolaemic anaemia, the benefit of a fast infusion rate may outweigh the risks of a transfusion reaction.

– A post-transfusion blood sample should be taken to check the success of the transfusion e.g. if the reason for transfusion was anaemia, the PCV/TP should be rechecked; if the reason for transfusion was hypoalbuminaemia, albumin should be rechecked. This should be repeated after a further 12 hours.

Transfusion Reactions

These can be **immunological or non-immunological.**

Signs associated with an immune mediated response include:
– agitation/restlessness/change in attitude
– nausea, vomiting, salivation
– urticaria with or without pruritus
– anaphylaxis
– pyrexia
– tachypnoea/dyspnoea
– tachycardia
– hypotension
– seizures
– haemolysis, jaundice, haemoglobinuria.

Non-immune related reactions include:
– hypocalcemia (this could be due to too much citrate binding blood calcium)
– circulatory overload
– hypothermia (blood not warmed prior to infusion)
– transmission of infectious diseases.

> **If a transfusion reaction is suspected: the infusion should be stopped and the vet contacted.**
>
> The vet may decide to dampen down the immune response by using corticosteroids, and if appropriate administer antihistamines. Dependent on the cost/benefit ratio, for a mild reaction the transfusion may continue but at a much **slower** rate. Otherwise, for a more severe reaction, no more of the blood product transfusion must be given.

Transfusion Volume Calculation

Intraoperative blood loss of greater than 20% of blood volume should be treated with blood products, usually replacing the same volume that has been lost (if whole blood is used). However, patients may require blood transfusions for other reasons, e.g. chronic anaemia. The calculation below requires knowledge of the donor blood PCV (for whole blood and packed red cells), the recipient's current PCV, and the desired PCV.

This equation is appropriate for all species, as long as the correct value for blood volume (e.g. 90 ml/kg for dogs, and 56 ml/kg for cats) is inserted:

$$\text{ml of donor blood required} = \text{recipient's blood volume} \times \frac{\text{desired recipient PCV} - \text{current recipient PCV}}{\text{donor PCV}}$$

NUTRITION FOR THE CRITICAL PATIENT

Whilst sorting out the critical patient's life-threatening issues, their nutrition is often overlooked. Ensuring adequate nutrition should be addressed as soon as possible after restoring haemodynamic stability, electrolyte and acid-base disturbances, and hydration status.

Whilst healthy patients may be able to metabolically adapt to a short fast, critically ill patients are unable to make these metabolic adaptations, and often end up in a negative calorie and nitrogen balance.

Feeding intervention should be instigated on day three of anorexia. This is because compromised immunity is detectable in cats by day four of anorexia, and metabolic changes in dogs by day three. Consequences of continued anorexia include infection, sepsis, organ failure, and poor wound healing. Indeed, the animal's history should be taken into account as anorexia may have been going on for several days at home e.g. nutrition may be implemented on day three of hospitalisation, but this is equivalent to day six of anorexia for the patient. Hyporexia (reduction in appetite) should also be considered, as inadequate nutritional intake may result in similar complications.

Nutrients

In critical care nutrition, **the three main macronutrients are protein, carbohydrates, and fatty acids.**

Carbohydrates

Carbohydrates are mostly **converted to glucose and used for energy.** Much controversy surrounds the illness energy requirement (IER) rationale, i.e. that an illness factor greatly increases the **resting energy requirement (RER)**. Calculating an illness energy requirement is currently less favoured because of the risk of overfeeding, leading to metabolic complications such as gastrointestinal intolerance, hepatic dysfunction, and hyperglycaemia. Current thinking is the RER in most critical patients is only moderately elevated, and can be calculated from the formulae below:

$$\text{Patients} > 2 \text{ kg: } 30 \times \text{bodyweight (kg)} + 70$$

$$\text{Patients} < 2 \text{ kg: } 70 \times \text{bodyweight (kg)}^{0.75}$$

For cats the formula is slightly different, as the above formula tends to overestimate feline calorie requirements.

$$\text{RER} = 40 \, (\text{Wt. in kg})$$

Protein Requirements

Protein is required for metabolic function, tissue growth, function and repair. The requirement for protein is significantly elevated in critical patients. Proteins should be easily digestible and so animal sources (e.g. egg and milk proteins) are often used for this reason.

Suggested protein requirements are 2–3 g/kg body weight for a dog, and 3 g/kg body weight for a cat.

Some animals with renal or hepatic dysfunction cannot tolerate a high protein load as they have trouble eliminating the protein. However, instead of restricting the protein, efforts should be made to help eliminate the protein levels, e.g. **fluid therapy to flush through kidneys.**

Micronutrients

In addition to calories, protein and water, there are micronutrients (at least 25 of them) e.g. fatty acids, vitamins, and minerals required to maintain healthy function and immunity. As most veterinary foods for nutritional support are balanced, deficiency should not occur. Electrolyte abnormalities are more common, however, with fluid losses.

Ways of Providing Nutrition

Enteral Nutrition

If the animal can and will eat this is the best way to provide nutrition, as the intestinal epithelium gets its nutrition (especially glutamine) from the nutrients passing along the gut wall. If the gut does not get its nutrition, the chance of bacterial translocation (bacteria moving from the gut lumen into the blood stream) and sepsis is much greater. This route is the cheapest, and if the animal is not eating by itself, coaxed feeding, appetite stimulants or some feeding tubes can be alternatives.

Coaxed feeding is the feeding of small, highly palatable, warm, smelly food in a stress-free environment. It is not the force feeding of a semiliquid diet from a syringe, which often stresses the animal and provides negative reinforcement for that animal to remain anorexic.

Appetite Stimulation

Diazepam (0.05–0.15 mg/kg IV or orally once a day) has been used with some success in dogs and cats as an appetite stimulant. It should not be relied upon as a long term measure, however. As a benzodiazepine, it can cause sedation or drowsiness, and can cause liver damage in cats. **Cyproheptadine and mirtazepine have fewer side effects** and may be more effective as an appetite stimulant.

Tube Feeding

Assisted feeding should be implemented if the patient is not voluntarily meeting 75% of its resting energy requirements (RER). Tube feeding is usually the most effective way of getting nutrition into a critically ill patient. In general, the more proximal the tube, the more physiological the feeding. In order from cranial to caudal:
- naso-oesophageal
- oesophagostomy
- gastrostomy
- jejunostomy.

Feeding tubes should be clearly labelled to avoid any mishaps, especially where there are concurrent oesophagostomy tubes (Figure 8) and central venous catheters, as the insertion sites are wrapped in the same neck dressing.

Parenteral Nutrition

This means that nutrition is delivered via the intravenous route and bypasses the gut. As it is always preferable to use the gut if possible, this route is only considered if enteral feeding is deemed hazardous or contraindicated e.g. the patient is at an increased risk of aspiration, such as depressed mentation. Parenteral nutrition can be used to supplement enteral nutrition if the patient is unable to meet 50% of its requirement via the digestive tract.

Solutions for parenteral nutrition contain a protein source, a carbohydrate source, and a fat source. **They must be prepared aseptically and delivered via a dedicated, central (usually jugular) venous catheter.**

Risks associated with parenteral nutrition include **thrombophlebitis of the catheterised vein** due to hyperosmolarity (hence the use of a central venous catheter), hyperglycaemia, hypertriglyceridaemia and hyperammonaemia.

Monitoring These Patients for Complications

The patient should be assessed every day to check they are receiving their RER or if intervention is required. **The nutritional monitoring of these patients includes twice daily weighing, body condition score, hydration status assessment, TPRs, and evaluation of demeanour.**

Animals with feeding tubes need to have the tube checked regularly to ensure they are patent, have not become dislodged, or caused a cellulitis in the area around the insertion site.

Gastrointestinal signs may occur after enteral feeding has started, manifesting as vomiting and diarrhoea. These are less likely if the feeding is started slowly, and the food initially diluted.

Metabolic derangements can be seen but are more common in parenterally fed patients, rather than the enteral route. These can be identified with blood tests such as glucose, total solids, triglycerides, urea, and electrolytes.

> The author would like to acknowledge Claire Dorey-Phillips who contributed the section on blood cross-matching.

Suggested Reading

- Davis, H., Jensen, T., Johnson, A., Knowles, P., Meyer, R., Rucinsky, R., Shafford, H., American Association of Feline Practicioners, & American Animal Hospital Association (2013). 2013 AAHA/AAFP fluid therapy guidelines for dogs and cats. *Journal of the American Animal Hospital Association*, 49(3), 149–159.

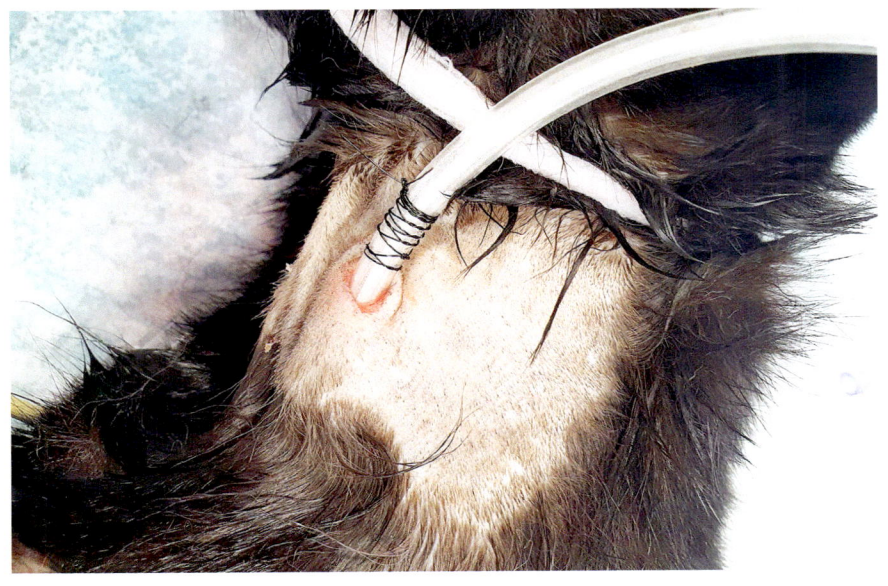

Figure 8. An oesophagostomy tube is usually placed on the left hand side of the neck.

Self-assessment

Test

1. Which of the following is a clinical sign of a non-immunological transfusion reaction?
    a. Urticaria.
    b. Hypocalcemia.
    c. Angioedema.
    d. Haemolysis.

2. What rate do current recommendations from the American Animal Hospital Association (AAHA) suggest as a starting rate in a normal health dog at the start of anaesthesia with crystalloid fluid therapy?
    a. 5 ml/kg/hr.
    b. 6 ml/kg/hr.
    c. 10 ml/kg/hr.
    d. 4 ml/kg/hr.

3. Fluid losses from vomiting are an example of what type of fluid loss?
    a. Extracellular fluid loss.
    b. Protein rich extracellular fluid loss.
    c. Whole blood loss.
    d. Pure water loss.

4. What is the percentage of NaCl in normal saline?
    a. 0.18%.
    b. 5%.
    c. 0.9%.
    d. 7.2%.

5. What is the maximum rate of potassium supplementation in a 10 kg dog?
    a. 2.5 mmol/hr.
    b. 5 mmol/hr.
    c. 7.5 mmol/hr.
    d. 10 mmol/hr.

6. What is the total maintenance volume of fluid therapy over 24 hours for a 25 kg dog?
    a. 1475 ml.
    b. 895 ml.
    c. 37 ml.
    d. 2.46 ml.

7. The maximum volume of blood donation that could be taken from a 6 kg cat is?
    a. 45 ml.
    b. 56 ml.
    c. 72 ml.
    d. 90 ml.

Answers on page 160

8. Which electrolyte is considered the 'osmotic skeleton' of the extracellular fluid?
    a. Potassium.
    b. Calcium.
    c. Sodium.
    d. Chloride.

9. Anatomically, from cranial to caudal, what is the correct order of feeding tube placement sites?
    a. Jejunostomy, oesophagostomy, naso-oesophageal, gastrostomy.
    b. Naso-oesophageal, gastrostomy, oesophagostomy, jejunostomy.
    c. Gastrostomy, jejunostomy, naso-oesophageal, oesophagostomy.
    d. Naso-oesophageal, oesophagostomy, gastrostomy, jejunostomy.

10. If refrigerated, a unit of packed red cells could be kept for how long?
    a. 6 hours.
    b. 4 days.
    c. 28 days.
    d. 42 days.

Clinical Case

A 3 kg cat is presented out of hours with inappetence. The vet palpates an abdominal mass and suggests an exploratory laparotomy planned for 10 hours time. On clinical exam, the cat has the following signs of dehydration:
- semi dry oral mucous membranes
- normal skin turgor
- moist eyes.

1. How dehydrated is the cat?

2. What does this percentage represent?

3. What is the fluid deficit in this cat?

4. The fluid deficit needs to be restored before surgery and maintenance fluid therapy provided over this time frame, as the patient is not eating. So starting with the maintenance rate; what is the maintenance rate for this cat?

Nursing Anaesthesia

5. Using the information above, what is the fluid therapy plan to rehydrate the cat before general anaesthesia?

6. The next morning the cat's hydration status is checked again, the cat is weighed and is now 3.15 kg and the vet feels that the cat is now normally hydrated, and the fluid deficit has been restored. The cat is going to be anaesthetised for the exploratory laparotomy, but what fluid rate should the cat be on during anaesthesia?

Correct Answers:

Test

1. b
2. a
3. a
4. c
5. b
6. a
7. c
8. c
9. d
10. d

Clinical Case

1. How dehydrated is the cat? 5%.

2. What does this percentage represent?
The percentage of bodyweight lost as water.

3. What is the fluid deficit in this cat?
5/100 × 3 kg = 0.15 kg = 0.15 l = 150 ml
(Remember the density of water is 1 g/ml).

4. What is the maintenance rate for this cat?
In the cat, the formula is 80 × body weight $(kg)^{0.75}$ and this gives the total volume of maintenance fluid for 24 hours.

Maintenance over 24 hours: $(80 \times 30)^{0.75}$ = 182 ml over 24 hours.

So this is the maintenance over 24 hours but the time frame of the fluid therapy plan in question is over 10 hours i.e. up until the point of the exploratory laparotomy.

10/24 × 182 ml = 76 ml over 10 hours.

5. what is the fluid therapy plan to rehydrate the cat before general anaesthesia?
If the 150 ml fluid deficit is paid back over 10 hours plus 76 ml for maintenance, these should be added together:

150 + 76 = 226 ml over 10 hours = 22.6 ml/hour.

6. What fluid rate should the cat be on during anaesthesia?
Following the AAHA guidelines, a starting rate of 3 ml/kg/hr should be used for the first hour then reduced by 25% every hour until the maintenance rate is reached. With the cat's new weight, the maintenance rate is $(80 \times 3.15)^{0.75}$ = 189 ml over 24 hours:

189/24 = 7.9 ml/hour and as the cat now weighs 3.15 kg, this is 2.5 ml/kg/hr.

So starting anaesthesia fluid therapy rate at 3 ml/kg/hr should be used but after 1 hour this should be dropped to 2.5 ml/kg/hr because this is the cat's maintenance rate and it should drop by 25% every hour, until maintenance is reached, and the maintenance rate is higher than the 25% reduction.

Notes

Analgesia

Nicki Grint

> **Chapter Summary:**
> - Pain assessment in different species. Understanding pain scoring.
> - The pathophysiology of pain.
> - The different analgesia options, including opioids, non-steroidal anti-inflammatory agents, local anaesthesia, and other agents such as α-2 agonists.
> - The use of constant rate infusions for analgesia.
> - Long term pain management and chronic pain.
> - Local anaesthesia: local blocks and epidurals.

The provision of effective pain relief to veterinary patients is crucial, not only for their welfare but to improve recovery times from surgery. To do this requires the ability to recognise pain, along with a knowledge of the pathophysiology of pain and which medications are best able to deal with it. The strategy for providing this pain relief is also important with options including multimodal analgesia, pre-emptive pain relief, local anaesthesia, and constant rate infusions (CRI).

PAIN ASSESSMENT

The first step in treating pain is to recognise its presence. In 2020, the International Academy for the Study of Pain (IASP) updated their definition of pain and added an addendum:

> "Verbal description is only one of several behaviours to express pain; inability to communicate does not negate the possibility that a human or a nonhuman animal experiences pain."

This encapsulates **the difficulty in assessing pain in animals as they cannot verbalise their pain** and we must rely on behavioural clues. The difficulty in assessing pain in animals results in one of two outcomes. Either analgesics are withheld because the animal is not showing overt signs of pain, or an assessor is overly anthropomorphic and assumes that because a human undergoing the same surgery requires a certain level of analgesia, the animal requires the same, and may administer excessive analgesics.

There is no gold standard pain assessment system; and **all rely on the interpretation/recognition of behaviours and so have a large subjective component** which is prone to observer error and bias. More objective measures such as physiological data (see Box 1) can be used as part of pain assessment (e.g. in the University of Melbourne Pain Scale (dogs) and Botucatu Scale (cats)) but are not reliable, as these are not specific enough to differentiate pain from other stressors e.g. anxiety, fear, or other pathologies.

> **Box 1. Physiological Signs Associated with Pain.** (Adapted from Muir & Gaynor, 2002).
> - Tachypnoea or panting.
> - Tachycardia.
> - Dilated pupils.
> - Hypertension.

Different Types of Pain Scoring Systems

The three main types of pain scores are known as visual analogue scales (VAS), numerical rating scales (NRS), and simple descriptive scales (SDS) as described in Table 1. The scales can be used to assign an overall pain score or used to compile composite scores (also known as categorical or multi-factorial). **A composite score is where there are multiple scales for different aspects of pain behaviour.** Scores are assigned in categories such as vocalisation and posture, and then added together to create a total score. Using composite scales often reminds the observer to look at several aspects of the animal's behaviour before assigning the pain score.

How to Use Pain Scoring Systems

Pain scales usually have an intervention level which guides the user as to when the animal requires additional analgesia.

Table 1. Visual analogue scales (VAS), numerical rating scales (NRS), and simple descriptive scales (SDS).

	VAS	NRS	SDS
Description	· Semiobjective scoring system. · A 100 mm straight horizontal line anchored with two phrases. · The observer places a mark on the line corresponding to the degree of pain.	· Semiobjective scoring system. · Pain score is assigned as a whole number. · Typically 0-10 is used.	· Semiobjective scoring system. · 4 or 5 categories of pain intensity. · Each descriptor is assigned a number
Example	No pain ⊢—X——⊣ Worst possible pain (100 mm)	No pain 0 1 2 X 3 4 5 Worst possible pain	1. No pain 2. Mild pain 3. Moderate pain X 4. Severe pain

If your clinical opinion is the animal is uncomfortable but the pain score has not reached the intervention level, analgesia should not be withheld for this reason.

A Dynamic and Interactive Approach

Whatever the pain scoring system, the observer must employ a dynamic and interactive approach. In any assessment it is not enough to merely observe the patient to assess pain but **must be interactive which means using palpation.** Firstly, the observer approaches the animal from outside the kennel to take note of any signs such as abnormal postures, restlessness, and attention to any wounds (e.g. licking, biting or chewing). The observer then opens the cage door and attracts the animal to the front of the cage, noting the animal's willingness to interact and move, and their general demeanour. Finally, the animal should be allowed out of the cage (if their condition allows) to move around. Observers should watch for signs such as reluctance to move, and lameness.

Then, importantly, the animal's painful focus (e.g. the surgical site) should be gently palpated and the animal's response (which watch out – could include turning and biting) noted (see Figure 1). **All of this information should be considered together when assigning a pain score.** Some published pain scoring systems suggest that if there is no painful focus, the palpation of a stifle should be used for consistent comparison.

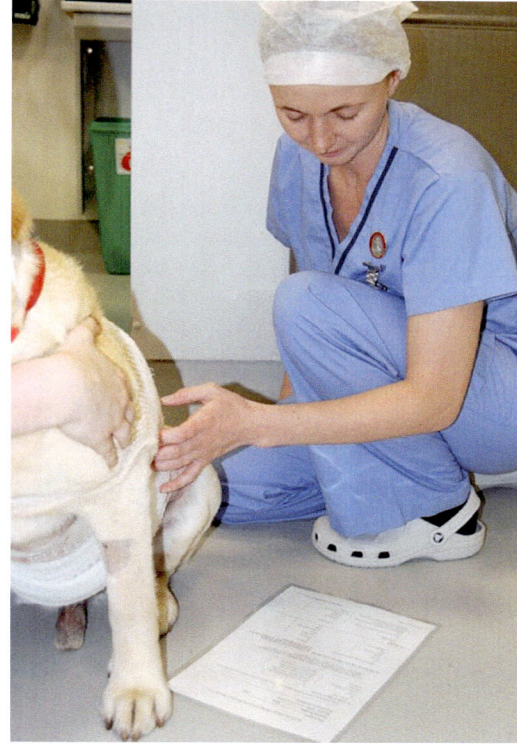

Figure 1. Nurse performing pain score.

Pain Assessment in Dogs

Table 2 includes behaviours to look for in dogs that are indicators of pain.

There are several published pain scores that are validated in dogs, but the one in common place use is the **Glasgow Composite Pain Scale.** It is a composite simple descriptive scale with six categories:
- posture
- activity
- vocalisation
- attention to wounds
- demeanour
- mobility
- response to touch.

Table 2. Some pain related behaviours observed in dogs.

Behavioural aspect	Dog
Vocalisation	Howls, barks, groans, whimpers, growls.
Facial expression	Furrowing of brow, fixed stare.
Self-awareness	Looks at painful area, licks, chews, or bites at it.
Locomotion	Limping or non-weight bearing on a painful limb.
Activity	Restless, slow to rise, reluctant to move.
Attitude	Poor response to owner with weak tail wag or can become aggressive with tendency to escape.
Appetite	Decreased, picky or absent.
Urination and bowel movements	Urine retention and constipation.
Grooming	Reduced.
Response to palpation	Vocalisation, aggression, withdrawing.
Posture	Abnormal positions may include dropped head, hunched, tucked in abdomen, "praying" position.

Table 3. Some pain related behaviours observed in cats.

Behavioural aspect	Cat
Changes	This could be an absence of a normal behaviour or a presence of a new one.
Facial expression	Fear slope, muzzle tension, orbital squeezing/eye squinting, hanging head, furrowed brow.
Posture	Hunched position or tense abdomen, shifting of weight or lying in an abnormal position.
Attention to wounds	Licking, chewing or scratching.
Vocalisation	Crying, hissing or growling or unusually quiet.
Response to palpation	Swish tail, flatten ears, cry, hiss or growl, bite or lash out.

The maximum score is 24, but where it is not appropriate to make the dog rise and leave the kennel, the maximum score is 20. **The analgesic intervention level is 6/24 or 5/20.**

Pain Assessment in Cats

Pain assessment in cats has lagged behind that of dogs. Cats tend to conceal pain more than dogs, which may be a reason analgesia is often suboptimal in this species.

When performing a dynamic and interactive assessment of the cat, there are three main phases of pain assessment: observation of the cat in the cage, interaction with the cat, and palpation of the painful area. The interactive portion of the assessment is often not be feasible in feral cats.

> There are **three pain scoring systems** validated in cats:
> - Glasgow Composite Measure Pain Scale for cats (Glasgow CMPS).
> - UNESP Botucatu multidimensional composite pain scale, (UNESP).
> - Feline Grimace Scale (University of Montreal).

The Glasgow composite pain score is a composite simple descriptive scale. Several of the categories have questions regarding presence or absence of behaviours but also include caricatures of two aspects of facial expression. **The authors suggest an analgesia intervention level of 5 out of 20.**

UNESP Botucatu scale is a composite descriptive scale. It has been validated in Brazilian, Portuguese, and English. It includes several categories including objective (blood pressure measurement) and subjective evaluations. **The authors suggest an intervention level of ≥8 out of 30.**

The Feline Grimace Scale concentrates solely on the cat's face. It scores five facial action units: whisker position, orbital tightening, ear position, head position, and muzzle tension. Each facial action unit is scored from 0 to 2. The score is then added up and divided by the total possible score (i.e. if you cannot score that facial action unit, it is left out). **The intervention level is >0.39.**

Pain Assessment in Small Mammals

Some behavioural signs associated with pain in small mammals include:
- **Rabbits:** hide, face back of cage, may become aggressive or docile, reduced appetite and grind teeth.
- **Guinea pig:** hides, lies recumbent, quiet, terrified, repetitive squealing, reduced appetite with increased respiratory rate.
- **Rats:** hiding or hunched, back arched and stretching (abdominal pain), aggressive or docile, reduced appetite, self-trauma, eating bedding, piloerection, lack of grooming, porphyrin staining (reddish-brown staining around eyes and nose) (Adapted from Grant, 2007).

Much work has been done on facial action units in various species (e.g. the Feline Grimace Scale above). Researchers at the University of Newcastle have published posters detailing pain assessment using facial expressions in rats, mice, and rabbits.

Difficulties in Pain Assessment

To recognise pain behaviours in an individual animal, it is **useful to know what the animal's normal behaviour is,** which is knowledge gained from the veterinary nurse's interaction with the patient in the kennels preoperatively. However, animals hospitalised away from their owner often do not exhibit normal behaviours in a strange environment. Small mammals housed in close proximity to their predators will also not exhibit normal behaviour. Difficulties in interpretation also stem from how different species exhibit different signs of pain behaviour. Even within a species, different breeds and individuals respond to pain in different ways. The obvious and well quoted example is the comparison of the Labrador still wagging its tail with a broken leg, compared to a Greyhound that screams during the premedication injection.

Postoperative pain scores can be confused by concomitant drug therapy. Just because an animal is sedated, it does not necessarily mean its analgesia is adequate. Take for example α-2 adrenergic agonists and opioids, where it is thought that the sedation caused by these drugs outlasts the analgesia. Observer variation also plays a part with some observers scoring consistently higher than others. This can to some extent be minimised if all observers use the same systematic approach to pain scoring.

Nociceptive Threshold Testing

The majority of pain assessment techniques are subjective. However, veterinary research has looked at nociceptive threshold testing as an objective tool to quantify an animal's nociceptive thresholds and see how they change after surgery and/or analgesia.

The technique involves application of a mechanical or thermal stimulus. For example, the mechanical test is the application of a blunt ended pin to a site next to the surgical site. The blunt ended pin is attached to a force or pressure metre. The blunt ended pin is then applied until the animal's reaction suggests they find it a noxious stimulus e.g. flinching, growling, snapping, lifting a leg. The force or pressure at which this occurs is the animal's nociceptive threshold. A baseline value is obtained before surgery. After surgery, if analgesia is insufficient the threshold goes down (i.e. the patient tolerates less stimulus before reacting). If analgesia is administered, the threshold increases.

This technique used to be used under Home Office licence, however, it is now legal for it to be used in clinical practice. However, it is best used in addition to pain scoring, rather than to replace it.

Physiology of Pain

Physiological Consequences of Pain

As well as being a welfare issue, animals should not be allowed to remain in pain, several physiological consequences occur which are listed in Box 2.

> **Box 2. Physiological Consequences of Pain.**
>
> - Increased sympathetic tone.
> - Increased systemic vascular resistance and preload.
> - Increased stroke volume.
> - Increased myocardial work.
> - Increased metabolic rate.
> - Altered clotting function.
> - Decreased gastrointestinal and urinary tone.
> - Increased ACTH, cortisol, ADH, renin, angiotensin.
> - Hyperglycaemia.
> - Increased protein muscle metabolism.
> - Retention of Na^+ and water.
> - Hypoventilation.

The International Academy for the Study of Pain (IASP) updated their definition of pain in 2020. The revised definition is: *"an unpleasant sensory and emotional experience associated with, or resembling that associated with, actual or potential tissue damage."*

The sensory component (detailed below) alone is nociception. For the term pain to be used there must be an emotional component as well.

The Pain Pathway

The pain pathway is illustrated in Figure 2. The conversion of a noxious stimulus (such as an extreme temperature or pressure) into an electrical stimulus is called **transduction,** and this is the first part of the pain pathway.

These electrical signals pass up nerves (either A delta or C-fibres) to a part of the spinal cord called the dorsal horn. This part of the pain pathway is called **transmission.**
- **Aδ-fibres** are fast conducting, small fibres which are myelinated for sharp, mechanical pain.
- **C-fibres** are slow conducting, unmyelinated fibres for longer lasting or dull, burning pain.

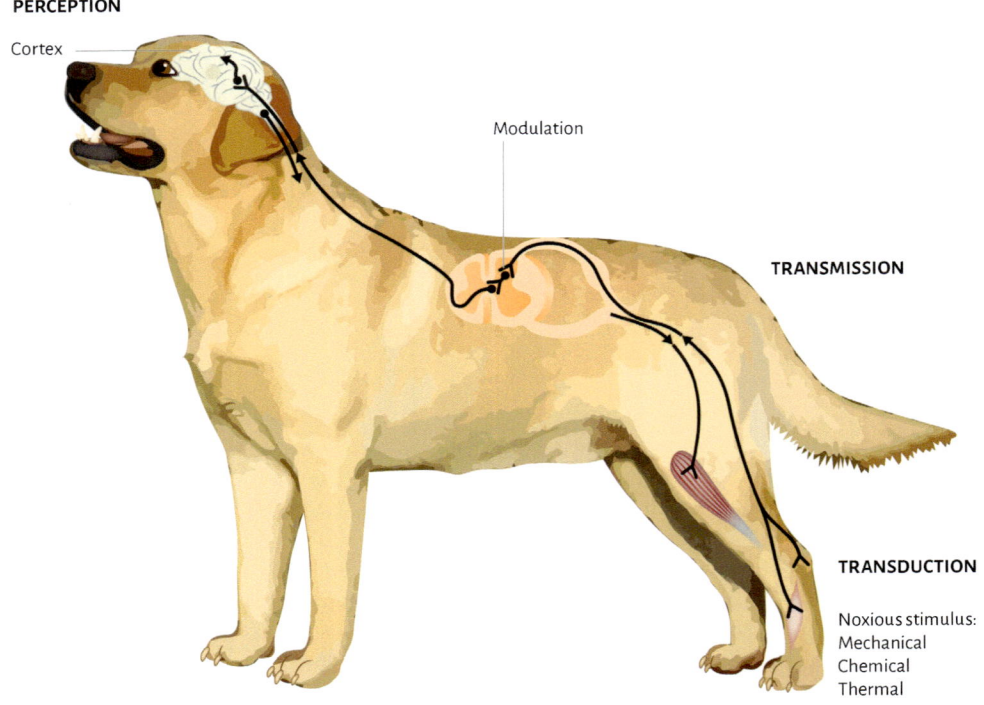

Figure 2. The pain pathway.

At the dorsal horn of the spinal cord, several things happen, including a reflex arc which makes the motor nerves (if the animal is conscious) move the muscles to remove the part of the body affected away from the noxious stimulus.

Also at the dorsal horn, a decision is made whether to pass the signal up the spinal cord to the brain, or not. This decision making is called **modulation.** When the signal is passed up to the brain and arrives at the cerebral cortex, this is when the animal becomes aware of the pain **(perception)**.

Types of Pain

Nociceptors

When tissue (skin, ligaments, viscera) is damaged this activates nociceptors (pain receptors). **Nociceptors respond to different noxious stimuli;** some respond to extremes of temperatures (thermoreceptors), some respond to extremes of pressure including incisions (mechanoreceptors) or chemicals (chemoreceptors). Some nociceptors are **unimodal** (i.e. only respond to one set of stimuli), and some nociceptors are **polymodal** and respond to more than one type of stimuli.

Nociceptors have a **firing threshold,** which is the threshold that triggers an electrical stimulus. The threshold might be a certain temperature or a pressure. **When tissue is damaged, this releases inflammatory mediators** such as prostaglandins and leukotrienes to form an inflammatory soup. These inflammatory mediators lower the firing thresholds and make nociceptors respond to less intense stimuli. **This lowering of the firing threshold contributes to the phenomena of allodynia and hyperalgesia.** In addition, silent nociceptors (usually dormant/inactive) can be recruited by the inflammatory soup.

Somatic and Visceral Pain

- **Somatic pain** is that arising from the skin or muscle.
- **Visceral pain** is that arising from the internal organs.

Visceral nociceptors are often polymodal C-fibres. They are sparsely distributed when compared to those in the skin (approx. 1:100). This means **visceral pain is difficult to localise because it is a diffuse sensation.** Visceral nociceptors also respond to different stimuli than those in the skin e.g. a sharp incisional stimuli is more painful for skin than viscera. **Stretching and distension** are often the major stimuli for visceral pain.

Acute versus Chronic Pain

- **Acute pain** is sudden onset and usually the result of a clearly defined cause such as an injury or surgery. Acute pain resolves with the healing of its underlying cause and is alleviated by analgesic drugs.
- **Chronic pain** persists for weeks or months, well past the course of the disease. Chronic pain is seldom totally alleviated by analgesics.

Analgesic Drugs

Opioids

Opioids are commonly used in small animals, and include morphine, pethidine, methadone, buprenorphine, butorphanol, fentanil, and alfentanil. They provide analgesia at modulation and perception sites on the pain pathway. These drugs all work on opioid receptors, of which there are several subtypes, including μ (mu), κ (kappa), and δ (delta). Different opioids act at different receptors, with the most effective analgesics being the pure μ-agonists such as morphine, methadone, and pethidine. Buprenorphine is a partial μ-agonist, and butorphanol is a κ-agonist and a μ-antagonist. Figure 3 demonstrates the difference between full and partial agonists.

The drugs are usually given in injectable form, and can be given intravenously (except pethidine), intramuscularly, subcutaneously, and epidurally. Some drugs are also readily absorbed across the mucous membranes. They are metabolized in the liver and excreted in the urine.

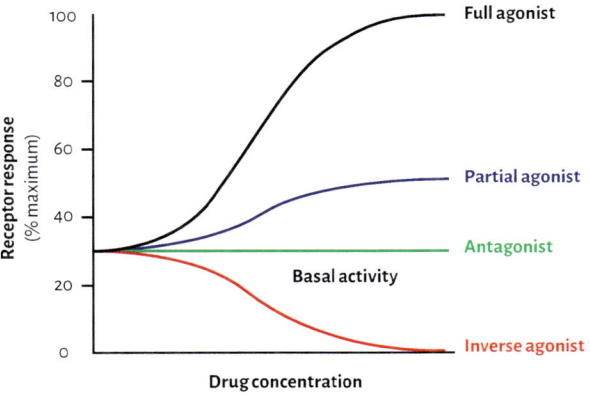

Figure 3. How full agonists compare against partial agonists.

Morphine, pethidine, buprenorphine, methadone, and butorphanol are commonly used for preanaesthetic medication, either by themselves, because they have good sedative properties, or in combination with acepromazine, the α-2 adrenergic agonists or benzodiazepines.

Injectable fentanil, alfentanil, and remifentanil tend to be used for analgesia when an animal is already anaesthetized, because they can have more profound effects on an animal's physiology. Patches containing either fentanil or buprenorphine are available to stick on to animal's skin, so the drug releases slowly across the skin over a period of a few days.

Most opioids decrease heart rate (especially fentanil and alfentanil). This is of little clinical relevance with morphine, methadone and buprenorphine, and pethidine tends to increase heart rate somewhat. At normal clinical doses, the opioids (except fentanil, remifentanil, and alfentanil) cause minimal respiratory depression. Some opioids are emetic (especially morphine) and vomiting may be contraindicated in certain clinical scenarios.

Non-steroidal Anti-inflammatory Drugs (NSAIDs)

NSAIDs work by blocking cyclo-oxygenase enzymes (COX). COX enzymes convert arachidonic acid to substances called prostaglandins (Figure 4). These prostaglandins are one of several substances which accumulate in areas of tissue injury and make the area red, swollen, warm and painful. By blocking these enzymes, NSAIDs provide analgesia by affecting the transduction part of the pain pathway.

As well as analgesia, other beneficial actions of NSAIDs include:
- anti-inflammatory
- antipyretic (decreases body temperature)
- anti-endotoxaemic.

Non-steroidal anti-inflammatory drugs should not be used in certain clinical situations:
- when a steroid has been used
- in renal failure
- hypovolaemic patients
- hypotensive patients
- evidence of gastrointestinal ulceration, vomiting or diarrhoea
- animals with a clotting dysfunction.

The rationale behind many of these reasons is that prostaglandins, as mentioned above, not only play a role in the inflammatory soup (caused by tissue damage), but are also part of the kidney and gut's homeostatic mechanisms. In times of poor perfusion to these organs (e.g. if animals are hypotensive or hypovolaemic) these prostaglandins help maintain function, and blocking them leads to serious consequences including intestinal ulceration and kidney dysfunction. Nonsteroidal anti-inflammatory drugs can also have an effect on clotting, as thromboxane A2 is a factor which helps in clotting and is also blocked when NSAIDs are administered.

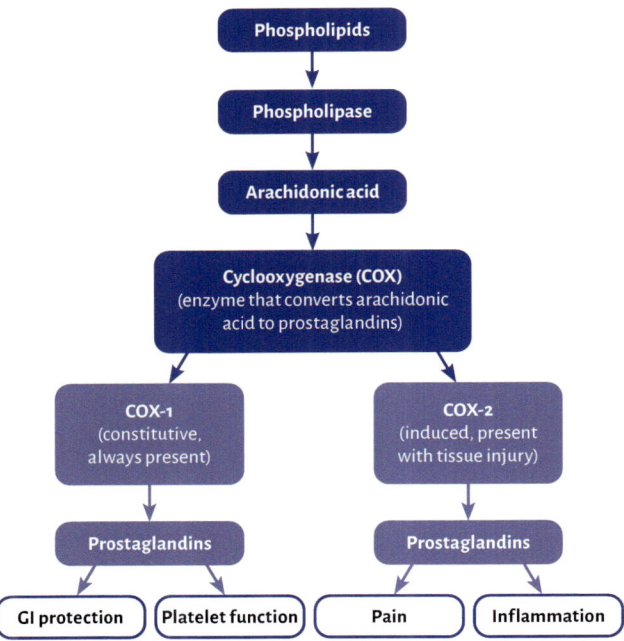

Figure 4. The COX pathway.

α-2 Adrenergic Agonists

This class of drugs provide good analgesia, mainly by affecting the modulation and perception part of the pain pathway. They can be given via the epidural route to provide analgesia, which helps alter pain transmission. Often, these drugs are given as part of the animal's preanaesthetic medication, although they are also suitable for use as CRIs either intraoperatively or whilst the animal is conscious.

Medetomidine (1 mg/ml) and dexmedetomidine (medetomidine's active isomer) (0.5 mg/ml) are α-2 adrenergic agonists used in small animal practice. These drugs are available in injectable form, and can be administered intravenously, intramuscularly, or subcutaneously. They are also readily absorbed via the mucous membranes.

These drugs bind to the α-2 adrenoceptors in an animal's central nervous system, to produce anxiolysis, deep sedation, and analgesia, along with some profound physiological effects. The drugs are metabolised in the liver and excreted in the urine. Atipamezole is an antagonist specifically for the antagonism of medetomidine and dexmedetomidine. However, when the sedative action of α-2 agonists is antagonized, this also stops any analgesia they provide. Also, the sedation α-2 agonists provide outlasts the analgesic effect, so just because an animal appears sedated does not mean they are pain free.

Ketamine

Although ketamine is a widely used induction agent, at sub-anaesthetic doses, it is a very effective analgesic. Because these doses are much smaller than those required to induce anaesthesia, the side effects of this drug are also limited. Ketamine works well in animals which have chronic pain (i.e. a painful condition which has lasted a long time), and may not be alleviated by normal doses of analgesic drugs. Its effectiveness against chronic pain is based on its action as an antagonist at NMDA (N-methyl-D-aspartate) receptors which are involved in the development of central sensitisation. Ketamine is also a useful analgesic for somatic pain (i.e. that associated with superficial tissues, skin etc.).

For analgesia ketamine can be given intramuscularly, subcutaneously, or intravenously. It is suitable for CRIs and can also be given by epidural injection. It is not very highly protein bound (30–50%). In the dog and horse, ketamine undergoes hepatic metabolism, and renal excretion. In the cat, it is excreted unchanged in the urine.

Local Anaesthetics

These drugs are the only ones which can produce a total absence of pain, all other drugs just reduce pain to a more tolerable level. These drugs block pain because they stop the nerves conducting the pain signals and work on the transmission part of the pain pathway.

To stop the transmission of the electrical impulses along nerves, the drugs block the sodium channels in the nerve fibres. Both sensory and motor nerves can be affected, so areas of the body are desensitised, but may also experience temporary loss of function and movement of that part of the body if the motor nerves are affected.

Examples of drugs in this class include lidocaine, bupivacaine, ropivacaine, mepivacaine, and procaine. Local anaesthetics are subdivided into two groups depending on their chemical structures; lidocaine, bupivacaine, mepivacaine and ropivacaine

all belong to the amide linked group, which undergo hepatic metabolism. Procaine belongs to the ester linked group; these drugs are broken down in the blood by enzymes. Lidocaine, bupivacaine, and ropivacaine are most commonly used in small animal practice.
- Lidocaine has a short onset of action (5–10 minutes) but also lasts for a limited amount of time (up to 1 hour).
- Bupivacaine has a longer onset (30 minutes) and duration (6–8 hours).
- Ropivacaine also has a similarly long onset and duration of action as bupivacaine, but often produces less motor blockade.

Local anaesthetic can be applied topically, such as in creams to desensitise the skin or drops for eyes to prevent corneal sensation. They can be injected subcutaneously to create a wheal, through which an instrument or catheter can be placed without the animal feeling it. They can also be injected into joints (intra-articular). Infiltration of local anaesthetic around specific nerves (perineural analgesia) supplying certain areas of the body can also be performed, e.g., intercostal nerve blocks, brachial plexus blocks, nerve blocks for dental extractions. Local anaesthetics can be injected into the epidural space to desensitise hind limbs, abdomens, tails etc. They can also be injected into the pleural cavity in the chest, and are a useful adjunct to provide pain relief for indwelling chest drains. Lidocaine only can also be used to provide analgesia when given intravenously as an infusion.

> **Care must be taken not to overdose local anaesthetics, as both central nervous system and cardiac complications may ensue.**

Pre-emptive Analgesia

To produce effective analgesia, **the aim should be to use a pre-emptive approach. The concept of pre-emptive analgesia is to have the analgesic agents on board before the painful stimulus starts.** Theoretically pre-emptive analgesia blocks the afferent input to the nervous system in order to prevent peripheral and central sensitisation. This decreases the amount of analgesia required postoperatively and also prevents long term problems associated with surgery such as abnormal sensitivity of the wound (allodynia and hyperalgesia).

Peripheral sensitisation is: *"the increased responsiveness and reduced threshold of nociceptive neurones in the periphery to the stimulation of their receptive field."* This is initiated when nociceptors are exposed to a noxious stimulus, which releases an inflammatory soup in the damaged tissues. These inflammatory mediators result in a lowered activation threshold and thus an increase in responsiveness of nociceptors.

Central sensitisation is defined as: *"an increased responsiveness of nociceptors in the central nervous system to either normal or subthreshold afferent input resulting in:*
- *hypersensitivity to stimuli*
- *responsiveness to non-noxious stimuli*
- *increased pain response evoked by stimuli outside the area of injury and expanded receptive field."*

With analgesia on board before the noxious input starts, this should make the analgesia more effective and reduce the need for postoperative analgesia. Different methods of ensuring this happens are proposed:
- Pain scoring systems: observer assessed in the veterinary field, patient-reported in the human field.
- Postoperative analgesia requirements: in the veterinary field postoperative analgesia is potentially guided by pain scores. In humans, requesting of analgesics or demand of a patient-controlled analgesia device (PCA); usually a syringe driver, controlling delivery of an opioid when the patient presses a button.

Theoretically, administering analgesia before the noxious input should result in lower pain scores postoperatively and less requirement for analgesia, compared to the patient that receives analgesia after the noxious input.

Lots of studies have been done in human and veterinary fields to see whether pre-emptive analgesia is more effective. All of the studies are preincisional versus postincisional (i.e. two groups of patients having the same surgery, with one group getting an analgesic drug before surgery and one group getting the same drug after surgery). The postoperative pain scores and analgesic requirements are then compared between the groups and theoretically the preincisional groups would have lower pain scores and postoperative analgesic requirements.

The evidence in human anaesthesia literature is equivocal, i.e. some studies show the preincisional group had lower pain scores, some studies the postincisional group had lower pain scores, and in some studies there was no real difference.

What could be the explanation for these equivocal results?
- Types of surgeries and type of analgesia used in the studies, and if the degree of afferent block (analgesia) is sufficient.
- Use of analgesia control groups: in human analgesia studies control groups with no analgesia cannot be used as this is unethical. Nor can human studies include doing a thoracotomy with just a paracetamol tablet for analgesia. People undergoing thoracotomy would have opioids, local blocks, CRIs of other analgesics etc.

This will make a comparison between groups that receive either preincisional and postincisional analgesic test drug difficult.
- How is postoperative pain monitored? In human studies, levels of postoperative pain are measured by self-reported pain scales and patient demands for analgesia. However, there are groups of people that are very stoic and do not want to ask for analgesia, nor report how much pain they are in, and then on the other hand, people who have low pain thresholds and report higher pain scores and require more analgesia. This could really confound results.

There have also been discussions surrounding what is termed as pre-emptive analgesia. It is not enough just to have drug bound before the noxious stimulus starts, but it is important to continue drugs bound to receptors throughout the primary and secondary phases of tissue injury (Box 3).

> **Box 3. The Primary and Secondary Phases of Injury.**
>
> - Primary phase of injury = noxious stimulation of the incision.
> - Secondary phase of injury = release of chemicals and enzymes from damaged tissues. This secondary phase extends well into the postoperative period.

However, several veterinary studies appear to prove the effectiveness of pre-emptive analgesia in dogs, cats and rats using various drug groups including NSAIDs, ketamine, and opioids. This was a real breakthrough in the field of pain research. The differences between the veterinary studies and the human studies, which means they may be a more valid investigation of this concept are that:
- The types of surgery and the afferent nerve block (i.e. degree of analgesia) were better matched.
- In earlier studies, no analgesia control groups were allowed, although as soon as animals were seen to be in pain, intervention analgesia was given.
- In these studies, usually one analgesic drug (often just the study drug) is used, and the drugs used for the anaesthetic protocol (e.g. preanaesthetic sedation and induction drug) are not inherently analgesic. Therefore, the effects of the timing of the analgesic drugs are seen more clearly.
- Pain scoring and therefore postoperative analgesia provision is performed by one trained observer in each study, who is unaware of the treatment groups.

Other benefits of providing pre-emptive analgesia include that many analgesics are also sedative and contribute to preanaesthetic medication. This calms and sedates the animal, facilitates intravenous catheter placement, and reduces amount of induction drug needed. Having centrally active analgesics on board during surgery smooths the anaesthetic and reduces the amount of volatile agent required.

There are occasional situations where it is more appropriate to give a specific analgesic drug after anaesthesia and surgery. Examples include:
- Emetic drugs in the preanaesthetic medication if vomiting is contraindicated for the patient's clinical situation, e.g. fragile eye, pharyngeal stick injury, gastric dilatation-volvulus. The drugs could be given intraoperatively as once the patient in unconscious they are not able to vomit.
- Non-steroidal anti-inflammatory drugs. These should be left until the patient has recovered from anaesthesia if hypotension or hypovolaemia through blood loss is a possibility during the anaesthetic.

However, it is important to remember, that even if one of these drugs was omitted from the pre-emptive analgesia plan, there should be other analgesic drugs in the multimodal approach to provide sufficient pre-emptive analgesia.

Multimodal Analgesia

The pain pathway is complex, involving multiple neurotransmitters and receptors. It is therefore extremely difficult to achieve effective analgesia by using a single class of analgesic drug alone. There are several drug groups that have analgesic properties, and it is good practice to try and include a drug from several different groups to optimise analgesia when anaesthetising a patient who is in pain or who is undergoing a painful surgery (Figure 5).

Using several drugs that target the pain pathway at several points mean it is possible to use lower doses of drugs to achieve the same or better effect than one very large dose of a drug such as an opioid. The benefit of using lower doses of drugs means a reduced risk of inducing the side effects of those drugs.

There may be a little overlap between parts of the pain pathway (e.g. α-2 adrenergic agonists when administered via an epidural have a local anaesthetic type effect) but in general, different analgesic drug groups act on the following parts of the pain pathway.

Transduction

Non-steroidal anti-inflammatory drugs (NSAIDs) reduce the formation of prostaglandins, part of the inflammatory

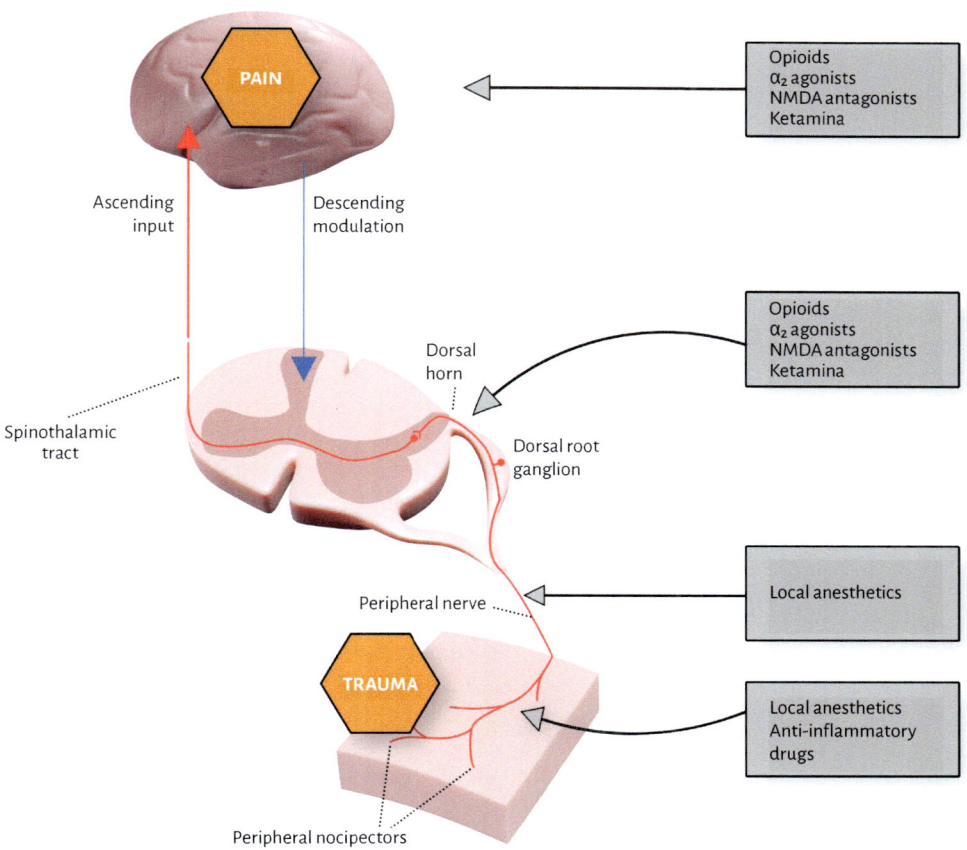

Figure 5. Where drugs work on the pain pathway.

soup which sensitizes nociceptors and lowers their firing thresholds.

Transmission

Local anaesthetics when injected perineurally. A local anaesthetic binds to the sodium channel and blocks the influx of sodium ions. This block stops nerve conductance and prevents further signals reaching the dorsal horn of the spinal cord.

Modulation

Modulation is a decision-making process in the dorsal horn of the spinal cord (and also in the brain stem) which decides the output from the dorsal horn. This output is dependent on various spinal mechanisms which either increase or decrease the activity of dorsal horn neurons. Such mechanisms include local excitatory and inhibitory inter-neurones, N-methyl-D-aspartate receptor activation (remember ketamine is an antagonist here), and descending influences from the brainstem, which can be both inhibitory and excitatory in nature and involve both opioid receptors and α-2 adrenergic receptors.

Perception

There are opioid, α-2 adrenergic agonists and NMDA receptors in the cerebral cortex of the brain so when drugs bind to these receptors, they produce analgesia (and often sedation).

Commonly Used Chronic Pain Drugs

Non-steroidal Anti-inflammatory Drugs

Non-steroidal anti-inflammatory drugs are used in cases of mild chronic pain, especially if there is an inflammatory component to the pain. Some animals need long term NSAID administration. To avoid side effects the following guidelines

should be adhered to:
- not to be used concurrently with steroids or other NSAIDs;
- to wean down to the lowest effective dose;
- to allow a sufficient wash out period before switching to another NSAID;
- to ask owners to monitor for gastrointestinal upsets and cease treatment pending veterinary advice if any seen.

In 2018, a new drug, grapiprant was released, indicated for use in osteoarthritis pain in dogs. Unlike classic NSAIDs, it works as an antagonist at the EP4 receptor for PGE2, which means it can provide analgesia for osteoarthritis without affecting the house keeping enzymes.

Paracetamol (acetaminophen)

This is a non-acidic NSAID which acts at the level of the spinal cord on COX enzymes, the opioid, serotoninergic, and cannabinoid systems. It is also antipyretic, and can be used more safely in dogs where COX inhibition is a concern (e.g. renal failure patients) than traditional NSAIDs, at a dose rate between 10 mg/kg (IV) up to 30 mg/kg (PO) BID or TID. Pardale-V™ is the licensed product in dogs, in which 400 mg paracetamol is combined with 9 mg codeine. In this formulation is it licensed for five days.

Use in the cat is contraindicated.

Pregabalin and Gabapentin

These drugs were originally produced as antiepileptics. Their mechanism of action seems to be by binding to calcium channels in the CNS, reducing the production of pro-nociceptive inputs and facilitating descending inhibitory pathways. They are useful for chronic and neuropathic pain in people. Usually, they are started in conjunction with an NSAID or opioid but are often used as a sole agent in the long term. Their major side effect is sedation. As they are metabolized in the liver and excreted by the kidneys, care should be taken in animals with dysfunction of these organs. These drugs are well tolerated long term, although in humans, a gradual tapering of dose is suggested to prevent status-epilepticus. This has not been documented in veterinary species so far.

Opioids

If NSAID type drugs are inadequate in controlling pain, opioids such as tramadol and oral transmucosal buprenorphine may be used. They work both at the μ-opioid receptors, 5HT receptors, and noradrenaline receptors. Tramadol needs to be metabolized to the active metabolite to exert analgesic effects at the μ-opioid receptor, and in acute pain models using nociceptive threshold testing, tramadol was shown to produce minimal analgesia in dogs which was likely due to the low levels of metabolite produced. The analgesic effect of tramadol in chronic pain may be through the non-opioid based mechanisms and therefore it may still be of use in these situations. Side effects include vomiting, diarrhoea, sedation, dysphoria, and lack of palatability (in cats).

Buprenorphine can be administered oral transmucosally in dogs and cats. It is particularly useful in cats, in which the bioavailability is very high. It can be used in dogs, but due to a lower bioavailability higher dose may be needed for sufficient effect. Case selection is important, both in terms of the lay people administering the drug at home, and the size of patient, as use in larger patients is expensive.

NMDA Antagonists

Amantidine is the main drug used in this group for chronic pain. It decreases central sensitization and is particularly useful in cases with neuropathic pain. It is not licensed in dogs or cats but has been used successfully in combination with NSAIDs for osteoarthritis pain.

Tricyclic Antidepressants

The supposed analgesic mechanisms for these drugs include blocking serotonin and noradrenaline reuptake in the CNS, increasing endogenous opioids, and altering the binding of substances at NMDA receptors. These drugs are particularly good at treating neuropathic pain. The drugs require hepatic and renal function to metabolise and eliminate them, and therefore care must be taken in patients with reduced function of these organ systems. Side effects include sedation, excitability, vomiting, weight gain, and arrythmias.

Monoclonal Antibodies

More recently, bedinvetmab (Librela®) was released for the alleviation of pain associated with osteoarthritis in dogs. It contains the active substance bedinvetmab. It is a solution for injection to be given subcutaneously once a month. Bedinvetmab is a monoclonal antibody designed to recognise and attach to a protein called nerve growth factor (NGF).

Once attached, it prevents NGF from attaching to its receptors on nerve cells and interrupts the transmission of pain signals. A drug with a similar mechanism of action (frunevetmab) is available for use in cats.

Constant Rate Infusions (CRIs) for Analgesia

Continuous or constant rate infusions (CRIs) are used to provide analgesia both intraoperatively and perioperatively for small animal patients. **The reason that some drugs are given continuously is to avoid the peaks and troughs in plasma levels which occur with repeat bolus injections.** This is especially important if the drug has a narrow therapeutic window, as the up-swings and down-swings associated with bolus dosing may produce toxic levels (at the peak of the upswings) or non-therapeutic levels (at the trough of the down swing). (Figure 6).

CRIs for analgesia are useful because the nurse does not have to wait to see signs of pain (as the previous dose wears off) before administering the next dose. Also, the patient's wellbeing is improved because the drugs are administered through an indwelling intravenous catheter, instead of disturbing the patient every four hours to repeat an intravenous injection, or even worse to repeatedly inject drugs into the muscle.

Often, before starting a constant rate infusion a loading dose of the particular drug is given. This is to quickly get plasma levels of the drug close to therapeutic levels (Figure 7). If the infusion is relied on solely, it takes approximately five half-lives of the drug before therapeutic levels are reached. (Half-life = Time taken for the plasma concentration to fall to 50% of its initial value) (See black line on Figure 8).

To maintain a therapeutic plasma level, infusion of the drug should be started to establish a steady state (Figure 9).

A steady state is where the rate of the drug administration is equal to the rate of drug elimination, so the levels in the blood do not accumulate or drop out of the therapeutic range.

Intravenous infusions require a well-secured intravenous catheter placed after aseptic preparation. A peripheral vein is usually appropriate for an analgesic CRI, although some CRIs of other drugs, e.g. high glucose content or total parenteral nutrition, require a larger bore central venous catheter.

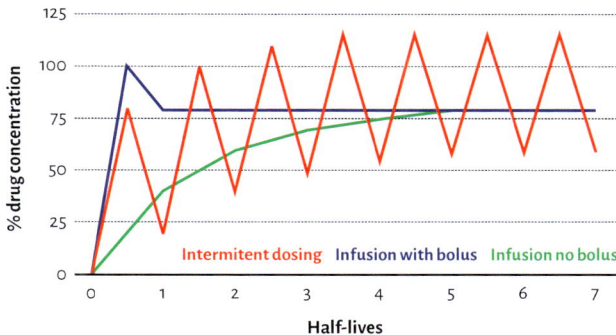

Figure 7. Giving a loading dose means that therapeutic concentrations are reached more quickly.

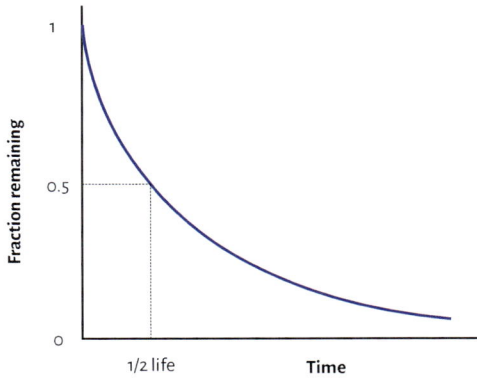

Figure 8. The half-life is the time taken for the plasma concentration to fall to 50% of its initial value.

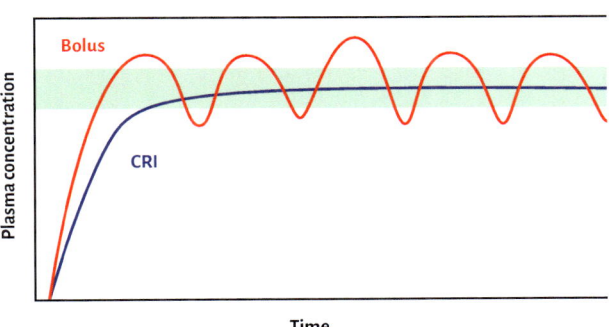

Figure 6. CRI versus bolus dose.

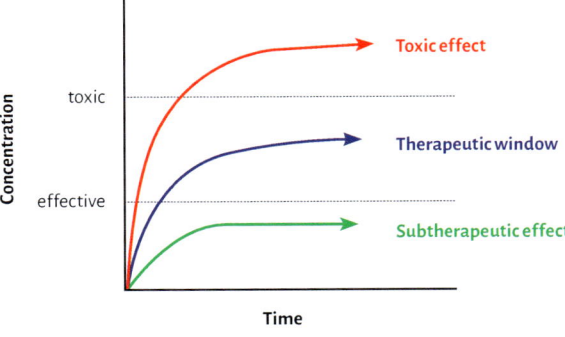

Figure 9. Administering an infusion at a steady state avoids toxic side effects or subtherapeutic levels.

The drug to be administered is usually dissolved in a crystalloid solution, either 0.9% sodium chloride or Hartmann's solution. The dose rate must be carefully controlled and therefore an infusion pump or a syringe driver is needed to ensure accurate administration. Finally, the drug in question needs to be drawn up after first checking the concentration of the solution and ensuring the solution's sterility.

Most importantly, a suitably qualified member of staff should monitor the patient, either under anaesthesia or in a ward situation. Infusions of these drugs alter how the animal responds to anaesthesia; and may alter their heart rate or their ability to ventilate. When the animal is conscious, attention needs to be paid to the catheter, to make sure that the animal is receiving the analgesics, and that rate is not too low (and the animal is still painful) or too high (and the animal is experiencing side effects).

Table 4 details some commonly used analgesic CRIs in small animal patients.

Table 4. Commonly used CRI rates for small animal analgesia.

Drug	Loading dose (slowly over 2–3 minutes IV)	Infusion rate (check whether per hr or per min)
Ketamine	0.5 mg kg^{-1}	10–20 µg kg^{-1} min^{-1}
Morphine	0.3 mg kg^{-1}	0.1–0.2 mg kg^{-1} hr^{-1}
Lidocaine	2 mg kg^{-1}	50–100 µg kg^{-1} min^{-1}
Fentanyl	1–5 µg kg^{-1}	2–5 µg kg^{-1} hr^{-1}
Alfentanil	0.5–1 µg kg^{-1}	0.5–1 µg kg^{-1} min^{-1}
Remifentanil	1 µg kg^{-1}	0.1–0.2 µg kg^{-1} min^{-1}
Medetomidine	5 µg kg^{-1}	1–2 µg kg^{-1} hr^{-1}
Dexmedetomidine	2 µg kg^{-1}	1 µg kg^{-1} hr^{-1}

NB: There are 1000 µg (micrograms) in a mg (milligram).

It is common to see combinations of some of the different analgesic drugs, such as morphine, lidocaine, and ketamine. These combinations are profoundly MAC sparing under anaesthesia, and postoperatively cause profound sedation. The author suggests running these combinations as separate infusions, so that the veterinary surgeon can turn one up or down without necessarily altering the others.

Many rates suggested in books are on a ml per kilogram basis, with instructions provided of how to make up the bag. Sometimes this is a wasteful approach, if say for example, the infusion is only required for a couple of hours.

1. The rate for the patient's weight should be calculated:
- Weight (kg) x infusion rate (mg kg^{-1} minute^{-1}) = mg minute^{-1}

2. Then converted from milligrams per minute to milligrams per hour (as this is what most syringe drivers or infusion pumps work in):
- Dose rate (mg min^{-1}) x 60 = dose rate (mg hour^{-1})

3. It should be decided how long the infusion is to continue:
- Dose rate (mg hour^{-1}) x number of hours = dose (mg)

This is the dose required to add into the bag or syringe of fluids.

4. To calculate the volume of drug the following formula can be used:
- Dose/concentration = volume

This shows how much drug needs to be added.

If this infusion is just piggybacking the animal's fluid therapy (an adjunct), i.e. via a separate line, then the drug can be added to a known volume (e.g. 500 ml bag or a 20 ml syringe of crystalloid).

If the drug volume is large, then the equivalent volume of fluid should be withdrawn from the bag or the syringe before adding in the drug.

5. The infusion rate to dial up on the syringe driver or fluid pump should be calculated:
- Volume of bag/syringe (ml) / number of hours (hr) = infusion rate (ml hr^{-1})

6. Where the infusion is also the patient's fluid therapy, their required fluid therapy rate should be calculated:
- Fluid therapy rate (ml kg^{-1} hr^{-1}) x body weight (kg) = fluid therapy rate (ml hr^{-1})

7. How many hours' worth of infusion that a bag will supply should be calculated:
- Volume of bag (ml)/fluid rate (ml hr^{-1}) = number of hours of infusion (hr)

This number of hours should be inserted into equation 3) to calculate the total dose needed for a particular bag, and then equation 4) for the volume. This volume of drug should be injected into the bag and the fluid administered at the fluid therapy rate chosen for the animal.

To calculate a rate from scratch, the following information is required:
- animal's weight
- the infusion rate
- the drug concentration
- duration of infusion
- whether or not the fluids making up the infusion also constitute the animal's intravenous fluid therapy.

All infusions should be fully and clearly labelled once made up, including drug added, amount of drug added, infusion rate, patient's name, date drawn up, and by whom. If for any reason, the animal's fluid therapy demands change, then the infusion should be discontinued and swapped for another fresh bag of crystalloids, whilst the deficit is corrected (e.g. it may need a bolus of fluids). If the overall rate changes, then this should be recalculated, and the infusion redrawn.

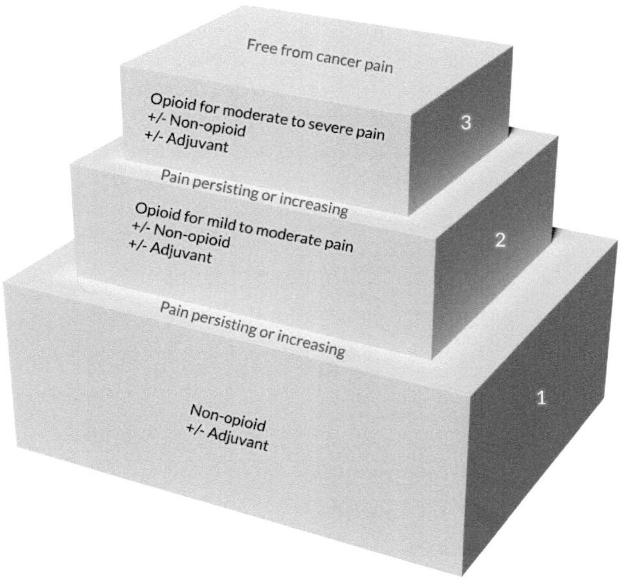

Figure 10. The World Health Organisation (WHO) pain ladder.

Chronic Pain

The Pain Ladder and Chronic Pain Drugs

Figure 10 shows the WHO (World Health Organisation) ladder for chronic pain relief in people. In dogs and cats, a similar approach is taken, **escalating the class of drugs as the severity of pain worsens.** Licensed products should always be used where possible, however, many drugs used to treat chronic pain in small animals are off-licence.
- Mild pain: non opioid (NSAIDs) +/- adjuvant.
- Mild to moderate pain: weak opioid +/-non-opioid +/-adjuvant.
- Moderate to severe pain: strong opioid +/- non-opioid +/-adjuvant.

Adjunctive Therapies

In addition to drugs, other therapies such as **acupuncture and physiotherapy** (including massage and hydrotherapy) can be incorporated into treatment plans. Acupuncture is an act of veterinary surgery in the UK. By inserting solid needles into either trigger points (painful knots in the muscle) or specific acupuncture points, pain relief is produced, mediated by endorphins and other opiates, and the suppression of transmission of signals along C-fibres. Electroacupuncture is a more intense alternative to the basic needling technique, where a low electric current is passed through paired acupuncture needles. Physiotherapy adjuncts can be added to a treatment plan under the direction of a registered physiotherapist to maintain and restore function.

Environmental modifications can be suggested to owners of patients with chronic pain, both to facilitate activities during daily living without causing discomfort and to improve the animal's affective state (mood).

Local Anaesthesia

The 2020 AAHA guidelines on dog and cat anaesthesia recommends that *"local anaesthetics should be used, insofar as possible, with every surgical procedure."* Local blocks are useful because they are the only class of analgesics which completely block pain sensation. In contrast, the drugs considered as analgesics, e.g. opioids and non-steroidal anti-inflammatory drugs are technically *hypoalgesics* in that they reduce pain sensations to a tolerable level.

For most of the blocks described below, no specialist equipment is required, other than a syringe, needle, and the local anaesthetic. For perineural injections of local anaesthetics, nerve location equipment can be used as a guide so long as a motor nerve accompanies the sensory branch.

Table 5 lists the maximum doses of local anaesthetic, however, many local nerve blocks also have a maximum volume of injectate. These are suggested volumes for large sized dolicocephalic dogs and should be reduced appropriately according to the size of the dog or cat.

When performing a block, blood drawback should always be checked for by aspirating prior to injecting, as local anaesthetics (with the exception of lidocaine in certain circumstances) should never be given intravascularly. Intravenous administration or overdose of local anaesthetics can cause cardiotoxic (peripheral vasodilation, hypotension, decreased myocardial contractility, and arrythmias) or neurotoxic (sedation, disorientation, ataxia, convulsions) side effects. **In addition, care should be taken not to insert the needle through infected tissue or into tissues containing tumour cells.**

Table 5. Dose ranges of commonly used local anaesthetic drugs.

Drug	Dose range	Onset of action	Duration of action
Lidocaine	2–4 mg/kg	10 min	1–2 hours
Bupivacaine	1–2 mg/kg	20–30 min	2–6 hours
Ropivacaine	0.1–2 mg/kg	2–20 min	2–6 hours

HEAD BLOCKS

Many of these blocks are used for dentals, mandibular and maxillary surgery. For the surgical removal of masses from the skin on the head or gums, these blocks provide excellent analgesia. Instead of injecting a wheal around the mass, which may disseminate tumour cells, the injection site is remote from the mass. When deciding which block to perform, it is important to remember the structures rostral to the injection site will be blocked. Infraorbital and mental nerve blocks may not desensitise teeth, unless the needles are inserted into the canals, however teeth are blocked if the more caudal blocks (maxillary and mandibular) are performed.

Infraorbital Nerve Block
The infraorbital foramen is midway between the rostrodorsal border of the zygomatic arch and canine root tip. Local anaesthetic injected here blocks the upper lip and nose (nasal planum and roof of nasal cavity), and skin rostroventral to the infraorbital foramen. Running a needle or catheter further up the infraorbital canal may block deeper structures. The maximum injection volume is 3 ml. (Figures 11 and 12).

Maxillary Nerve Block
Local anaesthetic is injected into the pterygopalatine fossa, between the rostral alar foramen and the maxillary foramen (entrance to the infraorbital canal). The nerve is blocked by inserting a needle under the rostral portion of the zygomatic arch directing it towards the maxillary foramen. This block desensitises the maxilla rostral to the block on the side of the injection. The maximum injection volume is 3 ml. This block can also be performed from an intra-oral approach, by injecting caudal to the dental arcade and palate on the relevant side. (Figures 11 and 12).

Mental Nerve Block
This nerve is blocked where the middle mental nerve exits the middle mental foramen (Figures 11 and 12). The middle mental foramen is biggest in dogs and carries the largest of the mental nerves. It is usually not possible to run a needle into the mental canal therefore the local anaesthetic is infiltrated where the nerve exits the foramen. This injection blocks the lower lip/chin rostral to the site of the block but not any teeth. The maximum volume of injection is 2 ml.

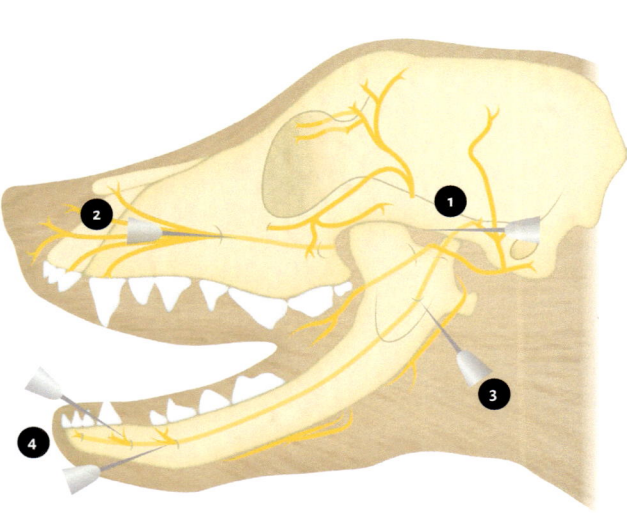

Figure 11. Maxillary (1), infraorbital (2), mandibular (3) and mental (4) nerve block in the dog.

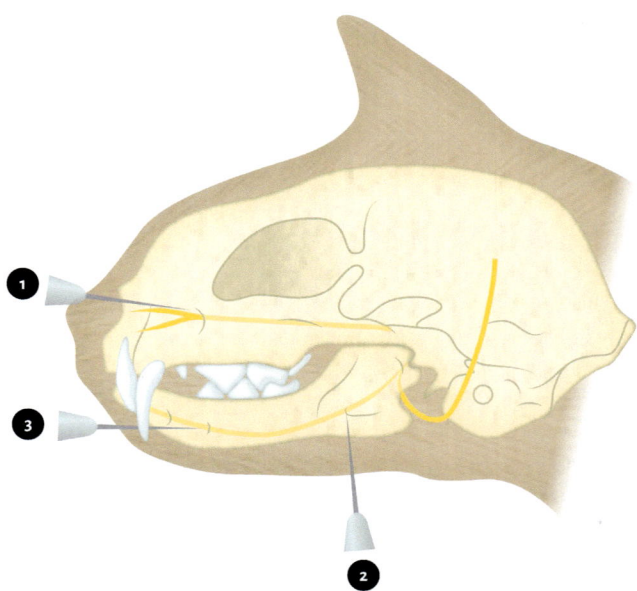

Figure 12. Infraorbital (1), mandibular (2) and mental (3) nerve block in the cat.

Mandibular Nerve Block

To block this nerve, the non-dependent hand should be placed inside the mouth to palpate the mandibular foramen (on the inside of the mandible). Then, the needle inserted percutaneously at the lower angle of the jaw, and advanced against the medial side of the mandible and directed towards the foramen. Often the needle can be guided whilst feeling the foramen and nerve from inside the mouth on the medial surface of the mandible. Local anaesthetic deposited here blocks the lower teeth, mandible, skin and mucosa of the lower lip. The maximum volume for injection is 2 ml. (Figures 11 and 12).

Retrobulbar Block

The retrobulbar block is another head block which is useful for ocular surgery. The retrobulbar block involves injecting local anaesthetic behind the globe. The injection blocks cranial nerves II, III, IV, V (ophthalmic and maxillary branches), and VI, which desensitises the globe, lids, conjunctiva, and much of the upper face, and also blocks the extra-ocular muscles and therefore produces a central eye. Some eyelid tone may remain from palpebral (cranial nerve VII) innervation.

There is a chance the globe can be punctured and so the author tends to reserve this block for enucleation surgeries. Even in these cases, a retrobulbar block is contraindicated if tumour and overt infection is the reason for enucleation, as the needle may disseminate tumour cells or infection to the back of the eye. Retrobulbar injections may produce traction on the optic nerve and therefore the technique is often avoided in shallow orbited cats, whose optic nerves (both in the injected eye and the contralateral one) may be affected by this tension.

A needle is inserted at 10 o'clock and 5 o'clock sites. The author uses a 21–23G needle, and slightly bends it whilst keeping it sterile before injection. The tip of the needle is bounced off the orbit until the tip sits behind the globe (Figure 13). Aspiration should be performed prior to injection, to check for blood but also for cerebrospinal fluid.

Auriculotemporal and Great Auricular Nerve Block

Blocking the auriculotemporal and great auricular nerve desensitizes the inner surface of the auricular cartilage and the external ear canal, which is ideal for ear surgeries such as total ear canal ablation. The auriculotemporal nerve is blocked by inserting a needle rostral to the vertical ear canal and directing it towards the base of the 'V' formed by the caudal aspect of the zygomatic arch and the vertical canal (Figure 14). The great auricular nerve is blocked by inserting a needle ventral to the wing of the atlas and caudal to the vertical ear canal and directing it parallel to the vertical canal (Figure 14). An alternative to this block is a splash block where local anaesthetic is squirted down the ear canal during surgery or injected around the surgical site prior to closure.

Limb Blocks

As orthopaedic surgery becomes more common place in general practice, most aspects of limbs can be desensitized with one of the following blocks.

Intra-articular Analgesia

This is a simple local anaesthetic block which can be done before or after any surgery involving a joint, including arthroscopy. As with all local anaesthetic blocks, it must be performed in a strictly aseptic manner to avoid introducing infection into the joint. Current recommendation is that this is performed as a one-off shot rather than a continuous infusion. As with all analgesia, pre-emptive administration is best, and so ideally the drug should be injected before surgery (often this can be performed once a joint tap has been performed with the same needle in place). Alternatively, it can be injected at the end of surgery just before the joint is closed, ensuring that saline flush is not performed immediately afterwards, otherwise the local analgesia is washed out of the joint.

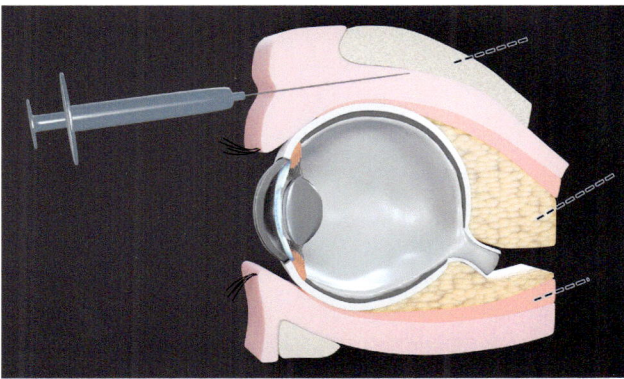

Figure 13. Retrobulbar block.

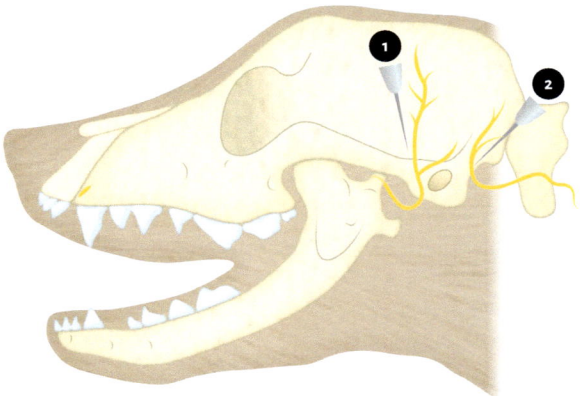

Figure 14. Greater auricular and auriculotemporal nerves can be blocked to provide analgesia for ear surgery. Auriculotemporal (1) and greater auricular (2).

Ropivacaine is the local anaesthetic of choice, but in animals with chronic joint disease, morphine can be added to the local anaesthetic. This is because with chronic joint inflammation, synovial opioid receptors are upregulated, and morphine should improve the quality and the duration of the analgesia.

Ring Block

Local anaesthetic agents can literally be injected to encircle the area of interest, e.g. a distal limb. **Local anaesthetics containing adrenaline should not be used,** as this may compromise the blood supply to the distal area. The local anaesthetic solution may be diluted to provide an easier volume to inject and reduce the risk of causing toxicity. It is important not to inject through inflamed or infected tissue as this may disseminate infection and is less effective due to altered pH of the tissue.

Intravenous Regional Analgesia

Intravenous regional analgesia (IVRA) is often used to desensitise distal limbs. Only lidocaine (without adrenaline) should be used with this technique, as it is the least cardiotoxic of the local anaesthetics. Local anaesthetic is injected distal to a tourniquet which is in place to keep the lidocaine in a discrete area (including the surgical site). The local block works for as long as the tourniquet is in place, as the drug does not return to the liver to be metabolised. **The tourniquet should not be left in place for more than 60–90 minutes.** An added bonus of this technique is that if the limb is exsanguinated, there is a bloodless field for surgery.

The step-by-step method for performing IVRA (using the exsanguination method) is outlined in Box 4.

> **Box 4. A Step by Step Guide to Performing IVRA (with exsanguination).**
>
> 1. The area of interest should be clipped and prepared and an IV catheter placed (facing downwards).
> 2. The limb should be exsanguinated from toe upwards by wrapping some cohesive bandage from the toe upwards, tying a tourniquet at the top, and then unwinding the bandage from the toe upwards.
> 3. Lidocaine should be injected into catheter (up to 4 mg/kg and flush), then the catheter can be removed.
> 4. Wait five minutes before starting surgery.
> 5. Do not remove the tourniquet until at least 15 minutes after the local anaesthetic is injected. If removing earlier than this, monitor the ECG should be monitored.

Digital Nerve Block

This block is useful for any pad or digital surgery, including digit amputation. The author often uses this block with sedation to suture pads, and without sedation to pull torn nails. A short needle should be inserted in the gap between the digits. This needs to be done in the inter-digital space either side of the affected digit. After aspiration to check for blood, inject a maximum volume of 0.5 ml on either side.

Epidural

Epidural (or extradural) analgesia is the administration of analgesic drug (including local anaesthetic) into the epidural space surrounding the spinal cord or cauda equina. Epidural injections are usually injected into the lumbo-sacral space (L7–S1) but the epidural space can be accessed at other points including more cranially, and between the coccygeal vertebrae. The remainder of this section pertains to lumbo-sacral epidurals.

Epidural analgesia is used to provide peri-operative analgesia for hind limb surgery, perineal, and tail surgery, as well as abdominal and thoracic surgery. Other drugs in addition to local anaesthetics which can be used include opioids (usually morphine), α-2 adrenergic agonists, and ketamine. The author uses opioid epidurals for thoracic surgeries, but often uses local anaesthetics for other surgical indications. Relative contraindications for epidurals are given in Box 5.

> **Box 5. Some Relative Contraindications to Epidural Injections.**
>
> - Obesity – difficult to find landmarks.
> - Pelvic injuries and fractures – if the anatomy is distorted and the lumbosacral space cannot be identified.
> - Coagulopathies.
> - Preexisting neuropathies.
> - Infection/dermatopathy of the skin over the injection site.

The volume of epidural injections should be reduced in the following cases:
- **obese animals:** the epidural space is only the same size as a lean dog, and therefore doses should be based on lean weight;
- **pregnant animals:** the increased intra-abdominal pressure and engorged epidural vessels promote forward flow of the injectate; and

— **elderly animals:** sclerosis of the intervertebral foramina reduces lateral flow of the injectate and therefore promotes forward flow.

For hindlimb surgery and abdominal surgery, 0.5 ml/kg volume should be used in the dog, and the author recommends a total of 0.5 ml per cat.

To locate the epidural space, first the craniodorsal iliac spines should be identified. An imaginary line can be drawn between these, which should intersect the dorsal spinous process of L7. Slightly caudal to this line is a dip between the L7 dorsal spinous process and the smaller sacral dorsal processes, i.e. the L7–S1 interspace. (Figure 15).

In most dogs the spinal cord terminates at about L6–7, whereas in cats it terminates at S1–3, and hitting CSF is more likely.

For epidurals the animal should be sedated or under anaesthesia. The animal should be placed in either sternal or lateral recumbency, but **it is important the animal is straight.** If in sternal, then the L7–S1 interspace is easiest to palpate with the legs frog-legged beneath the animal. Once the space is located, then the hind legs can be drawn forwards underneath the animal as this tenses the dorsal ligaments allowing a better popping sensation to be felt as the ligamentum flavum is penetrated. Other techniques to check for correct placement of the needle are suggested in Box 6.

Box 6. Checks Ensuring the Needle is in the Correct Space.

- A "popping" sensation is felt when advancing the needle.
- Lack of resistance to injection of a test injectate (air/saline).
- Air bubble technique (an air bubble at the top of the syringe should not compress when the drug is injected).
- Hanging drop technique (the stylet is removed from the needle after it has been passed through the skin and a drop of saline or drug is placed on top of the needle. As the needle advances into the epidural space, the negative pressure should "suck" the fluid in.

The landmarks should be located and then a scalpel blade used to make a nick in the skin. A spinal needle should be introduced through the skin nick with bevel facing forward, at 90° to skin. The needle should be advanced until a popping sensation is felt. The stylet should be withdrawn and the needle stabilised. The vet should aspirate to check for blood or cerebral spinal fluid. If aspiration is negative, then the drugs can be injected slowly.

Depending on the viscosity of the solution injected, many anaesthetists move the animal into the lateral recumbency which means the affected leg is dependent, encouraging a denser block on the affected side.

Saphenous, Common Peroneal, and Tibial Nerve Blocks

Blocking these nerves (Figure 16) provides analgesia for surgeries and injuries distal to the stifle. They are more commonly performed with a peripheral nerve stimulator.
- The saphenous nerve (branch of femoral nerve) is palpated in the femoral triangle on the medial aspect of the thigh. Pulsation of the artery helps guide needle placement, as injections should be aimed cranial to the artery.
- The common peroneal nerve (branch of the sciatic nerve) is blocked by injecting distally to the fibular head.
- The tibial nerve (branch of the sciatic nerve) is blocked by placing a needle deep to the medial and lateral heads of the gastrocnemius.

Radial, Ulnar and Median Nerve Blocks

Blocking these nerves desensitises the distal forelimb. Peripheral nerve stimulation can help identify the individual nerves.

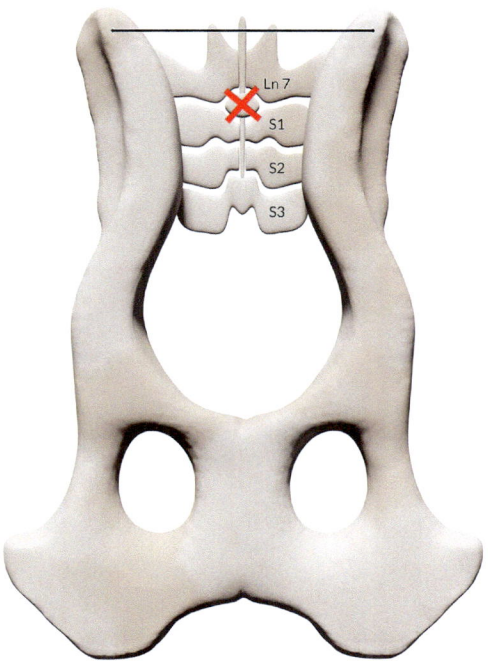

Figure 15. The cross indicates the palpable dip when locating the lumbosacral space.

In the cat, blocking the medial, ulnar and radial nerves desensitizes the fore paw (see Figure 17).

The radial nerve can be blocked by placing the needle subcutaneously dorsomedial to the carpus proximal to the joint. The medial and ulnar nerves are blocked by injecting medially and laterally to the accessory carpal pad on the palmar surface of the paw.

Blocking the radial, ulnar, median and musculotaneous nerves (Figure 18) in the dog will desensitize the forelimb distal to the elbow.

The radial nerve can be blocked by injecting proximal to the lateral epicondyle of the humerus and directing between the

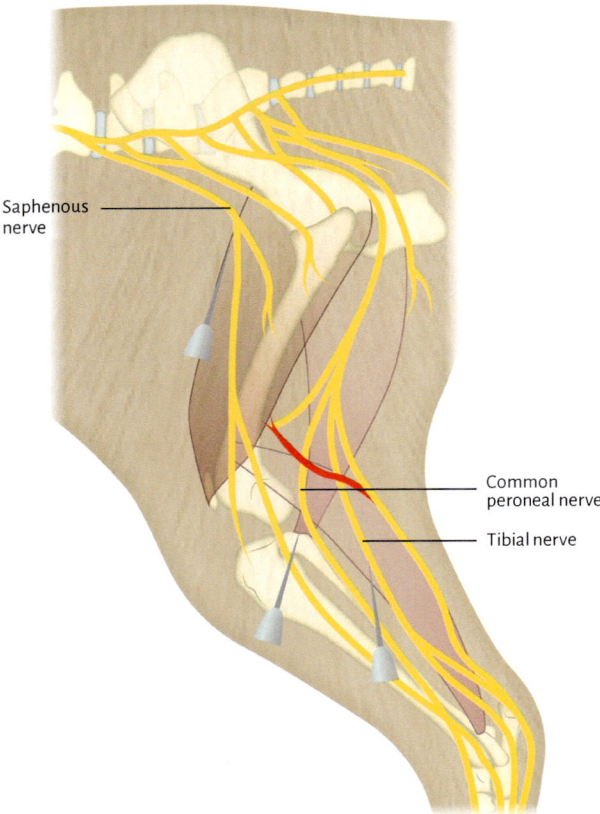

Figure 16. Saphenous, tibial, and common peroneal nerve blocks.

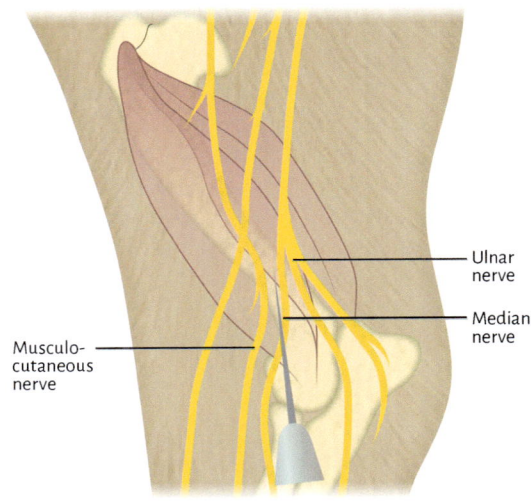

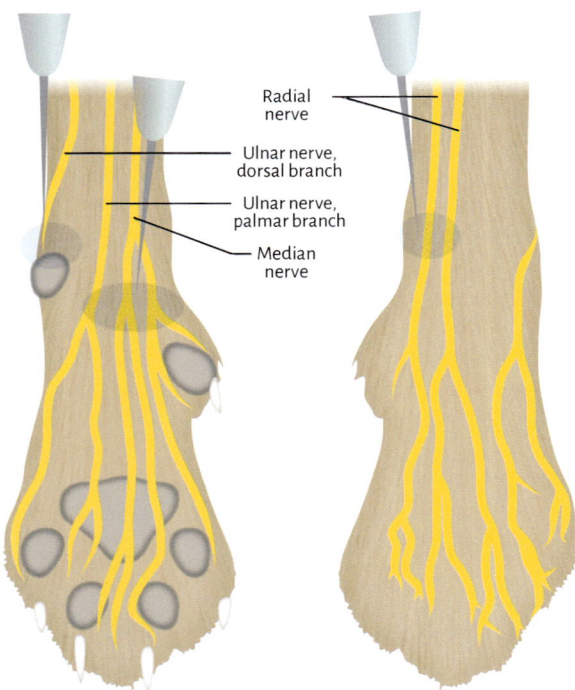

Figure 17. Radial, ulnar and median blocks in the cat.

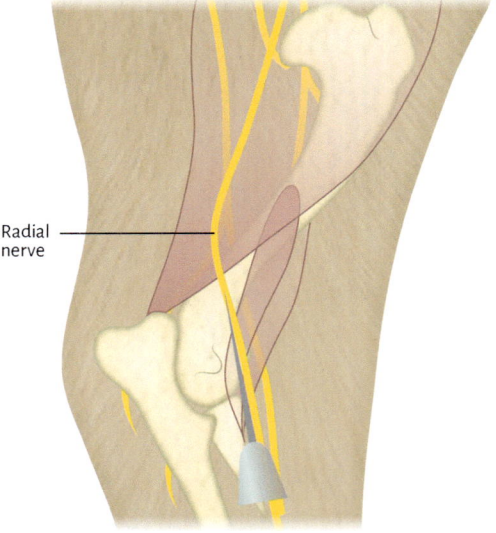

Figure 18. Blocking the radial, ulnar, median and musculocutaneous nerves in the dog will desensitize the forelimb distal to the elbow.

Nursing Anaesthesia

brachialis and lateral head of the triceps. The ulnar, median and musculocutaneous nerves are blocked by injecting proximal to the medial epicondyle of the humerus and directing between the biceps brachii and the medial head of the triceps.

Brachial Plexus Block

Blocking the nerves of the brachial plexus provides excellent analgesia for some forelimb surgeries and fracture repairs. The traditional brachial plexus block, injecting approximately 10–15 ml of local anaesthetic (for a 25 kg dog) into the axillary space at the level of the point of the shoulder blocks the lower forelimb, but not the shoulder or the proximal humerus (Figure 19).

The paravertebral brachial plexus technique produces a more complete blockade, including more proximally. Local anaesthetic is injected so the nerves of the brachial plexus are blocked as close as possible to the intervertebral foramina. The scapula should be shifted caudally to expose the large transverse process of the sixth cervical vertebrae and the first rib.

The ventral branches of C6 and C7 should be blocked as they cross the dorsal surface of the transverse process of the sixth cervical vertebrae. This is done by inserting a needle dorsal to the process and directing it towards the caudal and cranial margins. The ventral branches of C8 and T1 can be blocked on the lateral surface of the first rib by directing the needle to the cranial and ventral border of the dorsal part of the first rib.

Pneumothorax is a potential complication of both of these blocks and aspiration to check for air should be performed before each injection. Bilateral blocks should be avoided due to potential blockade of the phrenic nerve.

Thoracic Blocks

Intercostal Nerve Block

Intercostal nerve blocks are a useful analgesic adjunct for lateral thoracotomy surgeries but are also used to good effect to provide pain relief for rib fractures and chest tube placements.

The intercostal nerves are closely associated with the caudal borders of the ribs. For the chest wall there is much overlap of innervation, which means at least two blocks (cranial and caudal to the intercostal site that requires analgesia) (Figure 20).

To do this the needle should be aimed perpendicular to the body wall, sliding the needle through the skin and then off

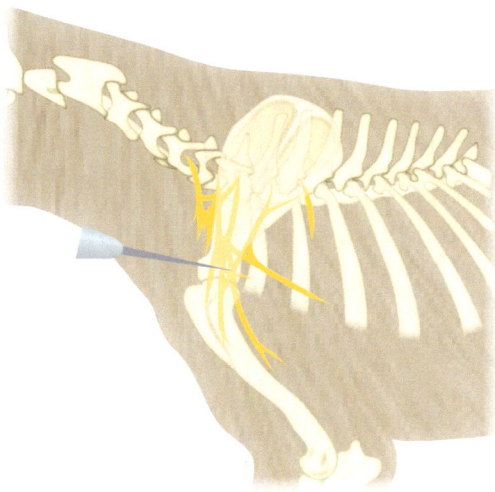

Figure 19. Brachial plexus block in the dog.

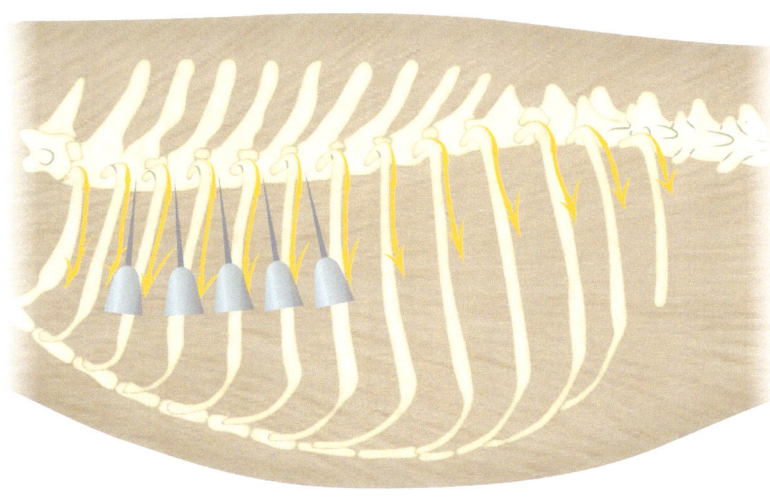

Figure 20. Intercostal nerve blocks are sited on the caudal edge of the ribs.

the caudal border of the rib and proximal to the incisional site. Injection should be as close to the intervertebral foramen as possible, as high up the intercostal nerve as possible so as to block the maximum number of branches. Aspiration should then be used to check the needle tip is not in the vascular component of the neurovascular bundle. ¼–1 ml should be injected per site, depending upon the animal's size.

INTERPLEURAL ANALGESIA

Interpleural analgesia is also useful post thoracotomy (lateral thoracotomy or sternotomy). This can be achieved by instilling local anaesthetic down an in-dwelling chest drain. Otherwise, a catheter can be placed into the pleural space percutaneously or under direct view before closure of a thoracotomy incision.

The author tends to instil the local anaesthetic down the chest drain whilst the animal is still under anaesthesia, and then rolls the animal so that the drug bathes the affected area (as long as this does not compromise the animal's ventilation). Interpleural anaesthesia can also provide pain relief for animals with indwelling chest drains. Analgesia of cranial abdominal organs and cranial mammary glands is also produced with local anaesthetics injected inter-pleurally, due to the stellate ganglion in the thorax which provides innervation to these organs.

Local Anaesthetic Techniques for Neutering

For ovariohysterectomy, local analgesia can be a line block (either before first incision or during abdominal wall closure) and intraperitoneal administration of a local anaesthetic in an aseptic manner just before abdominal closure. Local anaesthetics can also be applied to the ovarian ligaments and cervix before ligation.

Intratesticular injections of local anaesthetic may be of use if administered early enough in the surgical preparation to allow for diffusion into the spermatic cord. Additional sites for local anaesthetic injection include the prescrotal site for the skin incision and the spermatic cord just before clamp application.

Wound Soaker Catheters

These catheters can be implanted in any closed incision to provide excellent postoperative local analgesia. They are loosely tacked into place in the subcutis before skin closure and secured to the skin using a roman sandal suture. They are easily removed by pulling once the roman sandal suture is cut. Local anaesthetic is injected into the catheter and diffuses through a bacterial filter system (included in the catheter set) and injected in bolus doses or as a continuous rate infusion via an extension set to a syringe driver.

Transcutaneous Electrical Nerve Stimulation (TENS)

Local anaesthetic is placed using anatomical landmarks, whereas electrical nerve locators/stimulators are used to aid placement of regional nerve blocks, where the nerves have a motor component (i.e. muscle twitches are seen in areas served by the nerve).

TENS equipment uses an insulated needle (the insulated area allows for safe handling), which is longer than conventional hypodermic needles. The stimulator is set to deliver a repeated stimulus at 1 mA current. The needle is moved towards the anatomical location of the nerve until the greatest muscle twitching is observed distally, which suggests the tip of the needle is in the proximity of the nerve bundle. At this point the current is gradually reduced to 0.4 mA, and if the needle is close enough to the nerve bundle, muscle twitches are still seen. A very low current (<0.4 mA) check ensures the tip of the needle is not inside the nerve bundle itself before injecting the local anaesthetic.

If the nerve locator needle is left in place, reduced or absent twitches are observed a few minutes after local anaesthetic deposition.

Ultrasound guidance can be used to locate nerve trunks, because they usually run alongside arteries and veins, which are easily visualised.

REFERENCES

- 2022 AAHA Pain management guidelines. *J Am Anim Hosp Assoc*, 58:55–76.

Test

Answers on page 186

1. Which of the validated feline pain scales includes a physiological category?
    a. Glasgow Feline Composite Pain Scale.
    b. Feline Grimace Scale.
    c. Botucatu Pain Scale.
    d. Melbourne Pain Scale.

2. When using a peripheral nerve locator for a local block, what is the low current limit that should be checked to ensure the tip of the needle is not inside the nerve bundle itself before injecting the local anaesthetic?
    a. <0.2 mA.
    b. <0.4 mA.
    c. <0.6 mA.
    d. <0.8 mA.

3. When performing an intercostal nerve block, where should you aim for?
    a. The cranial aspect of the rib as dorsal as possible up the rib.
    b. The caudal aspect of the rib as dorsal as possible up the rib.
    c. The cranial aspect of the rib as ventral as possible down the rib.
    d. The caudal aspect of the rib as ventral as possible down the rib.

4. The Glasgow Canine Composite Pain Scale is an example of what types of pain scale?
    a. Visual analogue scale.
    b. Numerical rating scale.
    c. Simple descriptive scale.
    d. Grimace scale.

5. What three facial action units are featured in the Feline Grimace Scale but not the Glasgow Feline Pain Scale?
    a. Ear position, orbital tightening, whisker position.
    b. Head carriage, orbital tightening, muzzle tone.
    c. Whisker position, head carriage, ear position.
    d. Head carriage, whisker position, orbital tightening.

6. Which technique used to verify correct lumbosacral epidural needle placement is dependent on negative pressure being present in the epidural space?
    a. The "popping sensation" technique.
    b. Lack of resistance technique.
    c. Air bubble technique.
    d. Hanging drop technique.

7. The standard brachial plexus block (injected into the axilla) would be an appropriate local anaesthetic technique to desensitize the limb for what type of surgery?
    a. Elbow fracture repair.
    b. Bone graft taken from the humerus.
    c. Forequarter amputation (including scapula removal).
    d. Metatarsal plating.

8. A local analgesic injected perineurally works on which part of the pain pathway?
    a. Transduction.
    b. Transmission.
    c. Modulation.
    d. Perception.

9. Ketamine works as an antagonist against which receptor?
    a. α-2 adrenergic.
    b. μ-opioid.
    c. Seratogenergic.
    d. N-methyl-D-aspartate.

10. Which opioid is classed as a partial μ-agonist?
    a. Methadone.
    b. Pethidine.
    c. Buprenorphine.
    d. Butorphanol.

Clinical Case

A cross breed dog is being anaesthetised for an exploratory laparotomy to remove an intestinal foreign body. The dog has been vomiting for the past three days and a radiopaque foreign body is identified within the small intestine on radiography.

The vet plans a preanaesthetic medication of dexmedetomidine and methadone, anaesthetic induction with alfaxalone, and maintenance with isoflurane in oxygen. They request an intramuscular injection of ketamine just before the start of surgery, a paracetamol intravenous injection and a lidocaine continuous rate infusion.

1. Out of the protocol mentioned above, identify the drugs which are considered analgesic, and specify what drug groups they belong to which receptors they work on.

Self-assessment

2. You have been asked to calculate and draw up the lidocaine CRI using the following parameters:
- Body weight = 10 kg.
- Lidocaine CRI rate = 25 µg/kg/min.
- Concentration of lidocaine = 20 mg/ml.
- Duration of CRI = 5 hours.

What volume of lidocaine is needed for this CRI?

3. What are the benefits of lidocaine as a CRI for this particular case?

4. In order to respect the suggested dose limits of local anaesthetics, how else could local analgesia be employed in this case?

5. Why do you think the vet chose paracetamol instead of a typical NSAID (e.g. meloxicam or carprofen)?

Notes

Self-assessment

Correct Answers:

Test

1. c
2. b
3. b
4. c
5. d
6. d
7. a
8. b
9. d
10. c

Clinical Case

1. **Out of the protocol mentioned above, identify the drugs which are considered analgesic, and specify what drug groups they belong to which receptors they work on.**
   - Dexmedetomidine = α-2 adrenergic agonist.
   - Methadone = pure μ-opioid agonist.
   - Ketamine = NMDA antagonist.
   - Paracetamol = atypical NSAID.
   - Lidocaine = local anaesthetic.

2. **What volume of lidocaine is needed for this CRI?**
   - Convert μg into mg.
   - 1000 μg in 1 mg therefore CRI rate is 25/1000 = 0.025 mg/kg/min.
   - 10 x 0.025 mg/kg/min = 0.25 mg/min.
   - 0.25 mg/min x 60 min = 15 mg/hr.
   - 15 x 5 hr = 75 mg over 5 hours.
   - 75 mg/20 mg/ml = 3.75 ml lidocaine required for the CRI.

3. **What are the benefits of lidocaine as a CRI for this particular case?**
   As well as providing systemic analgesia, a lidocaine CRI is also prokinetic, anti-inflammatory and anti-endotoxic which may all be useful for patients having intestinal surgery.

4. **In order to respect the suggested dose limits of local anaesthetics, how else could local analgesia be employed in this case?**
   A line block, either infiltrated preincision or as the surgeon closes the linea alba could be used. A wound diffusion catheter could be used to similar effect and maintained to continue local analgesia in recovery. Intra-peritoneal local analgesia could also be considered by instilling local anaesthetic into the abdominal cavity at the end of surgery.

5. **Why do you think the vet chose paracetamol instead of a typical NSAID (e.g. meloxicam or carprofen)?**
   The prostaglandins that typical NSAIDs block are important in maintaining gut mucosal integrity and gut healing, and therefore not indicated for use around gut surgery. Also, the patient has been vomiting for several days and may be dehydrated, another contraindication for NSAID use.

Notes

Anaesthetic Considerations for Specific Conditions I

Nicki Grint

Chapter Summary:

- Normal neuromuscular physiology and the use of neuromuscular blocking drugs.
- The principles of intermittent positive pressure ventilation (IPPV), including patient selection for IPPV and choosing the correct settings.
- Anaesthetic considerations for thoracic surgery, head and neck surgery, the cardiac patient, the neurological patient and those with raised intracranial pressure.
- The difficulties of anaesthesia of patients undergoing magnetic resonance imaging (MRI).

NEUROMUSCULAR BLOCKADE

This is a technique sometimes used in veterinary anaesthesia, **to prevent normal neuromuscular function in an anaesthetised patient.** To understand neuromuscular blockade, requires an understanding of neuromuscular function. Figure 1 outlines the neuromuscular junction, which is the communication between the motor nerves and the muscles they supply. The neurotransmitter in these neuromuscular junctions is **acetylcholine, abbreviated to ACh.**

Terminology

- **Motor nerve terminal:** large nerves from the spinal cord carry impulses to the skeletal muscle. As it approaches the muscle, the nerves branch extensively, carrying stimuli to a vast number of muscle fibres that activate simultaneously for muscle contraction.
- **Motor end plate:** the neuromuscular junction, the postsynaptic muscle membrane is highly folded.
- **NAChR:** the folded postjunctional membrane has most nicotinic ACh receptors (NAChR) concentrated on the shoulders of its folds.
- **Acetylcholinesterase:** the crypts are important, as they harbour high levels of acetylcholinesterase, which is necessary to break down the transmitter, acetylcholine, once it has done its job and is recycled to form further acetylcholine.
- **Acetylcholine (ACh) vesicles:** when triggered, ACh is released from vesicles in presynaptic ends and cross the junction to stimulate receptors on the postsynaptic membrane. ACh molecules are contained in uniformly sized vesicles. When an impulse travels down the nerve and the nerve terminal is depolarized, the vesicles are discharged into the junctional cleft. When the ACh and receptor bind, it sets off an action potential and which causes muscle fibre contraction.
- **Synaptic cleft:** the gap between the nerve terminal and the motor end plate. ACh diffuses across the cleft to bind to the receptor. After activating the receptors, ACh in the

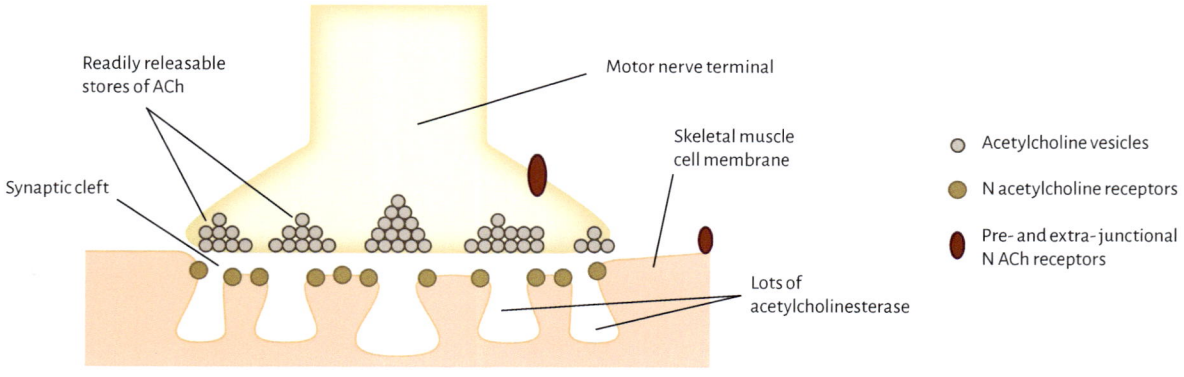

Figure 1. Neuromuscular junction structure.

junctional cleft is rapidly hydrolysed (broken down) by a cholinesterase enzyme. ACh's constituent parts (acetyl and choline) are recycled and taken back up into the presynaptic area to form more ACh.

The term NAChR (Figure 2) is used to differentiate these receptors from others (e.g. muscarinic) on which acetylcholine works.

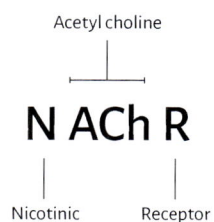

Figure 2. What does NAChR mean?

Muscarinic receptors are involved in many physiological functions including heart rate and force, contraction of smooth muscles, and the release of neurotransmitters.

Nicotinic AChRs are involved in a wide range of physiological processes and can be neuronal or muscle type. Muscle type nicotinic AChRs (those discussed here) are localised at neuromuscular junctions, where an electrical impulse from a neuron to a muscle cell signals contraction and is responsible for muscle tone and contraction. (Figure 3).

Each NAChR consists of five glycoprotein subunits which span the postsynaptic membrane. They consist of two alpha (α) subunits (identical), one beta (β) subunit, one delta (δ) subunit, and one gamma (γ) subunit. They are arranged in the form of a cylinder leaving a small pore in the centre, and the receptor spans the thickness of the cell membrane from outside to inside. Normally, one Ach molecule must bind to each of the two α subunits simultaneously, for channel activation to occur, i.e. two ACh molecules are required for one channel to open. Activation of the channel results in opening of a pore through which sodium and calcium move into the muscle cell and produce a current. When ACh detaches from the α subunits, the channel closes and current flow ceases.

Use of Neuromuscular Blocking Agents in an Anaesthetised Patient

There are several reasons for which neuromuscular blocking agents are used, these include:
- to facilitate endotracheal **intubation** (commonly used in human anaesthesia);
- to aid **muscle relaxation** for surgery;
- to facilitate **positive pressure ventilation;**
- to create a **central akinetic (non-moving) eye** for ophthalmological surgery; and
- as part of balanced anaesthesia.

Types of Neuromuscular Blocking Drugs

Neuromuscular blocking drugs are used to inhibit neuromuscular function and are divided into two broad groups:
1. **Depolarising** of which there is only one drug (suxamethonium, also called succinylcholine).
2. **Non-depolarising** of which there are two groups: aminosteroids and benzylisoquiniliniums.

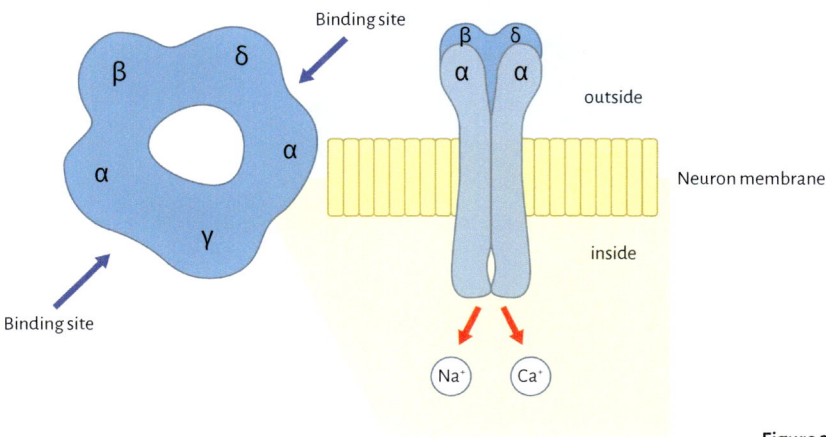

Figure 3. The structure of the NAChR.

Depolarising Neuromuscular Blocking Agents

Suxamethonium
Suxamethonium is simply two ACh molecules back to back. As suxamethonium molecules bind to masses of ACh receptors throughout the body, an initial depolarisation of all these receptors cause widespread muscle fasciculations (flickering contractions of the muscle bellies). This widespread muscle contraction is the main reason this drug has become less popular.

Non-depolarising Neuromuscular Blocking Agents

These are large polar molecules (i.e. they have a positive end (with N⁺ atom) and a negative end). It is the N⁺ atom that binds to the α subunit and does not allow acetylcholine molecules to bind to the receptors.

Only 75% of receptors need to be blocked to create an appropriate level of muscle relaxation for surgery.

There are two classes of this type of drug: aminosteroids and benzylisoquiniliniums.

Amino Steroids
These are pachycurare molecules, which are short and stocky. They are metabolised in the liver and produce active metabolites. They **do not cause histamine release.** Examples of this drug group include pancuronium, vecuronium, and rocuronium.

Benzylisoquiniliniums
These molecules are described as leptocurare molecules, which are long, and spindly. They are prone to degradation and broken down by hydrolysis and plasma esterases. When injected intravenously they can **cause histamine release.** Examples of these include atracurium, cisatracurium and mivacurium.

Effects of Neuromuscular Blockade on Muscles

After intravenous administration of a neuromuscular blocking drug, the body's skeletal muscles become paralysed (Figure 4).

Last to be blocked and first to return are the muscles associated with breathing. Nevertheless, the animal is not able to breath spontaneously and provision of **positive pressure ventilation is mandatory.**

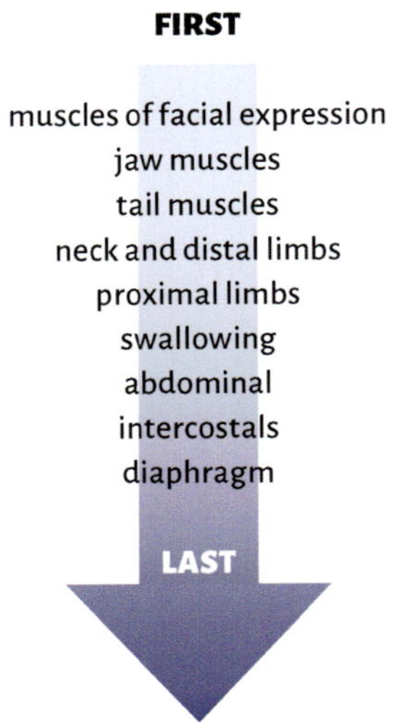

FIRST
muscles of facial expression
jaw muscles
tail muscles
neck and distal limbs
proximal limbs
swallowing
abdominal
intercostals
diaphragm
LAST

Figure 4. Order in which muscles are blocked in small animals.

This has a profound effect on how the patient's anaesthesia is monitored. It is difficult to monitor respiratory parameters as the animal cannot breathe spontaneously and their lungs are mechanically ventilated. Eye position or palpebral reflex are not helpful, as the eyes are central with no palpebral reflex because the extra ocular muscles are blocked. Jaw tone is relaxed, and no movement is evident, even if the patient is under really light anaesthesia.

Changes under anaesthesia that may be noted if a patient becomes too lightly anaesthetised:
- **Heart rate and blood pressure:** both increase as the patient gets lighter.
- **Lacrimation and salivation:** these are not governed by skeletal muscles, so may be observed if the patient is very light.
- **Diaphragmatic twitches:** may be observed if the patient is very light.

Monitoring the Degree of Neuromuscular Blockade

Monitoring for returning reflexes (e.g. eyes starting to rotate ventromedially again) is one option. It is preferable, however, to **use a peripheral nerve stimulator** (Figure 5). This equipment sends an electrical stimulus over a nerve which supplies a motor muscle unit. The peripheral nerve stimulator is attached once the animal is under anaesthesia but before the neuromuscular blocking drug is administered, to ensure stimulation of a peripheral nerve makes a muscle move (seen as twitches).

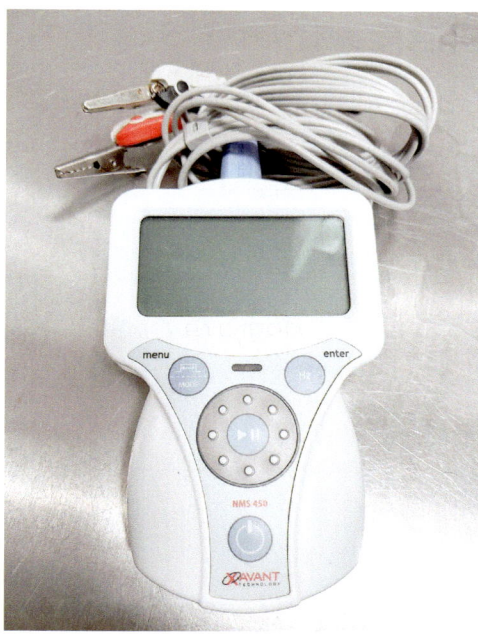

Figure 5. Peripheral nerve stimulator.

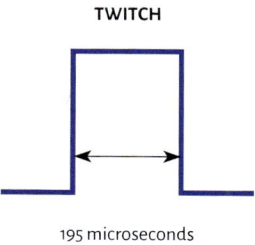

195 microseconds

Figure 6. Single twitch pattern.

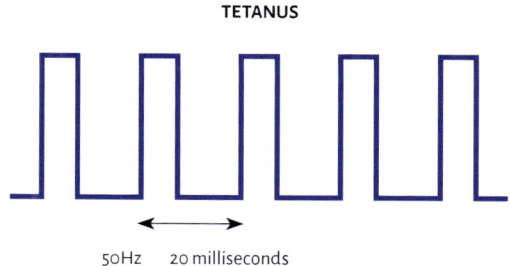

50Hz   20 milliseconds

Figure 7. Tetanic stimulus.

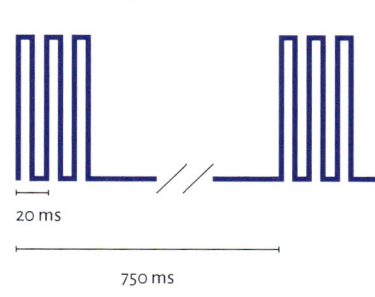

20 ms

750 ms

Figure 8. Double burst stimulus.

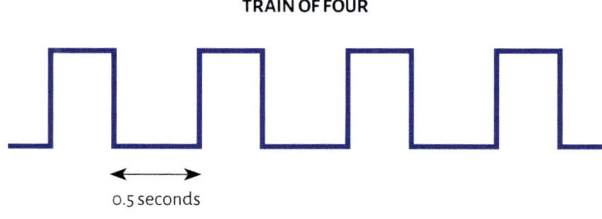

0.5 seconds

Figure 9. Train of four stimulus.

A peripheral nerve stimulator has two electrodes; one positive and one negative; and the positive electrode is always placed proximal to the nerve. There are several suitable nerves the anaesthetist can use for stimulation under anaesthesia; the choice often dictated by the surgical site (i.e. placing the monitor away from the surgical site).

Small animals:
- facial nerve
- ulnar nerve
- peroneal nerve.

Equine:
- peroneal nerve
- facial nerve.

Peripheral nerve stimulators have different types of settings which produce different twitch patterns.
- A **single twitch:** this is of limited use as fade cannot be seen. (Figure 6).
- **Tetanic stimulus** (50 Hz frequency – this means 50 twitches per second): the twitches are so fast it almost looks like one long contraction of the muscle. Fade can be seen with this twitch pattern (it looks like a gradually lessening degree of muscle contraction). (Figure 7).
- **Double burst stimulus** (two 50 Hz – i.e. 50 twitches per second – stimulations at 750 ms apart). Fade is evident with this pattern. (Figure 8).
- **Train of four** (2 Hz – i.e. two twitches per second – over two seconds). This is a commonly used pattern for monitoring neuromuscular blockade. (Figure 9).

What is Fade?

Fade is an unsustained tension in a muscle under neuromuscular blockade after a supramaximal stimulus (i.e. the electrical stimulus across the nerve supplying the muscle).

Fade is seen as decreasing twitch heights.

Fade is seen with non-depolarising neuromuscular blockade, but not usually with depolarising neuromuscular blockade. (Figure 10).

Once the patient is anaesthetised, and the peripheral nerve stimulator set up over an appropriate nerve, it should be ensured that the animal's lungs are ventilated and the neuromuscular blocking drug administered intravenously. After a couple of minutes, checking the twitches should be commenced and depending on the number of receptors blocked, fade may be observed.

Surgical relaxation requires 75% of receptors to be blocked, which correlates with the last twitch being lost (Figure 11).
- Non-depolarising neuromuscular blocking drugs cause twitch heights to decrease in a faded pattern as more receptors are bound.
- Depolarising neuromuscular blockers reduce twitch height but without fade, after the initial injection.

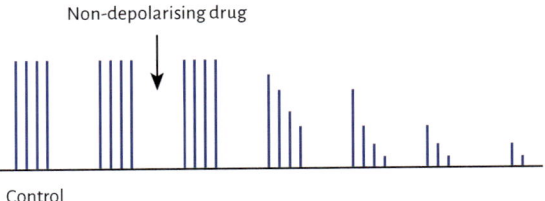

Figure 11. Illustration of how the train of four pattern changes after administration of a non-depolarising neuromuscular blocker.

Depending on the drug and dose, after a certain period of time (usually 30 minutes if the vet does not give a specific time) peripheral nerve stimulation should be checked every few minutes. If the twitches start to come back and increase in height, **administering half the original dose prolongs the duration of neuromuscular blockade by the same duration again.**

Measuring the Twitches

Clinically, the twitch response is seen or palpated. Certain peripheral nerve stimulators (often known as TOF watches) use acceleromyography to quantify the twitch heights and calculate a train of four ratio (a comparison of the height of the fourth twitch to the first twitch).

Once neuromuscular blockade is no longer required, the drugs can be left to wear off naturally (ensuring the train of four ratio is >0.9) or alternatively drugs can be administered to stop the action of the neuromuscular blocking drugs.

Depolarising drugs are antagonised with exogenous plasma cholinesterases (i.e. an injection of the enzymes responsible for breaking down these drugs). Non-depolarising drugs are antagonised by anticholinesterases. These drugs stop the acetylcholinesterase enzymes working (i.e. an anticholinesterase) to increase the amount of acetylcholine in the synaptic cleft.

The two commonly used anticholinesterases are **neostigmine and edrophonium.** Increasing acetylcholine concentrations at the muscarinic receptors causes physiological effects such as **bradycardia and bronchoconstriction.** To prevent this,

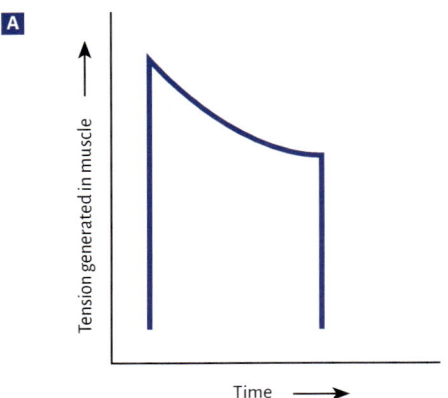

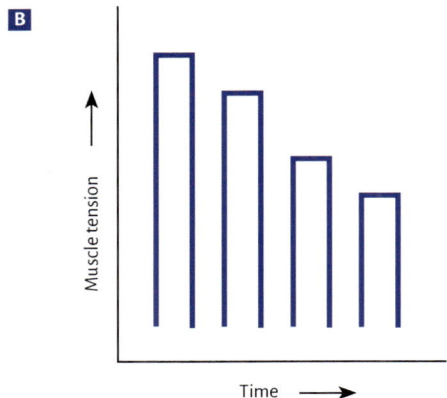

Figure 10. Fade is seen as decreasing twitch heights after administration of a non-depolarising neuromuscular blockade. **A.** Fade of muscle tension with tetanic stimulation e.g. at 50 Hz. **B.** Fade with train-of-four stimulation e.g. four successive stimuli at 2 Hz.

an anticholinergic, such as atropine or glycopyrrolate should be coadministered.

Suggamadex (a γ-cyclodextrin or sugar ring molecule) is a different type of reversal agent for rocuronium and vecuronium. It works by encapsulating the molecule and has the advantage over anticholinesterases of having no muscarinic effects and working in deep block, therefore it is not necessary to wait for twitches to return before giving the antagonist.

Ventilation

For spontaneous ventilation, **during inhalation the rib cage moves up and out, and the diaphragm flattens.** This creates a negative pressure in the interpleural space (a space between the visceral pleura lining the lungs, and the parietal pleura lining the inside of the rib cage). This negative pressure draws air from the atmosphere into the airways. **Exhalation is a passive action** due to the elastic recoil of the lung tissue.

Positive pressure ventilation is a term to describe when gas is delivered into the airways and lungs under positive pressure, producing positive airway pressure during inspiration.

In the majority of cases, animals spontaneously ventilate under anaesthesia, however there are some clinical situations (both in anaesthesia and intensive care) where positive pressure ventilation is beneficial or mandatory.
- Positive pressure ventilation must be provided when **neuromuscular blocking drugs** are used, as the drugs stop the muscles associated with ventilation from working.
- Some **potent opioids,** (such as fentanyl, alfentanil and remifentanil) produce respiratory depression and sometimes apnoea when injected, and therefore a means of ventilation must be available when these drugs are used.
- When the **thoracic cavity is open,** the interpleural negative pressure is lost and although the rib cage can still move, gases are not drawn into the airways. Positive pressure ventilation is therefore mandatory in these situations.
- Positive pressure ventilation can be used to **deepen the plane of anaesthesia** if an animal is taking very shallow breaths and not inhaling sufficient volatile agent.
- Ventilation can be useful in some body positions, such as **dorsal recovery,** and the **Trendelenburg position** (where the body is tilted so the hind limbs are higher than the head).
- **Hypercapnia** improves with appropriate lung ventilation. **Hypoxia** may be corrected by ventilation, but not in all situations.

Positive pressure ventilation is produced by **manual or mechanical ventilation.** Manual ventilation is ventilation of a patient's lungs by squeezing the reservoir bag of the breathing system to which the endotracheal tube (ETT) is connected; to do this the APL valve is closed. As a breath is delivered, the chest should be observed which should rise slightly more than a usual breath. A **slow respiratory rate of 10–20 bpm** should be aimed for. A slower respiratory rate allows the lungs to fully deflate in between breaths to avoid stacking where it is not possible to get one breath out of the lungs before the next breath is delivered. Manual ventilation can be safely performed in all breathing systems except for Mapelson A non-rebreathing systems such as the Lack.

Alternatively, a mechanical ventilator can be used to deliver tidal volumes to the patient's lungs.

The **advantages of mechanical ventilation** compared to manual ventilation include:
- **more accurate control** of variables to create stable physiological conditions;
- ventilating lungs with a constant rhythm depresses ventilation, provides narcosis and **improves operating conditions; and**
- using mechanical ventilation frees the anaesthetist for other duties.

The **disadvantages of mechanical ventilation** compared to manual ventilation include:
- disconnection or cuff deflation may go unnoticed: when manual ventilation is undertaken, it is easy to appreciate a disconnection or cuff deflation;
- mechanical failure can occur;
- over inflation of the lungs is more likely; and
- purchase and maintenance costs are high.

Mechanical ventilators are classified in terms of:
- **Method of cycling** (how the ventilator changes from inspiration to expiration): some ventilators are volume cycled, e.g. they apply a flow of gas until a specific tidal volume is delivered and then switch to expiratory phase. Others are pressure cycled; they apply a flow of gas until a certain airway pressure is reached, and then they switch to expiratory phase.
- **Expiratory cycling** (how the ventilator changes from expiration to inspiration): this is usually time cycled, i.e. the ventilator is set to wait a few seconds in the expiratory phase before applying the next breath.
- **Method of operation:** as the ventilator may generate flow by using the pressure gradient between the supply piped gas and the atmosphere or by means of a gas compressor turbine.
- **Electrical or pneumatic:** mechanical ventilators require electrical power and/or gas pressure to operate. They can be of three main types:
    1. Gas pressure to drive inspiratory flow and to supply **mechanical power** to operate valves and switches.

2. Gas pressure to drive inspiratory flow, but **electrically powered** valves and switches (this is a common set up).
3. Electrical power to drive turbines/compressors for inspiratory gas flow as well as to operate valves/switches.

The following can be used as initial settings but altered according to the end tidal carbon dioxide tension and the extent of thoracic excursions:
- breathing rate (10–20 bpm);
- tidal volume (inspiratory) (10–15 ml/kg). Remember tidal volume should be based on the lean body weight of the patient; and
- maximum peak inspiratory pressure (20 cm H_2O in dogs, 12 cm H_2O in cats). This is a safety feature to try and avoid overinflation of the patient's lungs.

An inspiratory:expiratory (I:E) ratio or an inspiratory time and expiratory time is often set. Physiologically it is more natural to have an **I:E ratio of 1:2, 1:2.5 or 1:3,** that is two, two and a half or three times more time spent in the expiratory phase compared to the inspiratory phase. Some ventilators ask for inspiratory time (in seconds) and expiratory time (in seconds) instead of a ratio. When working this out, it is important to ensure the respiratory rate is appropriate for the animal, and the I:E ratio is appropriate.

Complications

Ventilation is not without complications, not just for the respiratory system but on other body systems.

HYPOTENSION
Positive pressure applied in the thoracic cavity reduces venous return to the heart and in turn this **reduces cardiac output and thus blood pressure.** This is more likely if the patient is hypovolaemic.

VENTILATOR INDUCED LUNG INJURY
Overstretching the alveoli causes damage, producing barotrauma (too much pressure) or volutrauma (too much volume).

RENAL SIDE EFFECTS
Renal side effects can lead to a **transient reduced urine production.** This is an example of a syndrome related to inappropriate ADH release. The kidneys recognise that the cardiac output has reduced and in response to lowered renal blood flow, the kidneys release ADH (antidiuretic hormone) which causes the body to retain water, reducing the amount of urine produced.

ALTERED CARBON DIOXIDE TENSION
Overzealous ventilation reduces carbon dioxide tensions to low normocapnia or **hypocapnia.** This can cause **respiratory alkalosis and cerebral vasoconstriction.** Inefficient ventilation may result in hypercapnia, which in turn results in respiratory acidosis and cerebral vasodilation (amongst other changes).

OXYGEN TOXICITY
When high fractions of oxygen are inspired, oxygen free radicals such as superoxide and hydroxyl radicals are mopped up by free radical scavengers. If a patient is on a high fraction of inspired oxygen (>60%) for 12 hours or more, these free radical scavengers become overwhelmed, and damage is done to the alveolar basement membrane. Oxygen toxicity causes a variety of complications including **mild tracheobronchitis, absorptive atelectasis, and diffuse alveolar damage.**

Oxygen toxicity is more of an issue for ICU ventilation, where patients have their lungs ventilated for over 24 hours. To prevent oxygen toxicity, **the fraction of inspired oxygen should be reduced to under 60%** as soon as possible (or as low as possible whilst maintaining an SpO_2 over 95%).

ANAESTHESIA FOR THORACIC SURGERY

When the thoracic cavity is open, there is a loss of negative pressure in the pleural space, which means although the ribs move up and out, the lungs are unable to inflate. So, **intermittent positive pressure ventilation (IPPV) is needed to inflate the lungs** the moment chest cavity is open.

Monitoring During Thoracic Anaesthesia

Extensive monitoring is advisable because so many body systems are affected by the anaesthetic, primary disease, and surgery.
- **Capnography** indicates the efficiency of ventilation and lung excursions, disconnection from the ventilator, and obstruction of the ETT with blood, pus, etc.
- **Pulse oximetry** indicates haemoglobin saturation with oxygen and values may decrease if lung pathology is present. SpO_2 may decrease if there is obstruction of large airways with debris or the lung is being packed.
- **An electrocardiogram** is useful during thoracic anaesthesia as there are several nerves which run through the thoracic cavity and cause arrhythmias if tweaked by the surgeon. When cardiac surgery is performed, arrhythmias may occur if the surface of the heart is touched.

- **Blood pressure monitoring** is useful as some thoracic surgeries carry the potential for massive blood loss. When ventilation starts, a decrease in blood pressure may occur, and the surgeon may compress the vena cava which alters venous return to the heart. Blood pressure measurement can be direct or indirect. If available, direct pressure monitoring is preferable as it gives a beat to beat indication of blood pressure, and an arterial blood sample from the arterial catheter measures blood gases. Central venous pressure monitoring is also useful.

Pain Management for Thoracic Surgery

Pre-emptive, multimodal analgesia is ideal and used where possible.

A **base opioid is used for premedication,** with an intraoperative constant rate infusion (CRIs) of a more potent opioid (such as fentanyl or alfentanil) used to supplement opioid analgesia. The benefit of opioid CRIs is that they may cause respiratory depression/apnoea which decreases the animal's attempts to move their chest wall in between ventilated breaths.

Ketamine can be used either as a CRI or as bolus injections especially for thoracic opening and closure (as it is a good analgesic versus somatic pain, i.e. that arising from skin and thoracic wall).

Non-steroidal anti-inflammatory drugs are suitable for patients that are well hydrated, with normal renal function, no gastrointestinal disease, and no cardiovascular disease. However, if blood loss or hypotension is likely, these drugs should be avoided or administration delayed until the end of surgery. In dogs, paracetamol can be used as an alternative if typical NSAIDs are contraindicated.

α-2 adrenergic agonists, when used in preanaesthetic medication, can contribute to multimodal analgesia and be continued as a CRI. **Nitrous oxide** is relatively contraindicated in thoracic surgery. Often patients with lung pathology require higher concentrations of inspired oxygen, but also, if there is air in the pleural space then nitrous oxide rapidly expands into the pneumothorax and causes deterioration.

Any drugs administered to the patient long term for chronic pain relief, such as gabapentin, maropitant, or tramadol, will also contribute to analgesia.

There is a strong indication for local anaesthetic techniques in thoracic surgery. Techniques suitable for a lateral thoracotomy include intercostal nerve blocks, interpleural analgesia, wound diffusion catheters, and high epidurals with morphine. For sternotomy procedures, appropriate local anaesthetic techniques include interpleural blocks alongside incisional infiltration (either one off at the end of surgery or via a wound diffusion catheter), and a high epidural with morphine.

Thoracic Trauma

Trauma cases which need immediate surgical intervention include **flail chest** (multiple adjacent ribs are broken in multiple places, separating a segment, so a part of the chest wall moves independently from the rest of the chest wall), **punctured thorax,** or **uncontrolled intrathoracic bleeding.** In the emergency situation often only minimal stabilisation is possible. These patients are in pain, therefore **analgesia is essential,** usually with opioids such as methadone. In addition to welfare reasons, analgesia makes the animal easier to handle, and improves their ventilation if they have chest wall pain. Blood loss may be severe, and the volume of blood that is lost should be quantified where possible.

Control of ventilation should be gained as soon as possible, i.e. once the animal is anaesthetised. The only relative contraindication to this is a tension pneumothorax, as this is worsened by ventilation.

Chest wall trauma is often associated with concomitant injuries e.g. pulmonary contusions and cardiac contusions. **Pulmonary contusions are bruises of the lung,** caused by chest trauma, and as a result of damage to capillaries, blood and other fluids accumulate in the lung tissue. The excess fluid interferes with gas exchange, potentially leading to hypoxia. **Cardiac contusions are bruises in the heart muscle;** they represent focal damage to the heart which can cause arrhythmias.

Diaphragmatic Hernias

Diaphragmatic hernias may be **traumatic or congenital, and acute or chronic.** Some animals may be dyspnoeic, some asymptomatic. The most common abdominal organs to move through into the thorax are the **liver and the small intestine.** Where possible, the patient should be stabilised before continuing to anaesthesia, using fluids, analgesia (non-emetic opioid usually) and oxygen. If the stomach has entered the thorax, this may distend with air and require more urgent surgery.

Drug choices are affected by which organ is in the chest, as certain drugs cause some organs (e.g. spleen) to increase in size, causing further compromise of tidal volume. The patient should be monitored constantly after administration of premedication. Oxygen supplementation should be attempted so long as it can be achieved in a stress-free manner. Ventilation of the lungs should be started immediately after anaesthetic induction, rather than waiting until the abdominal cavity is open. The tidal volume is often compromised by the abdominal content in the chest, so a **smaller tidal volume with an increased respiratory rate** should be used to maintain the minute ventilation; this technique also avoids over inflating lungs that have been atelectic for a while, as this may predispose to pulmonary oedema once the ruptured diaphragm is corrected.

Once anaesthetised, the animal should be tipped so the abdominal contents fall caudally (a foam wedge is useful for this). The animal should be clipped in both lateral recumbencies if possible, as placing the patient into dorsal recumbency often leads to desaturation and should be left until as late as possible in the surgical preparation. The patient should be monitored from the time of preanaesthetic medication administration onwards into recovery.

Thymoma

Thymomas are the most common tumour in the thoracic cavity. They are a remnant of the thymus, an organ that usually disappears when an animal is young, but sometimes persists and can become neoplastic. Physical effects of the tumour, include their size which compromises tidal volume, compression of the trachea and vena cava, and wrapping around large blood vessels, which can produce major blood loss upon dissection.

Thymomas often cause myaesthenia gravis, an autoimmune reaction to acetylcholine receptors. Often myasthenia gravis patients are treated with anticholinesterases, these drugs may alter the duration of action of opioids and the response to neuromuscular blockers (so very low doses should be used to start with). Myaesthenia gravis can cause megaoesophagus through oesophageal muscular wall weakness, making **the animal prone to regurgitation** (and possibly aspiration pneumonia). Therefore, **the patient should be preoxygenated and anaesthesia induced in a head up fashion,** with suction available. (Figure 12).

Persistent Right Aortic Arch (PRAA)

This is a **restrictive lesion around the oesophagus,** and **paediatric patients** are most commonly anaesthetised to correct this condition. It is often recognised when the animal is weaned, as whilst milk fits past the restrictive lesion, solid food cannot. Therefore, paediatric considerations should be taken into account (see chapter 8), plus poor body condition. The oesophageal restriction makes the animal prone to

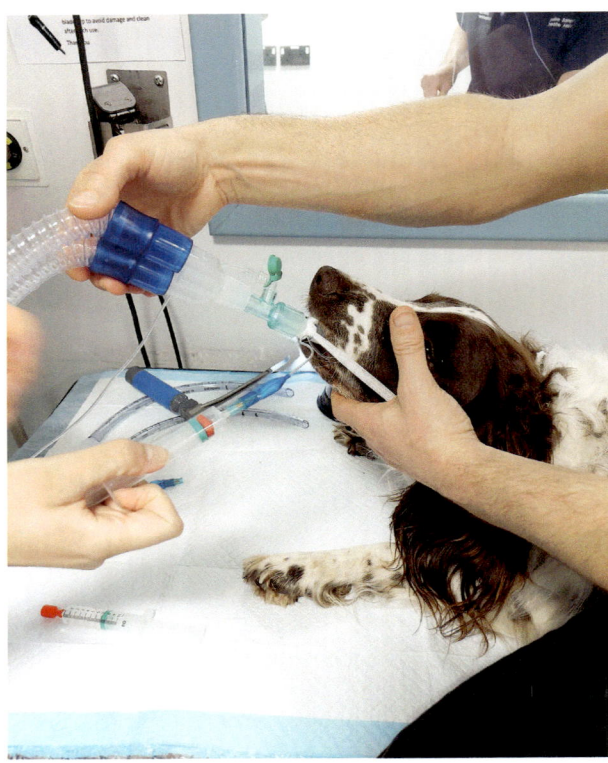

Figure 12. Head up induction. In a head up induction, the patient should be maintained in sternal recumbency with the head elevated above the chest until the ETT is placed, and cuff inflated.

regurgitation, and so **head up inductions** and suction are indicated. Patients may also have aspiration pneumonia and therefore preoxygenation, monitoring SpO$_2$ and oxygen supplementation in recovery may be warranted.

Pulmonary Lesions

Pulmonary lesions include abscesses, tumours, and foreign bodies; and the surgery involves localised resection or lung lobectomy. Oxygenation is often compromised, so preoxygenation, use of 100% oxygen during anaesthesia, and supplemental oxygen in recovery is suggested. Often the surgeon needs to pack the lung (including healthy lung) out of the way, which may alter blood pressure, carbon dioxide levels, and SpO$_2$. If the surgeon is performing a resection, the airway gases may be released into the atmosphere, and therefore total intravenous anaesthesia may be beneficial to reduce atmospheric contamination

When certain types of lesions (e.g. abscesses, tumours with necrotic centres) are disturbed, they may release pus into airways. Bronchial blocker tubes are helpful to avoid airway contamination with pus.

Pericardectomy

This surgery relieves pericardial effusion (fluid trapped between the pericardial sac and the heart muscle). If a large volume of blood is present in the pericardial sac (especially if the heart is tamponaded), this blood must be drained (usually under ultrasound guidance) before attempting anaesthesia.

The effusion may be associated with a **heart base tumour,** and therefore staging is required before anaesthesia for pericardectomy. Fluid therapy is needed to maintain venous return. Volatile agents produce a lot of myocardial depression and therefore MAC sparing drugs are warranted to reduce the percentage of volatile agent required.

Bradycardia should be avoided as this blunts the compensatory tachycardia mechanism, whereby the patient attempts to maintain cardiac output with an increased heart rate due to the reduced stroke volume of each beat. There may be major blood loss. An eye should be kept on blood soaked swabs and the suction bottle to calculate the volume lost. (Figures 13 and 14).

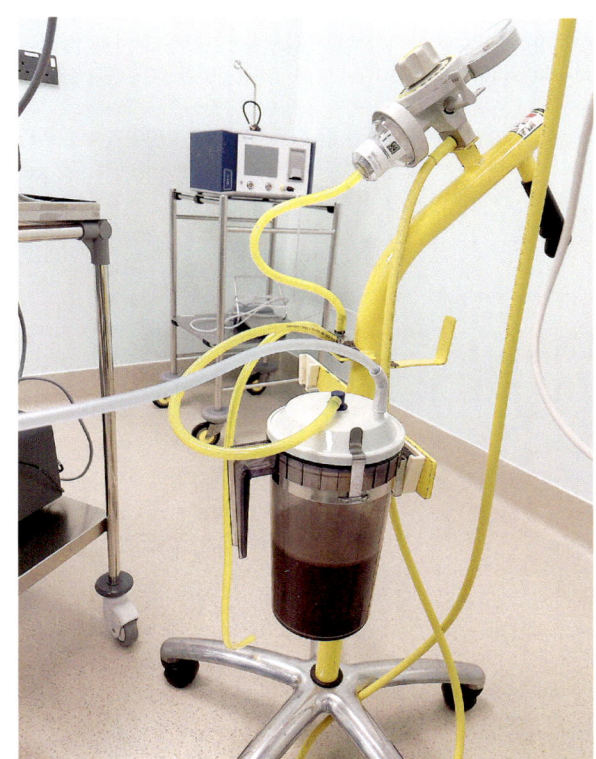

Figure 13. Blood loss.

Patent Ductus Arteriosus (PDA)

The patent ductus arteriosus (PDA) is a hole between the aorta and pulmonic artery, which represents a shunt between pulmonary and systemic circulation. It is often found and treated in young animals (requiring paediatric anaesthetic considerations) but when diagnosed later, left ventricular enlargement may be present. Diastolic pressure is often low (because of the connection of the systemic circulation with the much lower pressure respiratory circulation) and a priority is to **maintain blood pressure during anaesthesia.**

Correction techniques involve thoracotomy or interventional cardiology (implanting a metal plug into the PDA via the femoral artery). When performing a surgical ligation, a reflex bradycardia (Branham's sign) is often seen as a response to the increase in blood pressure (especially diastolic). If bradycardia persists then an anticholinergic, such as atropine should be administered. This is less likely to occur (but still possible) with the implant technique. The dissected area is often very vascular, with a small chance of sudden major blood loss.

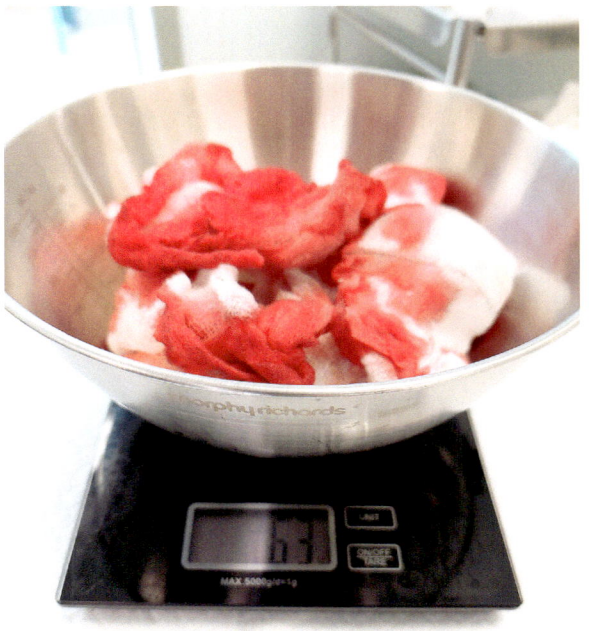

Figure 14. Blood soaked swabs.

Thoracoscopy

Thoracoscopy is a minimally invasive procedure which allows surgeons to examine the surface of the lungs and pleural lining. This usually involves placement of a thoracoscope in the thoracic cavity whilst inflating the pleural space with gas to aid visualisation. This insufflation of the pleural space can influence blood pressure, oxygenation, and tidal volume. Positive pressure ventilation is still needed. Thoracoscopy is usually less painful than thoracotomy, but if CO_2 is used as the insufflation gas, this can produce a stinging sensation. One lung ventilation is possible via a special ETT, which isolates one lung and causes the other to collapse.

Anaesthesia for Head and Neck Surgery

Head and neck surgery takes many forms from dental extractions to laryngeal tiebacks and maxillectomies. There are some general points to consider, along with additional considerations for specific cases.

The airway must be protected, but also shared with the surgeon. Often the tube cannot be secured around the back of the head as usual, but alternative methods are used. Sometimes it is necessary to direct an orotracheal ETT out of the way or gain access via an alternative route such as pharyngostomy (Figure 15).

Another consideration is the type of breathing system used. **Breathing systems with minimal drag are indicated** (in case the tube is not adequately secured), with APL valves and scavenge mounts located well away from the head.

Difficulty with Oral Access

There are a variety of clinical conditions which make endotracheal intubation difficult. The first to consider is **a patient with limited gape,** either through pain or functional difficulty opening the mouth. A thorough history and conscious examination helps to assess the presence or extent of a limited gape. If the latter is suspected, it should be ensured effective analgesia is included in the premedication +/- benzodiazepines for improved muscle relaxation. Preoxygenation is also worthwhile as well as setting up for difficult intubation.

Another example is **the presence of an oral tumour** (Figure 16) which may cause a potential obstruction. Preoxygenation prior to induction is advisable alongside preparation for a difficult intubation.

Preparation for a difficult endotracheal intubation should include (Figure 17):
- preoxygenation by mask for five minutes
- preparation of a range of ETT sizes plus stylet/urinary catheter
- laryngoscope with working light and appropriate length blade
- suction
- easy access to transtracheal oxygen
- easy access to a tracheostomy kit.

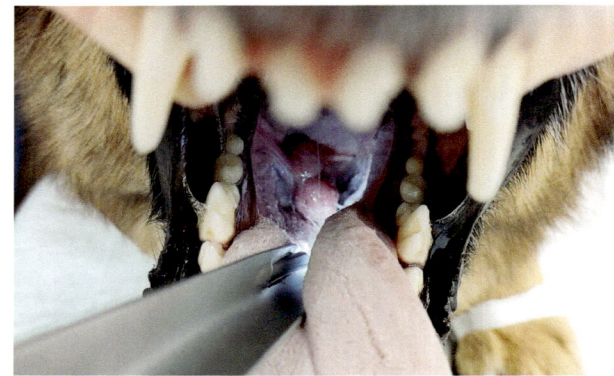

Figure 16. A tonsillar mass is lying in front of the larynx, potentially making endotracheal intubation more difficult.

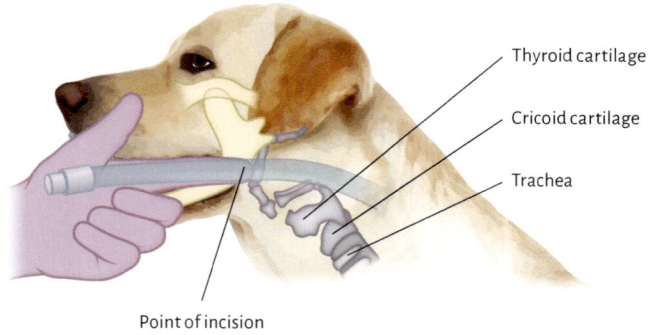
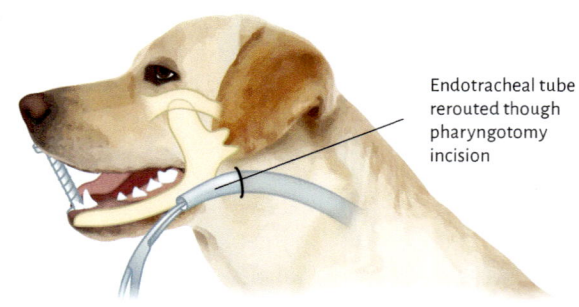

Figure 15. Pharyngostomy tube.

Nursing Anaesthesia

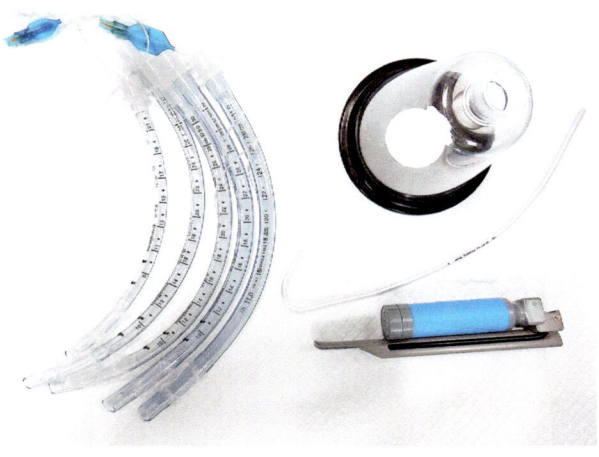

Figure 17. Difficult airway kit. Equipment should be prepared before induction to aid in a difficult intubation.

Airway Protection

During head surgery (e.g. jaw surgeries, dentals) it is important to **protect the airways** from the aspiration of water, saline, blood, tartar, pus or other cellular debris. The main way this is achieved is the use of **cuffed ETTs.**

It is important to **check cuffs before use,** by inflating them and leaving them inflated for several minutes to check for slow leaks. Also, when inflated the cuff profile should be checked to ensure it is normal and not eccentric (suggesting a weakness in one part of the cuff). ETTs are not as good at protecting the airway if the cuff is leaky.

Dental anaesthetics have been implicated in a high incidence of **tracheal rupture in cats, due to over inflation of ETT cuffs.** If cuffed tubes are used in cats, great care should be taken when inflating the cuffs and only sufficient air should be added to the pilot balloon to just stop a leak being heard when the reservoir bag of the breathing system is squeezed. In addition, **ETTs and breathing systems must be disconnected when turning the patient** during anaesthesia.

In addition to cuffed ETTs, **suction** at various points of anaesthesia aids in airway protection, i.e. at induction, during anaesthesia, and prior to endotracheal extubation.

Pharyngeal packs used during some jaw or dental procedures also aid airway protection; they soak up liquids and produce a barrier against solid debris. Options include a sponge or swab placed at the back of the throat around the ETT. The packs should be attached to the ETT to ensure removal at the end of anaesthesia. (Figure 18).

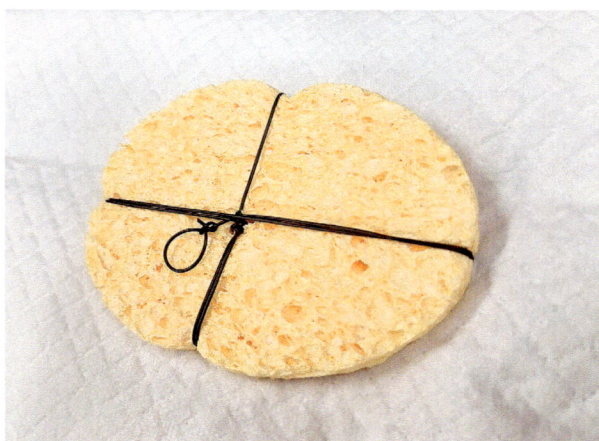

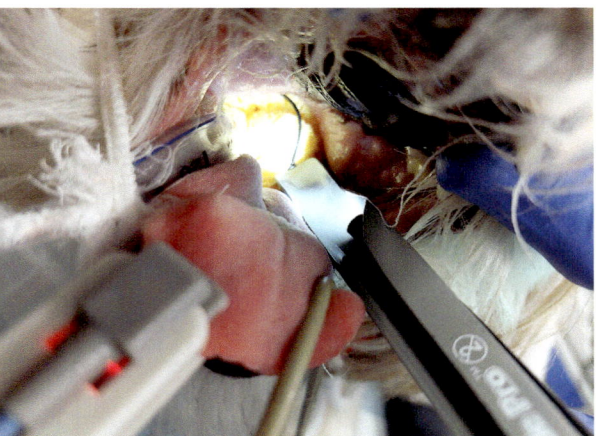

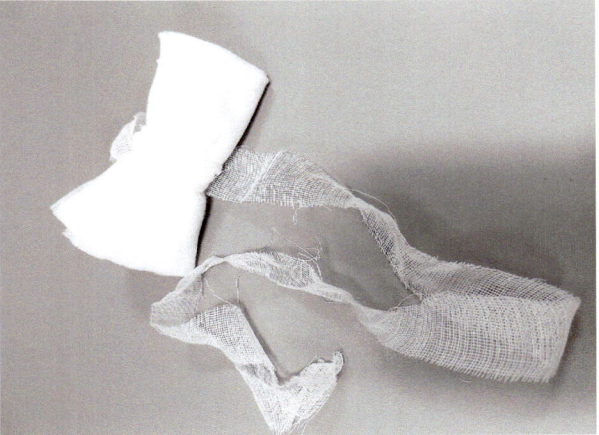

Figures 18. Different types of pharyngeal packs.

Staff involved with head and neck procedures can be at **an increased risk of exposure to volatile agents escaping from the oral cavity.** To reduce this incidence, the following approach is advised:
- use of cuffed ETTs;
- the vaporiser should not be switched on until the cuff is

inflated;
- total or partial intravenous anaesthesia (TIVA or PIVA) should be considered;
- high rates of ventilation should be ensured in the workspace;
- scavenging systems should be maintained well and regularly serviced;
- use of low flow rates; and
- keeping the patient attached to breathing system until most volatile agent has been exhaled at the end of the procedure.

Positioning for Certain Head and Neck Treatments

In certain head and neck investigations/surgeries, special positioning is required (e.g. flexed, extended, or rotated) but this can pose problems for the anaesthetist. Whenever a change of position is made, **the head and neck should be stabilised when any force is applied.** There is an increased risk of airway obstruction, breathing system disconnection, and inadvertent extubation.

When the body position is changed, the ETT and breathing system should be disconnected and then reconnected. This prevents shearing forces of the ETT cuff on tracheal mucosa. Vigilant monitoring of the rebreathing bag, and $ETCO_2$ trace quickly identify any accidental disconnection.

Good ETT security is needed to prevent endotracheal tubes coming out as a patient is moved or positioned. There is evidence that when the head and neck are flexed substantially, red rubber ETTs are more prone to kinking than silicone and plastic (Campoy et al., 2003). If kinking is likely, an armoured ETT is an option; these have a spiral of metal throughout the wall to resist kinking (Figure 19). There are some disadvantages to using these types of tubes; they are a little floppy to hold and more difficult to place, they cannot be shortened, their internal diameter is smaller than a regular ETT given the thickness of the wall, and they cause distortion to images in an MRI scan of the brain.

Mouth Gags

There are several publications that report the potential negative consequences of using mouth gags in cats for dental procedures. **This is a particular issue in the cat, whose cerebral blood supply comes solely from the maxillary artery** (whereas other species have additional routes of supply). Spring loaded gags generate a constant force which can contribute to bulging of soft tissue between the mandible and tympanic bulla decreasing maxillary blood flow. The decreased cerebral blood flow usually manifests as postprocedural blindness. Recommendations include limiting mouth opening with gags to a maximum of 30 mm, and if any wider gape is required, then periodic relaxation should be allowed for.

Dentals

These are often performed in older animals, with geriatric anaesthetic considerations to take into account. Airway protection is incredibly important for fluids and tartar, including cuffed ETTs and pharyngeal packs.

Prior to general anaesthesia the animal should be stabilised as much as possible; this includes intravenous fluid therapy for the dehydrated patient or those with concurrent chronic renal failure. Antibiosis should be considered if there is evidence of infection and patients with a decreased appetite should be fed up.

It is important to keep the patient warm, as hypothermia is a risk from the fluids associated with dental procedures. Pre-emptive, multimodal analgesia is required, and should include local nerve blocks if extractions are anticipated.

Pharyngeal Stick Injuries

Depending on the chronicity of the injury, **sequelae may be present which complicate anaesthesia.** For example, the dog may be dehydrated (from inability to eat/drink) or have debris in the pharynx making intubation difficult. Other concerns include potential pneumothorax/pneumomediastinum or subcutaneous emphysema. Once anaesthetised, removing the stick may cause additional problems (e.g. arrhythmias/blood

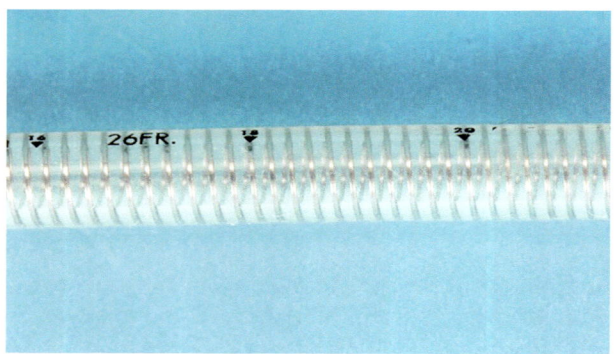

Figure 19. Armoured endotracheal tube.

loss) and if the surgeon explores the neck area, there are large blood vessels and nerves (including the vagus and sympathetic nerves) running through the neck. Postoperative swelling of pharynx is also a possibility.

Jaw Fractures

Jaw fractures are often due to trauma so the likelihood of **concomitant injuries** should be considered, e.g. head trauma and raised intracranial pressure. Depending on how chronic the injury is, whether the animal has been eating and drinking is a relevant question.

When planning the anaesthetic the requirements to **share the airway and airway protection** should be considered. Preoxygenation by mask and preparation for a difficult intubation are advisable. There may be blood loss during surgery, the blood volume lost in swabs and suction should be recorded, and the percentage of blood volume lost calculated to guide fluid therapy. Analgesia is paramount and a multimodal approach including local anaesthetic techniques should be used.

Certain jaw fractures are repaired by wiring the jaws. For these cases, **constant monitoring in recovery is essential,** in case of compromised airways (should the patient vomit without being able to open the mouth). To this end, scissors (if suture is the closure material or wire cutters (if wire is the closure material) should be kept next to the kennel.

Jaw Surgery for Neoplasia

Airway protection is required (due to blood and tumour tissue, including pus, if there is a necrotic centre). Sharing an airway with the surgeon is also a requirement. Blood loss should be anticipated especially for maxillectomies.

Patients with neoplasia may have metastasis. Therefore, the implications of the possibility of the following should be considered:
- local expansion (especially maxillary tumours)
- sites of metastasis (especially pulmonary sites)
- paraneoplastic syndromes (due to tumour cells producing hormones or cytokines which act as chemical signalling molecules or an immune response against the tumour).

Paraneoplastic syndromes include hypercalcemia of malignancy, anaemia, clotting dysfunctions, and cancer cachexia. Excellent analgesia is a must, including local anaesthetic techniques so long as this does not seed tumour cells into adjacent tissue.

Laryngeal Paralysis

This condition is often seen in older dogs and so geriatric considerations apply with regards to anaesthesia (see chapter 8). In this condition, one or both sides of the larynx are paralysed which produces an obstruction to breathing. The dog may present with stridorous sounds, with or without respiratory distress/cyanosis. Dogs are often stressed, which worsens their breathing, creating a vicious cycle.

These patients often present as hypoxic, hypercapnic, and hyperthermic; all of which make the animal prone to arrhythmias if not stabilised prior to anaesthesia.

If the patient is cyanotic, hyperthermic, and stressed, the patient needs to be cooled, calmed, and oxygenated. Ideally, an **intravenous catheter** should be placed and fluid therapy started, which also helps cool the patient and supports their renal function (as the patients are often elderly). Other **cooling therapies** include fans, cold towels, and alcohol spirit on paws. Body temperature should be monitored and cooling efforts stopped when the patient's body temperature is one degree centigrade above the target temperature, as there is always some overswing.

Preanaesthetic medication calms the patient; a non-emetic should be used as there is less laryngeal function to protect the airway from vomitus. **Acepromazine at a low dose** is often included as it is antiemetic and reduces body temperature (resetting the thermoregulatory centre of the brain as well as through vasodilation). At low doses, mild sedation is produced, which is desirable given the potential for airway obstruction.

Oxygen should be provided during stabilisation via mask, nasopharyngeal prongs, or flow by; whichever causes least stress to the patient. Sedation by itself may break the vicious cycle but progression to general anaesthetic may be required, allowing a slow recovery from anaesthesia once temperature is corrected, if corrective surgery is not to performed. Whilst under anaesthetic, diagnostic tests may be performed, e.g. examination of laryngeal function at induction and chest radiographs.

A general anaesthetic for surgical correction may be more straight forward if the dog has arrived cool and calm. If the patient appears stable, then the following should be considered when planning the anaesthetic:
- preanaesthetic medication including a non-emetic opioid +/- acepromazine
- reoxygenation by mask
- induction of anaesthesia with intravenous propofol or alfaxalone.

Once the ETT is in place, there should be few respiratory problems during anaesthesia as this is a disease of upper respiratory tract obstruction (which is bypassed once intubated). Sharing the airway with the surgeon is not an issue as the surgery is performed via the left lateral neck. However, the surgeon may request endotracheal extubation and reintubation towards the end of surgery to check laryngeal abduction.

Airway protection is of concern, especially as with limited laryngeal function there is a high risk of aspiration pneumonia. Therefore, in recovery close monitoring for postoperative swelling should be performed and administration of anti-inflammatory drugs e.g. NSAIDs (assuming adequate renal function) or steroids considered.

Brachycephalic Obstructive Airway Syndrome (BOAS)

Brachycephalic obstructive airway syndrome (BOAS) involves:
- elongated soft palate
- everted laryngeal ventricles
- stenotic nares
- hypoplastic trachea.

These dogs are prone to regurgitation and should have anaesthesia induced with their head up, until the endotracheal tube is placed, and the cuff inflated. If the dog is a known regurgitator, **intravenous omeprazole** is recommended the night before and the morning of anaesthesia. **Preoxygenation should be by mask** and preparations for a **difficult endotracheal intubation** made with a wide range of endotracheal tubes (a hypoplastic trachea is part of the syndrome, which means the tracheal lumen is narrower than expected for the size of dog). **Ocular lubrication** is important as these dogs often have eyes prone to exposure keratopathy.

During BOAS surgery, the endotracheal tube is directed out the side of the mouth, but most of the surgery is done with the endotracheal tube in place. However, endotracheal extubation may be required for laryngeal ventricle resection. Postoperatively the patient should be fully monitored until fully recovered from anaesthesia. An airway kit should be kept next to the patient's recovery kennel. (Figure 20).

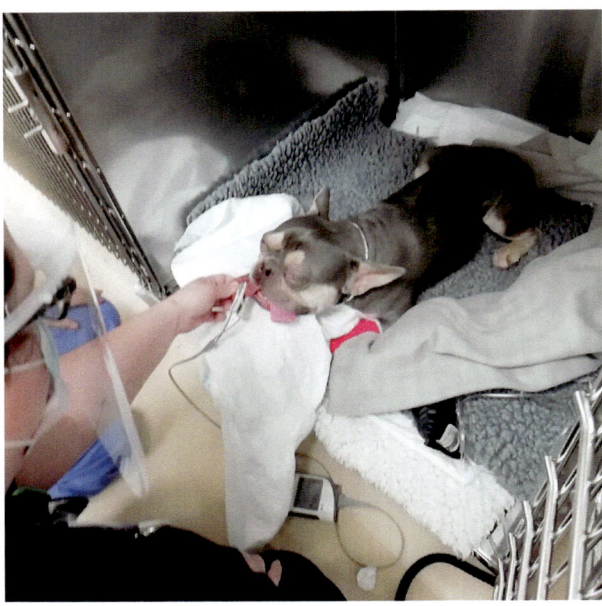

Figure 20. Patients with BOAS conformation should be monitored closely in recovery.

Anaesthesia for Cardiac Patients

One of the main aims in anaesthesia is to maintain an appropriate level of oxygen delivery to all tissues and keep the organs healthy and functioning. To ensure good oxygen delivery requires good cardiac output, good blood oxygenation, and good tissue perfusion.

Oxygen delivery = cardiac output (CO) x content of O_2 in the blood

Cardiac output is the amount of blood ejected from the heart in one minute. It is a product of heart rate and stroke volume (the volume of blood ejected from the heart with every beat).

Cardiac output = heart rate x stroke volume

Cardiac output influences blood pressure: if everything else stays the same, then a reduced cardiac output leads to reduced blood pressure, however, there are other factors in play, namely systemic vascular resistance.

Mean arterial blood pressure = cardiac output x systemic vascular resistance

Systemic vascular resistance (SVR) refers to the resistance to blood flow offered by all the systemic vasculature, excluding the pulmonary vasculature. Mechanisms that cause vasoconstriction increase SVR, and mechanisms that cause vasodilation decrease SVR. Although SVR is primarily determined by changes in blood vessel diameters, changes in blood viscosity also affect SVR.

From the formula above it is evident that if cardiac output stays the same, then an increase in SVR (vasoconstriction) leads to an increase in blood pressure. This is seen clinically after α-2 adrenergic agonist administration; blood pressure increases because of vasoconstriction.

Preload is defined as the initial stretching of the cardiac muscle cells prior to contraction. When venous return (i.e. volume of blood returning to the heart) is increased, the volume of the ventricles and the pressure in the ventricles at the end of filling are increased, which stretches the sarcomeres (unit of heart muscle), thereby increasing their preload.

Afterload is the amount of resistance the heart must overcome to open the aortic valve and push the blood volume out into the systemic circulation i.e. what the heart is beating against. Increased SVR (i.e. vasoconstriction) increases the afterload and conversely decreased SVR decreases the afterload.

Myocardial Oxygenation

Whilst oxygen delivery to vital organs such as the brain, kidneys, liver etc. is important, it is equally important the heart muscle itself is well supplied with oxygen, this is called **myocardial (heart muscle) oxygenation.**

Myocardial oxygenation is a balance between myocardial oxygen delivery and myocardial oxygen demand i.e. myocardial oxygenation decreases if delivery goes down or consumption goes up. If the myocardium becomes hypoxic, this can lead to abnormal heart rhythms as the heart muscle cannot contract efficiently.

Blood supply to the heart muscle happens during diastole (the relaxation phase of the cardiac cycle).

Heart Disease and Anaesthesia

Heart disease erodes cardiovascular functional reserve and therefore the stress of anaesthesia may mean the cardiovascular system cannot cope.

Also, cardiovascular disease may adversely affect other organ systems, which influences the anaesthetic. For example, a cat with hypertrophic cardiomyopathy (HCM) may present with pleural effusion secondary to heart failure, and thus the respiratory system is affected, causing dyspnoea which influences the anaesthetic.

Cardiovascular disease alters drug disposition and distribution, e.g. if a patient is in heart failure, often blood flow is diverted to their central compartment thus decreasing peripheral perfusion. In this situation subcutaneous or intramuscular injections are poorly absorbed.

Treatment of cardiovascular disease may include **drugs which may interact with anaesthetics,** e.g. ACE inhibitors cause vasodilation which may produce hypotension if administered in conjunction with certain anaesthetic drugs. Also, animals medicated with frusemide may have low potassium levels.

General Aims for Anaesthesia

Most cardiac drugs are administered as normal until the time of anaesthesia. In the 2020 guidelines for anaesthesia in dogs and cats, the American Animal Hospital Association suggested that cardiac medications such as frusemide and pimobendan are administered as usual (including the morning of anaesthesia) but **that antihypertensive drugs such as ACE inhibitors are not given on the morning of anaesthesia.**

Stressing the patient should be avoided, as this increases the patient's heart rate and limits the sedative effects of preanaesthetic medication (which then increases the required doses of induction agent and volatile agent).

To maximise the oxygen content of blood, oxygen should be administered before and after the anaesthetic, so long as this does not unduly stress the patient. (Figure 21).

Provision of adequate analgesia should be ensured. This prevents tachycardic responses to nociception during the

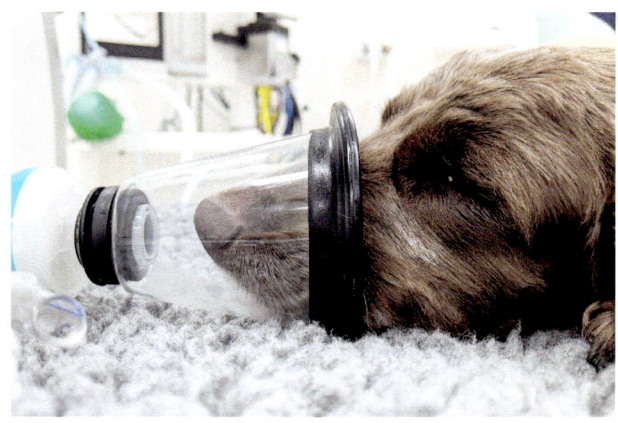

Figure 21. Preoxygenating a patient by face mask before inducting anaesthesia.

anaesthetic and lowers volatile agent requirements (and induction agent requirements if analgesics are included in the preanaesthetic medication). Both induction drugs and volatile agents can cause myocardial depression and so the lower dose used, the better. Whilst pre-emptive analgesia is always recommended, non-steroidal anti-inflammatory drugs may be held in patients with cardiac disease until the end of anaesthesia, as normotension cannot be guaranteed during the anaesthetic.

Overloading patients with fluid should be avoided and lower sodium isotonic fluids (such as Hartmann's solution) used as patients with heart disease do not cope well with a high sodium load.

Preanaesthetic Examination

To tailor an anaesthetic plan, it is important to know the specifics of cardiac disease, as the aims for anaesthesia differ depending on the cardiac disease present.

Clinical examination includes:
- mucous membrane colour, moistness, and capillary refill time
- auscultation of all four heart valves, noting grade and point of maximal intensity (PMI) of any murmurs (Figure 22)
- auscultation of lung fields
- if any irregular rhythm is auscultated, concurrent pulse palpation should be undertaken to identify any pulse deficits
- observation of respiratory rate and pattern
- assessment of peripheral pulse quality and rate.

If a murmur (often as a whooshing or swishing noise) is heard, the valve over which it is loudest (known as the point of maximal intensity (PMI)) and the grade (loudness) should be noted (see Table 1).

Table 1. Grading system for heart murmurs.

Grade	Murmur
I	Very soft murmur. Only heard in quiet surroundings after careful auscultation.
II	Soft murmur, but easily heard.
III	Moderate intensity murmur.
IV	Loud murmur, without a palpable precordial thrill.
V	Loud murmur with a palpable precordial thrill.
VI	Very loud murmur that can be heard with the stethoscope lifted away from the chest. Precordial thrill present.

The grade or loudness of the murmur does not necessarily correlate with the severity of the heart disease or risks associated with the anaesthetic. In addition to the clinical exam, a history should be taken including exercise tolerance (as this gives a good indication as to how well the animal's heart may cope with an anaesthetic) and whether the animal is coughing or has a distended belly (signs associated with congestive heart failure).

If a concern is flagged from the history or clinical exam e.g. a murmur, then further investigations are advisable, including:
- echocardiography
- thoracic radiographs to indicate heart size and state of lungs
- an electrocardiogram (ECG).

Once the type of heart disease is identified, the anaesthetic can be further tailored to meet the aims for anaesthesia.

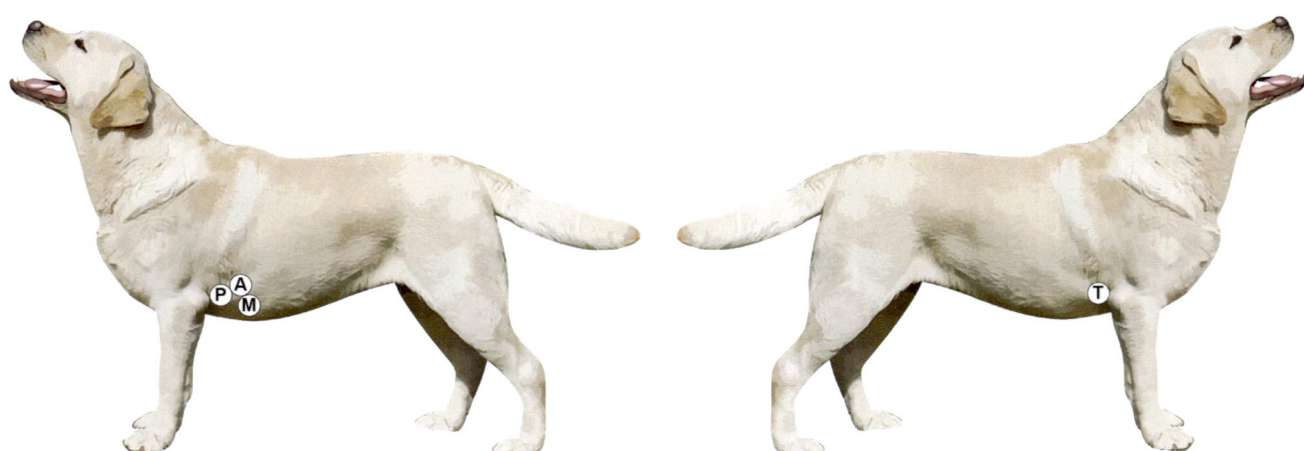

Figure 22. Pulmonic (P), aortic (A) and mitral (M) valves are auscultated on the left side of the chest, with the tricuspid (T) more audible on the right.

Specific Heart Conditions

Mitral Regurgitation

Mitral valve murmurs are often heard in Cavalier King Charles Spaniels and other small breeds. In geriatric patients mitral murmurs are often due to mitral valve endocardiosis (deposition of mucopolysaccharides causing nodular distortion of the valve leaflet), and other geriatric anaesthetic considerations must be taken into account. In these cases, there is regurgitant flow of blood back into the atria from the ventricle, reducing the forward flow of blood.

Aims for anaesthesia include:
- **Producing mild vasodilatation** to reduce the volume of blood that regurgitates back into the atrium and maximise the amount leaving the heart and entering the systemic circulation. When the systemic vascular resistance is reduced by administering a drug (such as acepromazine at a very low dose) to cause vasodilation, the blood takes the path of least resistance and more blood flows forward, out of the heart, rather than regurgitating back into the atrium.
- **Maintaining the heart rate at or slightly above pre-anaesthetic values** and avoiding bradycardia. The reason for avoiding bradycardia is with very low heart rates, there is a lot of time in between heart beats for the ventricle to fill with blood. This means the end diastolic volume increases, and the ventricle is sometimes so full that the mitral valve pushes back up into the atrium and becomes even more incompetent.

Hypertrophic Cardiomyopathy (HCM)

In the cat, hypertrophic cardiomyopathy (HCM) is a common sequela of hyperthyroidism, due to the effects of thyroid hormone on the heart muscle. The left ventricle is thickened, leading to a decrease in the volume of the heart chamber and to abnormal relaxation of the heart muscle. These changes cause tachycardia, resulting in decreased myocardial oxygenation. This can worsen heart function and lead to the development of arrhythmias. The heart muscle is sometimes so hypertrophied it creates an obstruction to the path the blood wants to take out of the heart into the aorta. This obstruction is worsened with increasing heart rate and contractility.

Aims for anaesthesia include:
- decrease heart rate
- suppression of ventricular arrhythmias
- maintaining filling pressures and
- maintaining or slightly increasing SVR by causing some vasoconstriction.

Lamont et al. (2002) suggests a low dose of an α-2 adrenergic agonist to produce a beneficial reduction in outflow obstruction in cats with left ventricular outflow tract obstruction. Very low doses of α-2 adrenergic agonists such as medetomidine or dexmedetomidine produce the suggested increase in SVR and bradycardia.

Pulmonic Stenosis

Pulmonic stenosis means a narrowed pulmonary valve limiting right ventricular outflow. In response to this right ventricular systolic pressure increases, often rendering the tricuspid valve inefficient. This condition is more commonly seen in Bulldogs and Boxers, and as brachycephalic breeds, airway management must be considered.

Aims of anaesthesia include:
- **maintain contractility:** the use of MAC sparing drugs limit the required amount of volatile agent (and therefore the effect on myocardial contractility);
- **maintain or reduce heart rate slightly,** avoiding tachycardia;
- **maintain preload** by giving some fluid therapy; and
- **avoid excessive IPPV pressures** as this makes it more difficult for the blood to flow out of the right side of the heart into the lungs.

Aortic Stenosis

This condition is more commonly seen in Boxers and Bull Terriers, where a stenotic valve limits the left ventricular outflow.

Aims for anaesthesia include:
- **avoid hypotension** by maintaining systemic vascular resistance i.e. try not to vasodilate or vasoconstrict;
- **maintain heart rate** within 20% of baseline; and
- avoid factors that reduce myocardial oxygenation.

Dilated Cardiomyopathy (DCM)

This condition is most commonly seen in large breed dogs. The large heart size can cause **atrial fibrillation** to occur, which is an irregularly irregular heart rhythm with a fibrillating baseline on ECG, where no P waves are generated.

Aims of anaesthesia include:
- maintain myocardial contractility and oxygenation;
- **avoid bradycardia** and maintain normal heart rate (the patient is often tachycardic to compensate for the poor stroke volume); and
- **maintain preload** with fluid therapy and avoid increases in afterload (i.e. vasoconstriction).

Anaesthesia for Neurological Patients

Neurology is a complex field which includes **pathologies of the brain and the spinal cord**. Anaesthesia may be required for patients with pathologies ranging from brain tumour surgery to imaging in patients with epilepsy, or head trauma. The following principles are applied across the board when considering anaesthesia for different cranial pathologies.

An important concept to understand before anaesthetising a patient with brain pathology, is the **Monro Kellie doctrine**.

The skull is a rigid bony box, which cannot expand. In most mammals, the intracranial space contains:
- brain parenchyma (84%)
- blood perfusing the brain (4%)
- cerebrospinal fluid (CSF) (12%).

If the volume of one component increases, it is compensated for by a decrease in another. The brain parenchyma cannot alter its volume easily, although the intracranial blood volume and intracranial CSF volume can alter a small amount (by moving out into the jugular veins and the subarachnoid space in the spinal cord respectively). There comes a point when the compensatory mechanisms are exhausted, there is an increase in intracranial volume, there is decompensation and the intracranial pressure then rises, often producing clinical signs (Figure 23).

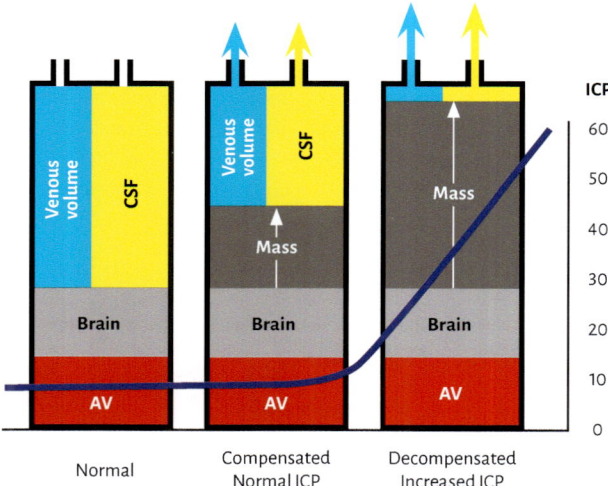

Figure 23. The Monro Kellie doctrine states that if the volume of one of the skull contents increases, it must be compensated for by a decrease in another. Initial compensation occurs, but once exhausted, there is an increase in intracranial volume, decompensation, and intracranial pressure (ICP) then rises. CSF: cerebrospinal fluid; AV: arterial volume.

The following clinical signs are indicative of raised intracranial pressure:
- **altered mentation** and changes in behaviour
- **cranial nerve deficits** including deafness, dysphagia (difficulty swallowing), dysphonia (altered voice), and visual disturbances
- **blindness,** changes in pupil size and reactivity, papilloedema
- **seizures**
- circulatory and respiratory changes (including the **Cushing's triad**).

The Cushing's triad (Figure 24) comprises three clinical signs which occur as a CNS hypoxic response in which there is massive sympathetic discharge. These three signs are:
- **systemic hypertension**
- **bradycardia**
- **irregular breathing patterns.**

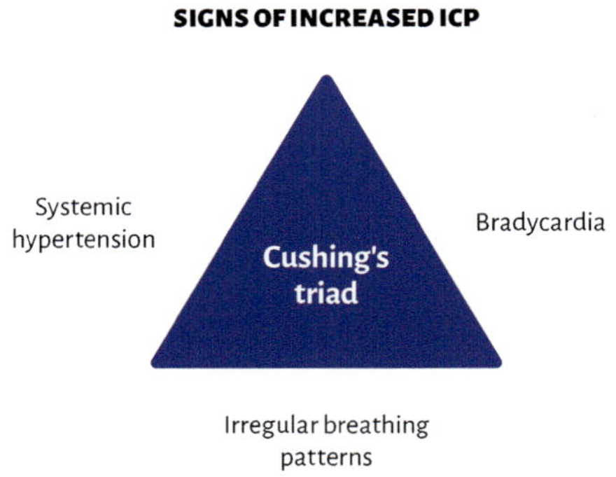

SIGNS OF INCREASED ICP

Figure 24. The Cushing's triad comprises three clinical signs which occur as a CNS hypoxic response.

Even if an elevated intracranial pressure does not produce clinical signs, it may negatively affect the perfusion of the brain. Intracranial pressure may be increased by several pathologies that affect one or more of the three skull contents (i.e. blood, CSF, or brain parenchyma). In addition, extra parenchymal swelling (e.g. abscesses or subdural haemorrhage) also increase intracranial pressure.
- **Brain parenchyma may increase in volume** due to oedema, haemorrhage, inflammation, or space occupying lesions.
- **Cerebrospinal fluid volume may increase** due to an increased production (e.g. choroid plexus tumour) or decreased drainage (e.g. due to space occupying lesions).
- **Blood volume increases** for a variety of reasons including increased central venous pressure or jugular pressure (remember blood from the cerebral vasculature tries to move into the jugular veins as an attempt to

compensate for increases in intracranial pressure) and the degree of vasodilation or vasoconstriction of the blood vessels in the brain.

The main influence anaesthesia has on intracranial pressure is on the blood volume in the skull. For example, how anaesthesia influences central venous pressure/jugular pressure should be considered:
- **The position of the patient's head** during anaesthesia and recovery; keeping the head raised at 30° will help drain blood out of the skull into the jugular vein.
- **Occlusion of the jugular vein** for blood sampling, placing jugular catheters, using collars etc. should be avoided.
- **Valsalva manoeuvres** (forced expiration against a closed glottis) such as vomiting, coughing, gagging, or sneezing should be avoided.
- **Peak inspiratory pressures should be kept lower** if performing IPPV as high inspiratory pressures may increase central venous pressures.

In addition, intracranial blood volume is affected by the degree of vasodilation or vasoconstriction (cerebral vasomotor tone). Cerebral vasomotor tone is normally responsive to several stimuli that may be influenced by anaesthesia (Figure 25).

The normal range for arterial blood pressure does not alter intracranial pressure, because the cerebral circulation is governed by autoregulation which maintains cerebral blood flow over a wide range of blood pressures.

Partial pressure of oxygen does have an influence on increasing cerebral blood flow (and therefor ICP) but only when PaO_2 is less than 60 mmHg (equivalent to SpO_2 of 90%) so by avoiding hypoxia, negative influences on ICP can be avoided. One of the biggest influences on cerebral blood flow and therefore ICP is $PaCO_2$. The graph (Figure 25) does not have a flat part like the other two stimuli, but shows a linear increase, and with every mmHg increase in $PaCO_2$, there is an increase in cerebral blood flow. To this end, ventilation of a patient's lungs is recommended to a low normocapnia if there is concern over raised ICP, in order to avoid worsening of ICP.

Patients with brain disease should be stabilised as much as possible before anaesthesia. Elevated intracranial pressure should be reduced to normal, or at least further elevations prevented. Cerebral autoregulation should be promoted by maintaining blood pressure and partial pressures of oxygen and carbon dioxide within normal limits. Seizure activity should be controlled in the perianaesthetic period.

There are several strategies to normalise a raised intracranial pressure, or at least to prevent further elevations. The use of **diuretics** (e.g. mannitol and/or frusemide) is often advocated to reduce the volume of the brain parenchyma, the blood and the CSF; however, **the patient's hydration status should be monitored closely.** Mannitol exerts its effects by drawing water from the interstitial space into the blood vessels, whilst this early plasma expansion reduces blood viscosity and this in turn improves regional cerebral microvascular flow and oxygenation. Two additional techniques to employ in an emergency, both require invasive measures; aspiration of CSF from the ventricles, and craniotomy and durotomy (making a small hole in the skull to relieve the pressure).

In obtunded patients preanaesthetic medication may not be necessary. If animals are still fairly bright, then preanaesthetic medication reduces anxiety and struggling. Recommended classes of drugs include **benzodiazepines** (these drugs also have antiseizure activity) and **opioids.** In nonpainful patients, high doses of opioids can depress ventilation, notably by decreasing the respiratory centre's response to elevated carbon dioxide tension, so high doses should be avoided, in addition to avoiding opioids which produce vomiting (this is a Valsalva manoeuvre).

Unless it causes the animal to struggle, **preoxygenation** (preferably by mask) is advocated.

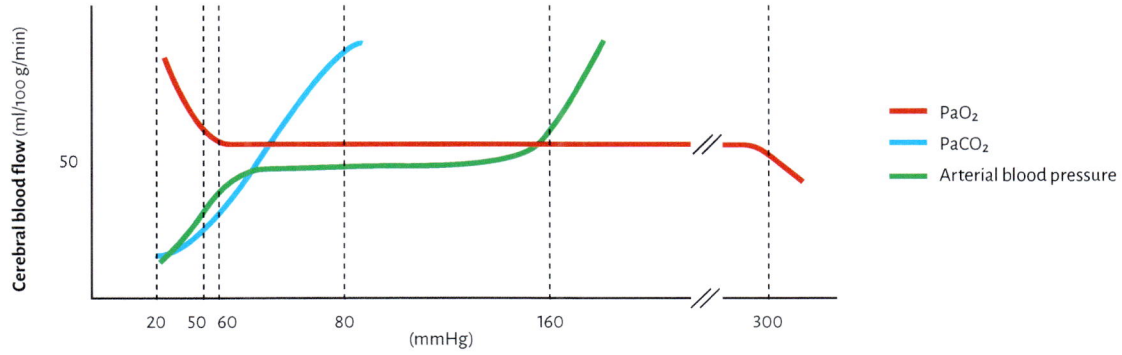

Figure 25. Cerebral vasomotor tone stimuli.

Coughing, gagging, and retching should be avoided during endotracheal intubation as they may increase central venous pressure and thus intracranial pressure. It should be ensured that the animal is at a suitable depth of anaesthesia and the larynx sprayed with local anaesthetic before intubation to help prevent coughing.

Different injectable induction agents have varying effects on cerebral blood flow and intracranial pressure. Both ketamine and etomidate maintain laryngeal and pharyngeal reflexes and therefore may make endotracheal intubation more difficult (coughing and gagging are Valsalva manoeuvres and raise ICP). Ketamine has also been reported to produce seizure like activity in some other species. Propofol, etomidate, and alfaxalone may decrease ICP.

Anaesthesia is usually maintained with inhaled volatile agents, although total, or even partial, intravenous anaesthesia with agents such as alfaxalone or propofol is also possible. **Sevoflurane and isoflurane are preferred** over halothane for maintenance of anaesthesia in brain cases as they produce less of an increase in ICP. Nitrous oxide, whilst useful as an analgesic, does increase intracranial pressure and may worsen the effects of air emboli should these occur during neurosurgery, for example a craniotomy.

The reason for neuroanaesthesia dictates the degree and type of analgesia needed. Pain should be controlled by analgesia, not only for welfare reasons, but also because uncontrolled pain adversely affects cerebral blood flow via sympathetic stimulation. A **multimodal, pre-emptive approach** should be used and analgesia continued into the postoperative period.

Analgesic drugs **not suitable** for some brain cases include:
- High dose opioids: may cause respiratory depression and elevated carbon dioxide tensions.
- Non-steroidal anti-inflammatory drugs: should not be used if glucocorticoids have been administered.
- Nitrous oxide: increases intracranial pressure.
- Ketamine: increases intracranial pressure and can produce seizure like activity.
- α-2 adrenergic agonists: can produce profound ventilatory and cardiovascular effects which affect cerebral vascular tone. They can cause vomiting in cats (a Valsalva manoeuvre).

Whilst intravenous fluid therapy is suggested to maintain blood pressure, over perfusion of the circulatory system may also increase central venous pressure with a secondary increase in intracranial pressure. Sufficient fluid therapy should be administered to **maintain an adequate circulating intravascular volume but avoid over perfusion.**

Animals must be carefully monitored during recovery from anaesthesia and elevating the animal's head should be considered. Allowing the animal to gag or cough on the endotracheal tube is deleterious to the animal if it still has raised intracranial pressure, so early endotracheal extubation is often indicated.

Cerebrospinal Fluid Sampling

A CSF sample can be aspirated from the cisterna magna or the subarachnoid space in the lumbosacral spine, as part of investigation of CNS disease. Cisternal punctures are more problematic for the anaesthetist as the head/neck is flexed which may kink the endotracheal tube. Cerebrospinal fluid sampling via cisternal puncture whilst an animal has an elevated intracranial pressure may produce herniation of the brain, especially of the cerebellum. If a lumbosacral puncture for CSF tap is performed under general anaesthesia, positioning necessitates pulling the animal's hind limbs forwards, which can compromise the animal's ability to ventilate effectively.

Magnetic Resonance Imaging (MRI) Scanning

Anaesthesia in the MRI environment poses other challenges to the anaesthetist as the animal lies in a long narrow tube and is not easily accessible, plus in cases of emergency the MRI facility is usually some way from the clinics or ICU. The presence of a **strong magnetic field attracts ferromagnetic objects** (ranging from laryngoscopes, scissors, oxygen cylinders to anaesthetic machines) potentially turning them into fast moving projectiles; therefore, all anaesthetic equipment which enters the MRI space must be MRI compatible. Small amounts of ferromagnetic substances e.g. the spring in the pilot balloon of an endotracheal tube, can cause anomalies in the MRI scan; whilst the electromagnetic fields may interfere with certain monitors and ventilators.

The intravenous contrast medium can be nephrotoxic. Anecdotally it may lighten the patient's depth of anaesthesia, and there are reports of it causing anaphylactoid type reactions in dogs (Girard & Leece, 2010).

Myelography

Myelography is the special radiographic technique by which **the spinal cord is outlined by a positive contrast medium injected into the subarachnoid space.** The injection of contrast agent into the subarachnoid space can be a challenge. The considerations for patient positioning for contrast injection/

dissemination are the same as for CSF sampling mentioned above.

After injection of contrast, alterations in respiratory rate and heart rate can occur and should be monitored for. Anecdotally, many patients become hypothermic during and after myelography. Seizure activity on recovery from anaesthesia is occasionally seen if the contrast has entered the cranial vault.

Anaesthesia of the Epileptic

Anticonvulsant drugs can act synergistically with sedatives and anaesthetic agents to depress the CNS and therefore doses of these drugs may be reduced. Some anticonvulsant drug classes alter the pharmacokinetics of drugs, especially phenobarbitone.

Epileptics may be prone to seizures around the time of anaesthesia with transitions between different levels of consciousness. Acepromazine is often maligned as causing seizures. This is not supported by the relevant literature (Drynan et al., 2012) (McConnell et al., 2007) (Tobias et al., 2006).

Spinal Patients

Imaging may be required to investigate spinal pathology. There are several modalities available, most require the patient to be anaesthetized rather than sedated:
  – radiography: plain or myelogram
  – computed tomography +/- myelogram
  – magnetic resonance imaging.

Intravenous access is recommended for all cases, no matter which imaging modality is chosen; the procedures are often long and therefore fluid therapy is recommended. Preanaesthetic medication varies depending on the case, but analgesia should always be included if the patient is painful or surgical treatment anticipated. Calming the patient with preanaesthetic medication also facilitates safe moving of the patient, which may be vital for patients with unstable spines.

Induction of anaesthesia is usually induced using an intravenous agent such as propofol or alfaxalone, given slowly and to effect. Cervical spinal cases benefit from a head flat endotracheal intubation following preoxygenation (Figure 26).

Maintenance of anaesthesia is usually by volatile agent anaesthesia (+/- analgesic continuous rate infusions). During spinal surgery, ventilation of the lungs may be useful.

Providing adequate analgesia is paramount, which is best supplied **with a multimodal, pre-emptive analgesia plan.**

Perioperative nursing is also important as spinal cases often have chronic pain and require careful postoperative analgesic management. Positioning during anaesthesia, especially for cervical spine patients, requires careful consideration, whilst **monitoring needs to be thorough and should include blood pressure, capnography, pulse oximetry, body temperature, and electrocardiogram.**

Serious perianaesthetic complications may occur, including dysrhythmias, haemorrhage, air emboli, and respiratory arrest. Bladder function is affected in some spinal patients and **placement of an indwelling urinary catheter** helps improve perioperative comfort in the recumbent patient.

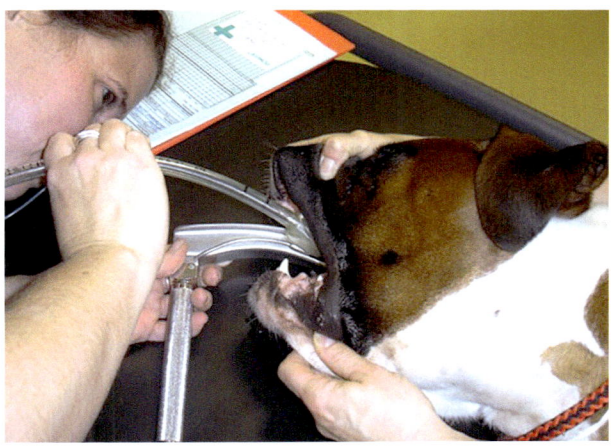

Figure 26. Keeping the head flat during endotracheal intubation prevents exerting forces which may damage the spinal cord.

REFERENCES

■ Campoy et al. (2003) Kinking of endotracheal tubes during maxima flexion of the atlanto-occipital joint in dogs. *J Small Anim Pract*, 44, 3–7.
■ Drynan et al. (2012) Incidence of seizures associated with the use of acepromazine in dogs undergoing myelography. *JVECCS*, 22, 262–266.
■ Girard & Leece (2010) Suspected anaphylactoid reaction following intravenous administration of a gadolinium-based contrast agent in three dogs undergoing magnetic resonance imaging. *VAA*, 37, 352–6.
■ Lamont et al. (2002) Doppler echocardiographic effects of medetomidine on dynamic left ventricular outflow tract obstruction in cats. *J Am Vet Med Assoc.* 221, 1276–1281.
■ McConnell et al. (2007) Administration of acepromazine maleate to 31 dogs with a history of seizures. *JVECCS*, 17, 262–267.
■ Tobias et al. (2006) A retrospective study on the use of acepromacine maleate in dogs with seizures. *JAAHA*, 42, 283–289.

Self-assessment

Test

Answers on page 212

1. Which of the following drugs will increase the concentration of acetylcholine in the synaptic cleft?
   a. Suggamadex.
   b. Suxamethonium.
   c. Atracurium.
   d. Neostigmine.

2. For positive pressure ventilation, which of the following is the most physiological setting, for the inspiratory to expiratory ratio?
   a. 1:3.
   b. 1:6.
   c. 1:9.
   d. 1:12.

3. In the neuromuscular junction, acetylcholinesterase is stored in:
   a. The motor nerve terminal.
   b. The synaptic cleft.
   c. The peaks of the muscle end plate.
   d. The troughs of the muscle end plate.

4. During positive pressure ventilation, which of the following monitors indicate the efficiency of the ventilation?
   a. Electrocardiogram.
   b. Pulse oximetry.
   c. Capnography.
   d. Arterial blood pressure.

5. The ventilatory pattern suggested for anaesthetics in patients with a ruptured diaphragm is:
   a. High frequency, low volume.
   b. Low frequency, low volume.
   c. Low frequency, high volume.
   d. High frequency, high volume.

6. A patent ductus arteriosus is a communication between:
   a. The vena cava and aorta.
   b. The pulmonary vein and vena cava.
   c. The pulmonary artery and aorta.
   d. The pulmonary vein and pulmonary artery.

7. Spring loaded mouth gag use in the cat can have negative consequences because of compression of the:
   a. Mental artery.
   b. Maxillary artery.
   c. Mandibular artery.
   d. Medial artery.

8. Vasoconstriction is primarily associated with:
   a. Increased preload.
   b. Decreased preload.
   c. Increased afterload.
   d. Decreased afterload.

9. Which of these is a component of the Cushing's triad?
   a. Tachycardia.
   b. Hypercapnia.
   c. Hypotension.
   d. Irregular respiratory pattern.

10. The Valsalva manoeuvre is defined as:
    a. Forced expiration against a closed glottis.
    b. Maintenance of cerebral blood flow across a range of different arterial blood pressures.
    c. Aspiration of CSF from a ventricle to lower intracranial pressure.
    d. Outlining the spinal cord by injection contrast into the subarachnoid space.

Clinical Case

A 7-year-old Pekingese dog (6 kg) requires anaesthesia for a thoracotomy to remove a left caudal lung lobe (aspirates suggest primary pulmonary carcinoma). The surgeon plans a left lateral thoracotomy via the fifth intercostal space. The dog has mitral valve disease and is stable on treatment with benazepril and frusemide. She has a markedly brachycephalic conformation. Think about the anaesthetic considerations for this case and make a note of them.

1. What clinical signs are likely to be present or tests are indicated prior to anaesthetising this dog?

2. How can the anaesthesia be approached in terms of the dog's brachycephalic conformation?

3. The owners call to ask whether the dog should be given the heart medication the morning of anaesthesia. What is the recommendation?

4. Where can the point of maximal intensity be heard on a mitral valve murmur?

5. What are the aims of anaesthesia for mitral valve disease?

6. What local anaesthetic techniques would be appropriate for this case?

7. The total dose of bupivacaine for use in this case is 2 mg/kg. What volume of 0.25% bupivacaine is available to be split between all of these local anaesthetic techniques?

8. What initial settings would you set on the ventilator?
   - Tidal volume (ml).
   - Inspiratory time (s).
   - Expiratory time (s).
   - Maximum peak inspiratory pressure (mmHg).

9. Atracurium is being used as a neuromuscular blocking drug for this anaesthetic. What are the possible anatomical sites of peripheral nerve stimulation in the dog and which twitch patterns can be used to indicate fade?

10. Other than a peripheral nerve stimulator, what other monitoring modalities are important in this case? Justify your choices.

Self-assessment

CORRECT ANSWERS:

TEST

1. d
2. a
3. d
4. c
5. a
6. c
7. b
8. c
9. d
10. a

CLINICAL CASE

1. **What clinical signs are likely to be present or tests are indicated prior to anaesthetising this dog?**
   Thoracic imaging such as computed tomography or radiography provide an idea about the size of the lung tumour (which provides an idea about the possibility of hypoxaemia, and restriction of tidal volume). Assessment of the other lung fields for evidence of pulmonary oedema (to check for congestive heart failure) would be beneficial. Preanaesthetic blood tests should include potassium, as long-term frusemide administration may cause hypokalaemia. The owner should be asked for further information including exercise tolerance (related to cardiac disease) and evidence of regurgitation (related to brachycephalic conformation).

2. **How can the anaesthesia be approached in terms of the dog's brachycephalic conformation?**
   If the dog is a suspected regurgitator (common in brachycephalic animals), omeprazole should be administered the night before and on the morning of anaesthesia. A head up position should be used to help prevent regurgitation during induction of anaesthesia. Preoxygenation should be by mask and preparation of equipment for a difficult intubation should be made (including a wide range of endotracheal tubes). Regular ophthalmic lubrication intra and postoperatively is indicated as the breed is exophthalmic.

3. **The owners call to ask whether the dog should be given the heart medication the morning of anaesthesia. What is the recommendation?**
   Frusemide can be given on the morning of anaesthesia, but the ACE inhibitor should not be given as the vasodilation caused may promote hypotension.

4. **Where can the point of maximal intensity be heard on a mitral valve murmur?**
   On the left-hand side of the chest, as the most caudal of the left-hand side valves. It is heard over the apex beat (where the heartbeat is palpable when placing a hand on the chest wall).

5. **What are the aims of anaesthesia for mitral valve disease?**
   Producing a mild vasodilatation to reduce the amount of blood that regurgitates back into the atrium and maximise the amount of blood that wants to leave the heart and go into the systemic circulation. The heart rate should be maintained at or slightly above preanaesthetic values and bradycardia avoided to avoid over filling the ventricle at the end of diastole.

6. **What local anaesthetic techniques would be appropriate for this case?**
   An intercostal nerve block, blocking two ribs in front and two ribs behind the proposed incision site, and interpleural local analgesia (instilled down the chest drain postsurgery). Incisional infiltration is also a possibility. A high epidural could be considered; the author suggests with morphine only.

7. **The total dose of bupivacaine for use in this case is 2 mg/kg. What volume of 0.25% bupivacaine is available to be split between all of these local anaesthetic techniques?**

   6 kg × 2 mg/kg = 12 mg
   0.25% solution is 2.5 mg/ml
   12 mg / 2.5 mg/ml = 4.8 ml total volume

8. **What initial settings would you set on the ventilator?**
   The following are suggestions; however, slightly different values may have been calculated by the reader.
   - **Tidal volume:** the author would start with the lower end of the 10–15 mg/kg range as the lung tumour may be taking up some tidal volume, so a starting value of 6 kg × 10 ml/kg = 60 ml could be used.
   - **Inspiratory and expiratory times:** these need to be calculated to administer an appropriate respiratory rate (e.g. 15 bpm). That means that each breath would last 4 seconds (60/15). Inspiratory and expiratory times then need to be split so that they fit with a ratio of between 1:2 and 1:3. If a 1 second inspiratory time and 3 second expiratory time were chosen, then that would be an appropriate ratio and respiratory rate.
   - **Maximum peak inspiratory pressure** is usually set at 20 mmHg in the dog.

9. **Atracurium is being used as a neuromuscular blocking drug for this anaesthetic. What are the possible anatomical sites of peripheral nerve stimulation in the dog and which twitch patterns can be used to indicate fade?**

Anatomical sites are facial, peroneal, and ulnar nerves. Twitch patterns are train of four, double burst stimulus and tetanic stimulus.

10. **Other than a peripheral nerve stimulator, what other monitoring modalities are important in this case? Justify your choices.**

Capnography indicates the efficiency of ventilation and lung excursions, disconnection from ventilator, and obstruction of the endotracheal tube. Pulse oximetry indicates saturation of haemoglobin with oxygen and values may decrease because of the lung pathology. SpO_2 may decrease further if healthy lung is packed away while the surgeon performs the lung lobectomy. An electrocardiogram is useful during thoracic anaesthesia as there are several nerves which run through the thoracic cavity which can cause arrhythmias if tweaked. Blood pressure monitoring (ideally direct) is useful because of the potential for blood loss, the dog's cardiac disease, and the influence of positive pressure ventilation on blood pressure.

Anaesthetic Considerations for Specific Conditions II

Nicki Grint

Chapter Summary:

- Pregnancy and anaesthesia.
- Anaesthetia for caesarean section.
- Anaesthesia of paediatric and neonatal patients.
- Anaesthesia for the geriatric patient.
- Anaesthesia for liver dysfunction.
- Chronic renal failure and anaesthesia.
- Anaesthesia for endocrinopathies.

The paediatric patient has different physiological requirements to the geriatric patient, whilst pregnancy, endocrinopathies, and organ dysfunction alter the patient's tolerance of anaesthesia. This chapter explains these differences and how best to anaesthetise the patient without worsening their condition.

PREGNANCY AND ANAESTHESIA

The anaesthesia of pregnant animals comes with many special considerations, mainly because of the major physiological changes associated with pregnancy; indeed, the risks of anaesthetising a pregnant animal differ, depending on the trimester of gestation. In the **first third of pregnancy (first trimester)** one of the main risks is **embryotoxicity**. Unfortunately, most veterinary drugs are not tested in pregnant animals and are therefore rarely licenced for use in pregnant animals.

When an animal in early pregnancy requires anaesthesia and the proposed drugs are used in humans, the datasheets of the human versions should be studied to check for contraindications in pregnancy.

In the second trimester, the main risk is placental separation.

The **third trimester is associated with major physiological changes** and is also the trimester when anaesthesia is most often required, i.e. caesarean section.

Physiological Changes in the Third Trimester

The dam's cardiac output and blood volume increase to meet the needs of the growing placenta. For the blood volume both plasma volume and red cell mass increase, but the plasma volume increases proportionally more, resulting in **a dilutional anaemia** (Figure 1). **Albumin levels also are decreased** in pregnant animals.

Cardiac reserve decreases therefore animals with preexisting cardiac disease may decompensate. A pregnant animal's **systemic vascular resistance decreases,** and this vasodilation contributes to the potential for **hypotension.** There is also a physical contribution to this hypotension; the large gravid (pregnant) uterus puts pressure on the great vessels running along the dorsum e.g. the vena cava and aorta. When the patient is placed in dorsal recumbency, the uterus compresses these vessels, reducing venous return and therefore cardiac output.

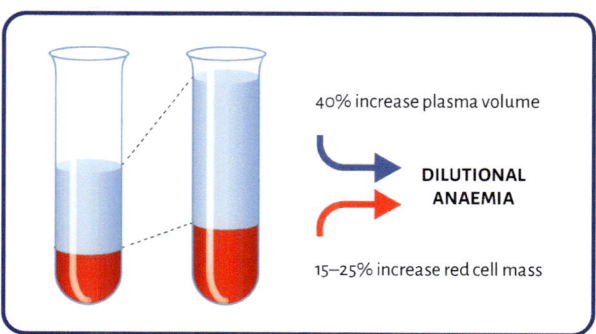

Figure 1. Both plasma volume and red cell mass increase, but plasma volume increases proportionally more, resulting in a dilutional anaemia.

In pregnancy the animal's **minute volume is increased.** In addition to oxygen consumption increasing, the animal's metabolic oxygen requirement also increases. There is a decrease in functional residual capacity (FRC). **The FRC is the volume of gas left in the lungs at the end of a normal breath** as the lungs do not empty completely during exhalation. Functional residual capacity represents the interbreath store of alveolar oxygen and so if an animal has a decreased FRC, they are more likely to suffer from desaturation (i.e. become hypoxaemic). The pregnant animal has a reduced FRC because of the gravid uterus pushing forward and compressing the diaphragm which limits lung capacity and volume. Therefore, both a decreased FRC and increased metabolic oxygen requirement **warrant oxygen supplementation before and after anaesthesia.**

The gravid uterus places pressure on the stomach and alters its position; in turn this alters the angle at which the oesophagus enters the stomach, making the **oesophageal sphincter incompetent.** Progesterone (one of the main hormones of pregnancy) also decreases the tone of the oesophageal sphincter and slows the digestive process, keeping food in the stomach for longer. Overall, this means that **the animal is more prone to regurgitation.** In addition, many caesarean sections are not elective and therefore the patient may not be starved.

In patients prone to regurgitation, it is good practice to use a head up induction where the patient is kept in sternal recumbency with their head up until their trachea is intubated and the tube's cuff is inflated. This technique uses gravity to avoid stomach contents moving up into the oesophagus and potentially pharynx whilst the airway is unprotected.

Because of the increase in cardiac output, more blood flows through the kidneys (i.e. renal blood flow). In turn, glomerular filtration rate (the flow rate of filtered fluid through the kidney) increases. **Urea and creatinine concentrations therefore decrease** because of dilution.

Anaesthesia for Nonpregnancy Reasons

Anaesthetising a pregnant patient when the foetuses are staying put (i.e. a nonpregnancy related anaesthetic) is an easier task because there is less concern if drugs cross the placenta because maternal physiology metabolises the drugs, with **the main aim during anaesthesia being to maintain placenta and foetal oxygenation.**

- Maintenance of oxygenation using:
    - preoxygenation
    - oxygen supplementation in recovery
    - measurement of SpO_2.
- Carbon dioxide levels should be maintained within normal limits: carbon dioxide has effects on vasodilation and vasoconstriction and ensuring it remains at normal levels it is advisable to avoid foetal acidaemia.
- Blood pressure should be maintained with a systolic value >90 mmHg.
- Teratogenic drugs should be avoided, which are drugs that cause developmental malformations.
- Drugs that induce labour (known as ecbolic drugs) should be avoided. Xylazine (an α-2 adrenergic agonist) is a veterinary drug that is a known ecbolic, and is therefore best avoided.

Anaesthesia for Caesarean Sections

Anaesthesia for caesarean sections can be stressful because there is more than one patient to anaesthetise, and the dam (the principal concern) has altered physiology. In caesarean sections the foetuses are delivered from the uterus and need to process the anaesthetic drugs themselves.

The general aims of anaesthesia are:
- **maintain placental blood flow and delivery of oxygen** until the foetuses are delivered; and
- **use short acting drugs or drugs which do not cross the placental barrier,** to reduce the amount of anaesthetic drug transferred to the foetus. There is also a small amount of drug transfer via the milk.

Drugs crossing the placenta depend on:
- thickness of tissue
- ionisation
- lipid solubility
- foetal concentration
- maternal concentration
- foetal metabolism.

For caesarean section in veterinary species, there are two main options for chemical restraint:
- In large animals, such as cattle and sheep, sedation plus **local anaesthesia** (e.g. an epidural, paravertebral, inverted L block or line block) is more common.
- In small animals, **general anaesthesia** is more practical, but the use of injectable drugs mean more crosses the placenta.

Preanaesthetic Medication

Provision of preanaesthetic medication for caesarean sections is becoming more common. The benefits of premedication include:
- **pre-emptive analgesia,** when appropriate drugs are used;

- **reduction of the amount of induction and volatile agent required,** thus reducing cardiovascular and respiratory depression;
- **smoothing the anaesthetic** and avoiding responses to surgical stimulation (which could include regurgitation if the patient becomes light); and
- **smoother recovery** from anaesthesia.

However, most drugs cross the placenta to the foetuses, which may cause respiratory depression, cardiovascular depression, and a lower **APGAR (appearance, pulse, grimace, activity, and respiration) score** (see Table 1).

The current WSAVA guidelines suggest **use of IM or IV opioid ± acepromazine at the lower end of the dose range** for elective caesarean section stating that: "an opioid normally provides adequate sedation for venous access however acepromazine can be used if the dam is difficult to manage and requires more sedation than an opioid alone can provide."

Their recommendation **for emergency caesarean sections is fentanyl IV (3–5 µg/kg).**

In a retrospective study (Romagnoli et al., 2019) of emergency caesarean sections, comparing the use of systemic methadone 0.3 mg/kg premedication, epidural methadone 0.1 mg/kg or epidural lidocaine 4.4 mg/kg in bitches undergoing caesarean section, heart rate, respiratory rate, and APGAR scores did not differ between groups.

In another study (Vilar et al., 2018) morphine was used to premedicate bitches for elective caesarean section before comparing different maintenance protocols. At 60 minutes after delivery, the APGAR scores showed a normal viability in 94% of puppies.

> Therefore, there is evidence that a low dose of pre-emptive opioid analgesia does not influence the viability outcome of neonates.

In the UK, the license for buprenorphine specifically states that the drug should not be used for caesarean section. Morphine is unlicensed in the dog and cat, **which leaves pethidine and methadone,** which are currently licenced for dogs and cats in the UK.

Pethidine is not as commonly stocked as other opioids and therefore the alternative is **methadone administered at a low dose (0.1–0.2 mg/kg).** A benefit of both of drugs is they are pure mu (µ) agonists and the **effects are antagonised in the neonate (using naloxone)** if respiratory depression is observed.

Table 1. APGAR is a scoring system which indicates neonatal viability.

Parameter/Score	0	1	2
Heart rate	<180 bpm	180–220 bpm	>220 bpm
Respiratory effort	No crying <6 br/min	Mild crying 6–15 br/min	Crying >15 br/min
Reflex irritability	Absent	Grimace	Vigorous
Motility	Flaccid	Some flexions	Active motion
Mucous membrane colour	Cyanotic	Pale	Pink

Score 7–10 = no distress; 4–6 = moderate distress; 0–3 = severe distress. A version of modified APGAR score (Veronesi et al., 2009).

In addition to the use of pre-emptive opioid as suggested above, further opioids can be administered to the dam after the offspring are removed from the uterus.

Non-steroidal anti-inflammatory drugs (NSAIDs) can be administered **at the end of anaesthesia,** partially because hypotension may occur during the anaesthetic. The WSAVA recommend a **one off dose of NSAID is appropriate** but that until further studies are conducted, multiple doses are not warranted. **Paracetamol** can be safely given to dogs after a caesarean section.

Local anaesthetic is appropriate for caesarean sections, with line blocks preincision or at closure into the abdominal wall/skin; or alternatively, an epidural can be given. The use of morphine alone or a morphine and lidocaine epidural avoids prolonged postoperative motor blockade.

Providing appropriate analgesia is important, not just for welfare reasons, but so the dam is comfortable enough to feed the neonates. Untreated pain also causes uterine vasoconstriction and reduced blood flow, and reduced milk production.

Preparation and Anaesthetic Induction

The patient should be started on intravenous fluid therapy at a standard rate of 5 ml/kg/hr (dog) and 3 ml/kg/hr (cat), unless the patient is hypotensive or dehydrated and requires fluid boluses. Whilst setting up for anaesthesia, as much of the belly as possible should be clipped prior to induction, to reduce time spent under anaesthesia.

The patient should be preoxygenated if possible, to maintain placental blood oxygenation, but also because the dam is prone to desaturation because of reduced FRC. A **head up induction** is advisable, (especially if the surgery is an emergency and no starvation possible) due to the risk of regurgitation.

Short acting, titratable drugs are required to induce anaesthesia. Both **alfaxalone and propofol** are safe for induction of anaesthesia in bitches undergoing emergency caesarean section. In one study (Doebeli et al., 2013) found puppy survival was similar after the use of these drugs, although alfaxalone was associated with better neonatal vitality during the first 60 minutes after delivery.

Maintenance of Anaesthesia

A cuffed endotracheal tube should be used to protect the airway if regurgitation occurs. Positive pressure ventilation may be needed, and if the tube is uncuffed, sufficient pressure may not be achievable and staff in theatre exposed to volatile agent pollution.

For a swift recovery from general anaesthesia a low solubility, volatile agent such as **isoflurane or sevoflurane** should be used. Minimum alveolar concentration (MAC) is decreased in pregnant animals and therefore it may be possible to reduce the vaporiser settings.

The dam's abdomen should be clipped with the patient in both lateral recumbencies, if possible, as this avoids placing her into dorsal recumbency until the last possible moment.

Once in **dorsal recumbency,** the gravid uterus put pressures on the diaphragm (causing hypoventilation and a reduced FRC) and vena cava/aorta (causing decreased venous return). The vena cava is most easily compressed, as it is a vein and therefore thinner walled, and it lies to the right, so **tilting the animal slightly to the left** is suggested. (Figure 2).

Anaesthesia of Paediatric and Neonatal Patients

Anaesthesia of a very young animal may be required to correct a congenital abnormality or for a condition unrelated to their age. Whatever the reason, the physiological differences associated with neonates and paediatrics mean there are additional considerations for anaesthesia techniques.

There are different cut off points for **what is considered a neonate or paediatric patient.** In the literature a consensus appears to be:
- <4 weeks is neonate
- 4–12 weeks is paediatric
- <12 weeks is juvenile.

After 12 weeks of age, there is less concern about paediatric factors as the majority of circulatory, ventilatory, thermoregulation, hepatic, and renal functions are well developed. Up until 12 weeks of age, several of the organ systems are underdeveloped which must be considered when planning an anaesthetic.

Neonatal and Paediatric Physiology

Respiratory System

A paediatric patient has two to three times the tissue oxygen demand of an adult, and a higher respiratory rate. **The FRC is**

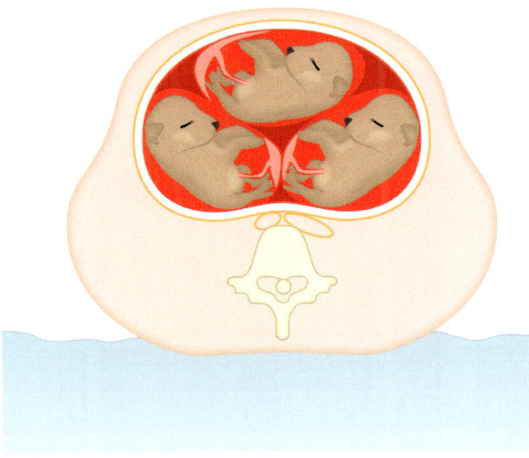 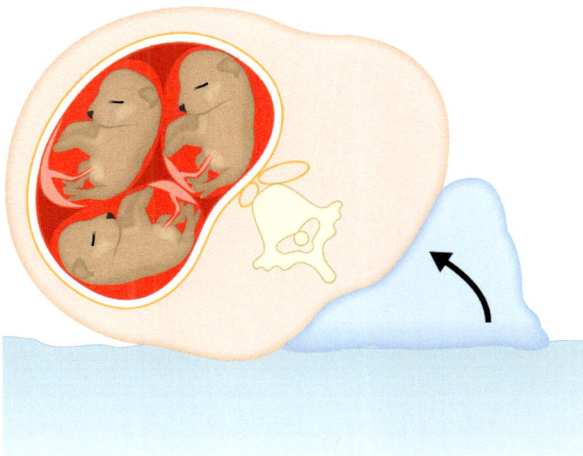

Figure 2. Tilting the animal slightly to the left minimises aortocaval compression.

also lower in paediatric patients compared to adults. This is because the chest wall in a neonate is very compliant and is easily pulled in by the inward forces created by the elastic recoil of the lung.

In relation to the oral cavity, the tongue is relatively large, yet the diameter of the airway narrow, i.e. it is possible to fit a larger endotracheal tube into the trachea of an adult 8 kg Jack Russell Terrier than would be possible in an 8 kg German Shepherd puppy.

Cardiovascular System

When an animal is born, its **cardiovascular system needs to transition from foetal** (where oxygen is supplied across the placenta from the mother) **to adult** (where the neonate must fend for itself, and blood moves through the lungs to pick up oxygen) (see Figure 3).

In utero, the foetal blood does not need to go through the lungs to pick up oxygen, as the oxygen is provided by the placenta. Instead, there are **two shunts which allow blood to go from the right side of the heart to the left without going through the lungs.** These is the **foramen ovale** which moves blood from the right atrium of the heart to the left atrium and the **ductus arteriosus** which moves blood from the pulmonary artery to the aorta.

When the neonatal animal takes their first breath and the lungs fill with air, oxygen makes the pulmonary blood vessels vasodilate, decreasing the pulmonary vascular resistance (PVR) to a value lower than the systemic vascular resistance (SVR). This causes blood from the right side of the heart to take a path through the lungs, reducing blood flow through the PDA and foramen ovale, which close over the first few days of life.

The shunts are not fully sealed for the first few days of life. If it is necessary to anaesthetise a patient at this very young age, **increases in PVR should be avoided,** which may increase the resistance to blood flow through the lungs and encourage blood to flow through the shunts again. As there is no oxygenation from the maternal side to fall back on, the patient can become hypoxic. Ventilating a neonate with high peak inspiratory pressures, is one potential cause of increased PVR.

The myocardium is stiff in neonates and therefore they cannot increase stroke volume if an increase cardiac output is required and maintenance of cardiac output is heart rate dependent. Therefore, **in this age range, it is best to avoid drugs that produce bradycardia.**

Hepatic Physiology

The neonate and paediatric patient have an immature microsomal enzyme system until they are 8–12 weeks old, which means they are **slow to metabolise drugs.** Glycogen storage is minimal, and they have **poor gluconeogenic** (making new glucose) **ability** which means these young animals are **prone to hypoglycaemia.** Neonates and paediatric patients also tend to have **lower albumin levels.**

Renal Physiology

The neonate and paediatric patient's total body water and extra cellular fluid volume is higher than an adult, meaning their

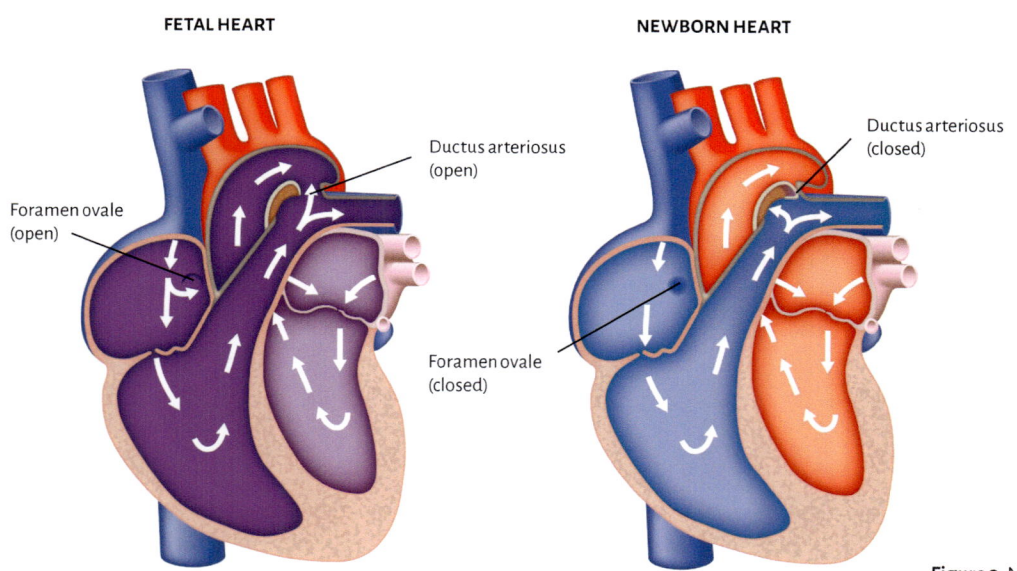

Figure 3. Neonatal heart circulation.

daily water requirement is higher. The animal's renal function is reduced up until 6–8 weeks of age meaning they have:
- poor ability to concentrate urine
- poor ability to excrete a water load
- poor acid-base regulation.

Thermoregulation

These animals are born with **little subcutaneous fat,** and together with poor thermoregulatory capabilities and an immature control of vasomotor tone (i.e. limited control of vasodilation and vasoconstriction) they are **prone to hypothermia.** This is compounded by prolonged preanaesthetic starvation, as metabolism generates body heat. Also, their small size means they have a high surface area to volume ratio, making them **more prone to heat loss.**

Dealing with Drugs

Neonates and paediatric patients may appear resistant **to non-depolarising neuromuscular blocking drugs,** but these drugs have a prolonged action so a low dose should be used to start with and titrated up to an adequate level of muscle relaxation for surgery.

Renal and hepatic clearance of drugs can be prolonged, so use of **lower doses** of drugs should be considered, and indeed with some drugs (such as opioid analgesics) **repeat doses should be administered based on pain scoring** (rather than giving every four hours), since the duration of action may be longer than anticipated.

Due to the increased extra cellular fluid volume, **water soluble drugs (e.g. ketamine) may require higher doses.** Lower albumin concentrations mean the patient **is more prone to overdose with highly protein bound drugs.** There is also **less subcutaneous fat for redistribution of drugs.**

Preanaesthetic Preparation

Neonates and paediatric patients should have **limited starvation** as they are prone to **hypoglycaemia,** plus prolonged starvation promotes **hypothermia.** Current AAHA recommendations are that **animals under eight weeks of age or 2 kg in body weight should be starved for only 1–2 hours.** A blood sample is indicated, prior to anaesthetic induction, to check for hypoglycaemia.

Animals should be weighed accurately and appropriately sized equipment prepared, including catheters and endotracheal tubes. The patient's temperature should be checked and care taken to **prevent hypothermia.** As these animals are small it is also easy to overheat them, so the monitoring aspect is equally important to **avoid hyperthermia.**

Pain and Analgesia

The physiology of neonatal and paediatric patients is constantly developing until they reach maturity; their central nervous system, including their ability to process pain is no exception. There is a lot of evidence **that subjecting neonatal animals to pain during this time is detrimental to them,** worsening their response to pain later in life.

From the 1940s to the 1980s there was a widely held belief that newborn babies lacked the neuroanatomical and neuroendocrine components necessary to perceive pain. During this period, newborns often received inadequate anaesthesia and analgesia for painful procedures. For example, newborn babies often underwent painful surgeries without the use of opioids. The Liverpool technique named after the institution and hospital where it was developed, used an oxygen nitrous oxide inhaled mixture, muscle relaxant and volatile agent to anaesthetise newborns for even lengthy painful procedures without injectable analgesics (Subramaniam, 2019). The rationale being the belief that neonates lacked the capacity to feel pain and were sensitive to the deleterious effects of opioid analgesics. Thankfully, these beliefs and practices changed with research breakthroughs in the 1980s.

Research undertaken in the 1980s demonstrated the foetus has developed the necessary anatomic, neurophysiological, and hormonal components to perceive pain. These findings in basic research were complemented by clinical research which demonstrated that **outcomes were worse for newborns and infants not adequately treated with analgesia during painful procedures.**

Pain Assessment in Neonates

The majority of pain assessment tools rely on observing behavioural cues for pain. This may invalidate these tools in neonatal puppies and kittens as their repertoire of behaviours is not the same as their adult counterparts. Currently there are **no validated pain scoring systems designed for use in puppies or kittens,** therefore the following approaches should be considered:
- An **anthropomorphic approach:** if the procedure or condition the neonate is experiencing is expected to be painful, then analgesia is warranted.
- **Pain assessment tools** (especially composite ones where there are different categories) validated in adult dogs and cats guide the observer to consider different aspects

of the neonate's behaviour, giving a more thorough evaluation of the patient.
- The response of the puppy or kitten to **palpation of the painful area** of the body should be considered.
- When attempting to assess pain post surgically in neonates, **observation or preanaesthetic pain free behaviour** is vital for comparison to postsurgery behaviour.
- If behaviours in the neonate are pain related, then these should **diminish after appropriate analgesia administration.**

So, if a young animal is undergoing a painful procedure or is suffering from a painful condition, **providing analgesia to avoid permanent changes to their pain perception is vital.**

Opioids are an appropriate choice, although ideally drugs that do not produce bradycardia should be chosen. Avoidance of bradycardia is a reason to not use α-2 adrenergic agonists.

Ketamine is a useful analgesic for somatic pain, but it is water soluble and therefore an adult dose may not have the same effect in the neonate.

Local anaesthetic techniques are appropriate, provided the dose and volume of drug used is accurate. In babies, the spinal cord ends more caudally in neonates compared to older children and therefore there is more chance of dural puncture and CSF coming out of the needle. As the myelination is not complete in neonates, **lower concentrations of local anaesthetics are effective** and high concentrations of local anaesthetic, such as 0.5% bupivacaine or 0.5% ropivacaine, are not recommended in babies and children. Instead, **larger volumes of more dilute local anaesthetics are more commonly used** to cover several spinal segments of interest.

Non-steroidal anti-inflammatory drugs can be used in certain ages of puppies and kittens, but the data sheet for each drug should be checked as the minimum ages and weights differ.

Preanaesthetic Medication

There is little need to control or sedate neonates and induction of and recovery from anaesthesia are usually smooth, so it could be argued minimal preanaesthetic medication is required. However, it is worthwhile giving some preanaesthetic medication as this reduces the amounts of other drugs needed and provides pre-emptive analgesia for painful procedures.

Short acting drugs are preferable, as renal and hepatic clearance is slower, and drugs that produce bradycardia should be avoided. Benzodiazepines can also be used as they may produce some sedation in neonates (in healthy adult animals they tend to produce excitement). (Figure 4).

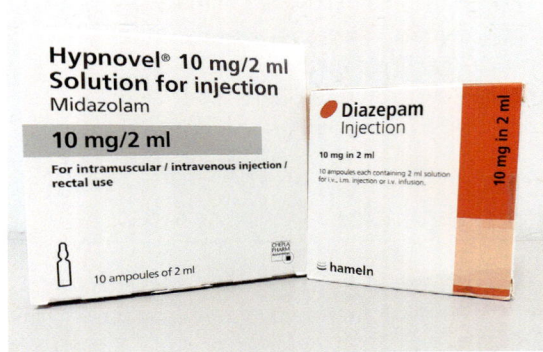

Figure 4. Benzodiazepines.

Induction of Anaesthesia

Intravenous access should be secured and the patient should be preoxygenated by mask.

Induction of anaesthesia is either via intravenous injectable drugs or inhalational induction. If the latter is chosen, **sevoflurane** is preferable as it is less irritant to the mucous membranes and has a more pleasant taste compared to isoflurane.

The patient's trachea should be intubated with an endotracheal tube (cuffed or uncuffed). When an uncuffed tube is used, a larger diameter tube can be fitted with less chance of damaging tracheal cartilages but there is less airway protection. **Excessively long tubes should be cut to an appropriate length** to avoid increased breathing system dead space.

Maintenance of Anaesthesia

Inhalational maintenance is preferable to total intravenous anaesthesia as there is less injectable drug to metabolise. A low solubility volatile agent such as sevoflurane or isoflurane is appropriate, as this low solubility leads to fast recoveries from anaesthesia.

A breathing system with low drag, resistance, and dead space should be selected; usually an Ayre's T-piece with a Jackson Rees modification or Mapleson D T-piece. As the chest wall is more compliant there is less effect on blood pressure if IPPV is performed.

Fluid therapy must be administered with accuracy so drip pumps or paediatric burettes should be used to avoid over or under hydration. As neonates have a stiff myocardium, they are not as responsive to fluid loading, and any blood loss is more likely to be significant.

Because of the physiological differences in neonates, as thorough monitoring as possible is suggested but this may be difficult because of the small size of the animals. **Intermittent blood glucose monitoring is useful in lengthy anaesthetics.**

Recovery from Anaesthesia

Gag reflexes are less developed in paediatric patients so **endotracheal tubes may be left in place for longer without swallowing.** Supplementary oxygen should be given, if possible, especially if the patient is shivering. Food should be offered as soon as the patient can sit up and maintain their own airway. Temperature monitoring should be continued and warming performed as necessary. Fluid therapy should be continued until good oral intake, and pain assessed for pain to be managed effectively.

ANAESTHETISING THE GERIATRIC PATIENT

Increasing age does not necessarily increase the risk of anaesthesia, as ageing itself is not a disease; **but ageing does increase the chance of comorbidities** and also reduces the functional capacity of some organ systems. The term geriatric is often suggested as over 10 years of age in dogs and over 12 years of age in cats. However, different breeds age differently, and therefore a better approach is to use a **cut off of >80% of anticipated lifespan.**

Age Related Changes

Ageing is a multifactorial, all-encompassing process, which **decreases an animal's capacity for adaptation and reduces functional capacity of organ systems.**

Central Nervous System (CNS) Changes

Geriatric animals have a progressive reduction in CNS activity, with reduced amounts of neurotransmitters and receptors. This means **lower doses of sedative, induction, and maintenance drugs** achieve the same level of sedation as expected in a younger animal. Their visual and auditory acuity may be reduced and this needs to be factored into nursing plans. **Thermoregulatory ability is also reduced,** meaning the animal is unable to keep themselves warm, or cool themselves as efficiently as younger animals.

Cardiovascular Changes

Cardiac performance decreases gradually with age; amongst these changes the following may occur:
- **Reduced baroreceptor activity,** which means a slower response to changes in blood pressure.
- **Increased vagal tone,** which leads to a slower heart rate which in turn leads to a reduced cardiac output and slower circulation time.
- Cardiac output becomes preload dependant.
- Animals are more **prone to hypotension or volume overload.**
- Older animals may have **chronic valvular disease** (e.g. mitral valve or tricuspid valve endocardiosis is a disease in dogs characterized by progressive myxomatous degeneration of the atrioventricular valves).
- Autonomic responses are slower.
- Exercise tolerance tests are influenced by other disease processes e.g. arthritis.

Respiratory Changes

The lung loses elasticity with age and the small airways close at a higher lung volume. This tends to lead to **a reduction in the vital capacity** (volume of the lung available for maximal inspiration and exhalation) **and functional residual capacity** (FRC).

There is **an increased risk of atelectasis and ventilation perfusion mismatch** (Figure 5) (where part of the lung receives oxygen without blood flow or blood flow without oxygen). This means there is a greater risk of hypoxia and hypercapnia. There is also an increased incidence of respiratory tract pathologies including those which decrease capacity for diffusion of oxygen from the alveoli into the blood stream.

Chest wall compliance (expandability) is decreased, therefore positive pressure ventilation has a greater effect on venous return. The trachea and larynx are increased in diameter in the geriatric, leading to **increased anatomical dead space.** Protective laryngeal reflexes may be diminished, making **aspiration of any regurgitated material more likely.**

Renal Changes

As an animal ages, there is a reduced number of nephrons (the functional unit in the kidney). In addition, because kidneys receive approximately 25% of cardiac output, renal blood flow also decreases with reduced cardiac output. With age there is a reduction in renal mass. Overall, this means **the animal's kidneys have a reduced ability to correct for fluid, electrolyte, and acid-base derangements,** and therefore fluid therapy is beneficial in geriatric patients.

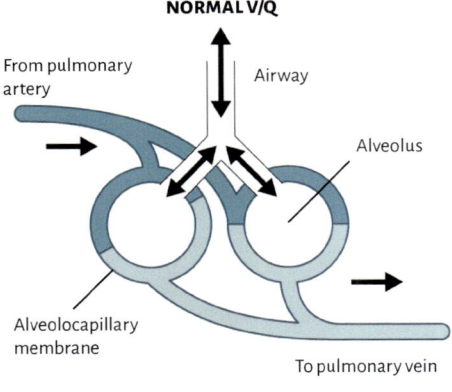
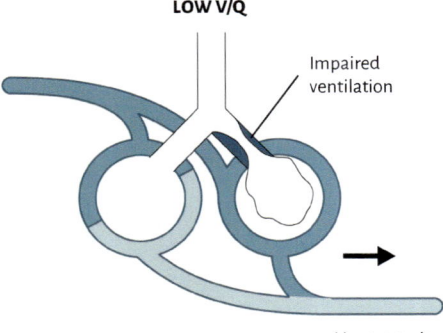
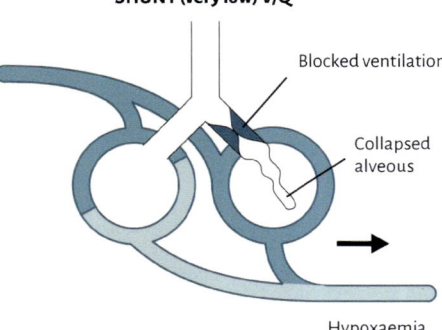
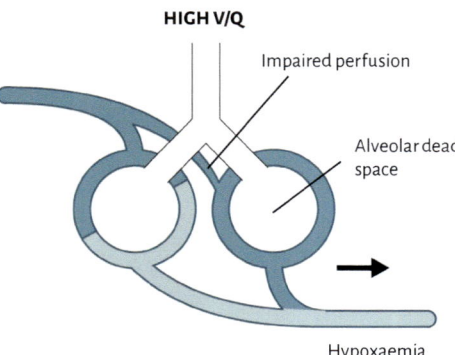

Figure 5. A ventilation perfusion mismatch is where part of the lung receives oxygen without blood flow or blood flow without oxygen. The V/Q ratio refers to the ratio of ventilation to perfusion: V = the flow of air that reaches the alveoli through the alveolar duct; Q = the flow of blood that reaches the alveoli through the capillary beds.

However, they are **more prone to fluid overload,** so any geriatric patient on fluids must be monitored carefully.

Hepatic Changes

The liver also receives 25% of cardiac output and so as cardiac output decreases there is reduced liver blood flow and there is reduced hepatic function leading to **slower drug metabolism.** The liver generates a lot of body heat as an exothermic (a chemical change that is accompanied by a liberation of heat) by product of metabolism. So, if the liver is not functioning well the animal is more **prone to hypothermia.** Geriatric patients also have **reduced albumin formation, which influences binding of protein bound drugs.**

Altered Drug Disposition

- **Less muscle mass:** meaning less mass is available for intramuscular injections.
- **Increased adipose tissue:** some intramuscular injections may end up intrafat if the needle is not long enough.
- **Decreased albumin:** less drug is bound, and more drug is free (active). Induction agents must be given slowly to effect to avoid overdose.
- **Decreased total body water:** lower doses of water soluble drugs (e.g. ketamine) should be used to achieve the same effect as in a younger dog with a lower dose.
- The minimum alveolar concentration **(MAC) values** of volatile agents **decrease** by 30%.
- **Decreased hepatic elimination** means the effect of drugs may be prolonged.
- **Decreased renal reserve,** and so drugs relying on renal clearance have a prolonged duration of action.
- **Extradural (epidural) injections spread more cranially.** When a drug is injected into the epidural space, most spreads cranially but some moves into the epidural cuffs that accompany the spinal nerves as they leave the spinal cord through the foramen between the vertebrae (Figure 6). In geriatric animals, these intervertebral foramina become narrowed, so for the same volume of epidural drug injected, less moves sideways into the epidural cuffs and more moves cranially. Therefore, a reduction in volume is beneficial.

Comorbidities

Some diseases that are more common in older animals include some endocrinopathies:
- canine hypothyroidism
- Cushing's disease
- diabetes mellitus
- feline hyperthyroidism.

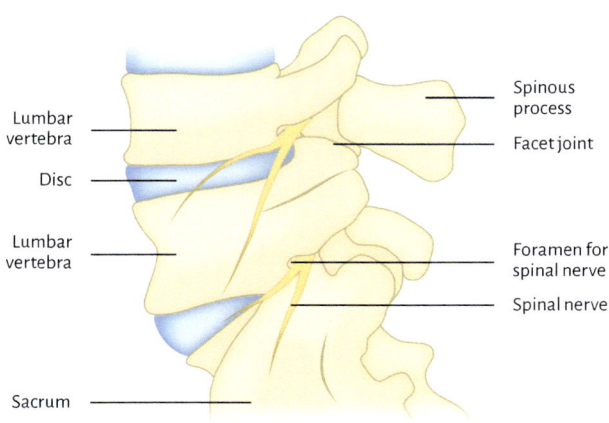

Figure 6. Epidural cuffs accompany the spinal nerves as they leave the spinal cord through the intervertebral foramina.

Other Factors

Stabilisation

If the case is elective and time allows (up to two weeks), **the patient should ideally be stabilised prior to anaesthesia.** This may include dieting (although not crash dieting), administration of antitussives, mucolytics, and/or bronchodilators to produce wide, clean, dry airways if there is a history of airway disease.

If there is evidence of renal disease, dietary protein restriction may be beneficial; whilst low protein diets and multivitamins may be beneficial for patients with hepatic dysfunction.

Patient Handling

Many patients are **visually and/or hearing impaired** and this should be factored into the nursing plan. Geriatric animals may be more anxious and more likely to have more **emergence delirium.** If emergence delirium is observed, it is important to ensure pain is controlled, and additional small doses of sedative drugs can be administered, as well as a member of staff sitting with the animal to provide comfort and reassurance.

Care should be taken positioning elderly patients whilst under anaesthesia; including good padding to prevent inception of decubital ulcers, and gentle positioning of limbs as the animals may be arthritic.

Anaesthesia

Lower doses of preanaesthetic medication are likely to be required, with shorter acting drugs preferred due to the patient's slower metabolism. Benzodiazepines may be sedative in geriatric patients (unlike in younger adult patients when they can cause excitement).

Intravenous access should be secured to allow accurate administration of the induction agent and any further drugs which are required. Fluid therapy is also indicated in the older patient, even if urea is normal on preanaesthetic bloods (75% of nephrons need to be lost before urea starts to increase).

Prior to induction, **the patient should be preoxygenated for three to five minutes via a mask,** unless this stresses the animal. **Short acting induction agents should be used, injected slowly and to effect to avoid overdosing.**

To maintain anaesthesia, **low solubility volatile agents such as isoflurane or sevoflurane are preferred.** Fluid therapy should be continued throughout anaesthesia. These animals may need ventilatory support (if aberrations in SpO_2 or $ETCO_2$ are seen). Again, multi modal analgesia should be administered, but renal function should be checked before administering any NSAIDs.

Given all the changes to the physiology of the body systems, monitoring must be thorough.

Recovery from Anaesthesia

The bladder should be emptied before allowing the patient to recover from anaesthesia. It is important to ensure good analgesia and assess pain before repeat dosing as the duration of action of drugs may be prolonged in geriatric patients. Good nursing care considers anxiety, reduced visual and auditory acuity, to help calm the geriatric patient. Where clinically appropriate, the animal should be returned to their owner, provided they are alert, comfortable, normothermic, and have had sufficient fluid therapy.

ANAESTHESIA FOR LIVER DYSFUNCTION

A major consideration for anaesthesia is how organ dysfunction impacts anaesthetic management of the patient, and how **a poorly considered anaesthetic can make organ dysfunction worse.**

The Effect of Liver Dysfunction on Anaesthesia

The liver has lots of functions, and if it is not working properly, anaesthesia is affected in several ways:
- **Hypoproteinaemia:** the liver is a site of production of several plasma proteins, including albumin, so if protein production is decreased, the following may occur:
    - **Ascites** (fluid accumulation in the abdomen) which can compromise ventilation and reduce the functional residual capacity.
    - **Peripheral oedema,** which can make it difficult to get peripheral intravenous access.
    - Reduced **plasma oncotic pressure.** Oncotic pressure, or colloid osmotic pressure, is a form of osmotic pressure induced by proteins, notably albumin, in the plasma in blood vessels that draws water into the intravascular space from the interstitial space.
    - **Drug binding:** many anaesthetic drugs bind to albumin; the less albumin available, the less drug is bound, and the more is free and active.
- **Anaemia:** there are several reasons a patient with liver dysfunction may be anaemic.
    - **Erythropoietin:** the liver is one of the sites of production of erythropoietin, a hormone that stimulates red blood cell production.
    - **Clotting abnormalities:** blood loss anaemia due to clotting abnormalities which occur due to liver dysfunction.
    - **Oxygen carrying capacity:** moderate to severe anaemia influences the patient's blood-oxygen carrying capacity and anaesthetic requirements (e.g. a lower MAC value of volatile agents).
    - **Detection of cyanosis:** moderate to severe anaemia influences the ability of the human eye to detect cyanosis. Cyanosis (blue discoloration) can be seen by the human eye when the deoxygenated haemoglobin level is above 5 g/dL. However, if the patient is anaemic, their haemoglobin concentration in total (i.e. oxygenated and deoxygenated) may not even reach 5 g/dl, so even if the patient is extremely hypoxic, the person responsible may not be able to see the blue discoloration.
- **Hypocalcemia:** reduction in total serum calcium can result from a decrease in albumin secondary to liver disease. Hypocalcemia predisposes to muscle weakness and arrhythmias. Monitoring the electrocardiogram during anaesthesia and being prepared to ventilate the lungs, in case of ventilatory muscle weakness is also advised.
- **Hypoglycaemia:** the liver is key to glucose homeostasis. Any disruption of its metabolism, structural integrity, or intracellular dynamics may alter the liver's ability to maintain normal glucose homeostasis. Hypoglycaemia causes systemic effects e.g. neuronal damage, immunosuppression, and muscle weakness.
- **Hypothermia:** the liver is one of the main exothermic organs in the body, and therefore the patient may be prone to hypothermia.
- **Clotting disorders:** within the liver, hepatocytes are involved in the synthesis of most blood coagulation factors, which means blood may not clot properly.
- **Hepatic encephalopathy:** a condition that occurs when the liver is too diseased or damaged to properly process ammonia. In this disorder, ammonia builds up in the blood and affects the brain leading to dullness, depression and seizures. This disorder must be corrected before anaesthesia takes place.
- **Bacteraemia:** the liver is also responsible for filtering bacteria out of the blood stream and so there is an increased risk of bacteraemia; therefore thorough skin preparation prior to intravenous catheter placement should be ensured.
- **Jaundice:** some liver diseases produce jaundice (also known as icterus) and this yellow discoloration can obscure other mucous membrane colour, e.g. pallor, cyanosis.
- **Hepatomegaly:** some liver diseases such as hepatitis or hepatic tumours cause hepatomegaly (an enlarged liver). As the liver sits just behind the diaphragm, when enlarged it may limit thoracic excursion and reduce the ability of the animal to ventilate and oxygenate properly, predisposing to hypoxia and hypercapnia.
- **Gastrointestinal disturbances:** some patients with liver disease have gastrointestinal signs e.g. vomiting and diarrhoea. If this is apparent in the patient's history, it is important to check for dehydration, hypovolaemia, electrolyte, and pH abnormalities.
- **Drug biotransformation:** the liver is the site of biotransformation of many anaesthetic drugs, and so their metabolism may be slower, and recovery from anaesthesia delayed. With postoperative analgesia, the administration of top ups based on pain assessment rather than a strict dosing regimen should be considered. It is important to take into account that if prodrugs are given, formation of the active drug is delayed.

The Effect of Anaesthesia on the Liver

If an organ with poor function is challenged with poor perfusion and oxygen delivery, its function will only worsen; so, both aspects require attention during an anaesthetic:
- ensuring adequate oxygenation
- measuring and maintaining blood pressure.

Different drugs have varying effects on hepatic blood flow. **All volatile agents decrease the arterial blood pressure and**

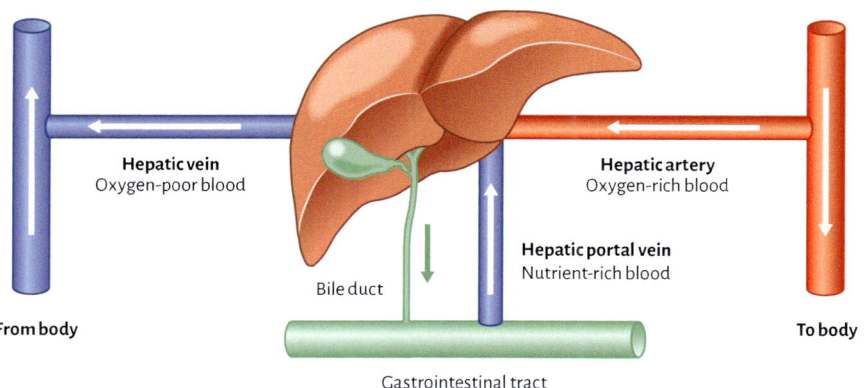

Figure 7. Hepatic blood flow.

therefore portal flow, although there appears to be little difference between sevoflurane, desflurane, or isoflurane. Intravenous anaesthetics have a modest impact on hepatic blood flow; etomidate decreases hepatic blood flow secondary to increased hepatic arterial vascular resistance and reduced blood pressure. **Propofol increases hepatic blood flow,** probably through a significant vasodilator effect. Ketamine has little impact on hepatic blood flow.

Some drugs have reportedly caused hepatotoxic effects, although these are mainly anecdotal. Older volatile agents such as halothane and enflurane were associated with hepatotoxicity in humans. Several case reports have appeared in the literature linking isoflurane/sevoflurane and liver damage but there were mitigating factors including postoperative hypoxia and hypotension, which make a definite link unlikely.

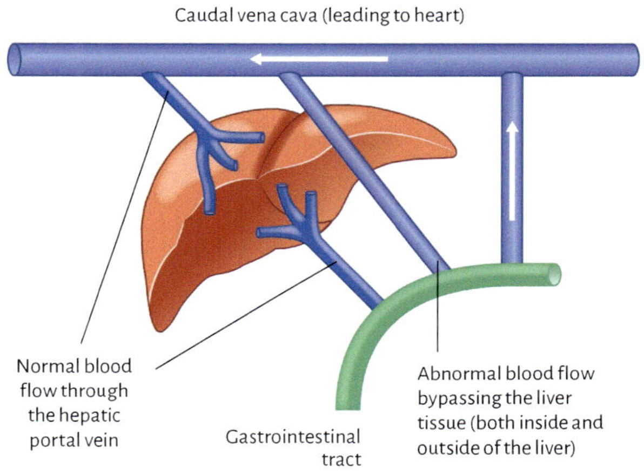

Figure 8. A portosystemic shunt is an aberrant blood vessel, bypassing the liver.

Liver Conditions and Anaesthesia

Portosystemic Shunt Anaesthesia

A portosystemic shunt (PSS) is an abnormal vein which bypasses the liver (shunting) and connects the blood supply returning from the intestines to the vein returning blood to the heart (Figure 8). Portosystemic shunts can either be congenital (present at birth) or acquired (usually through liver disease). **Most of the PSS that present in practice are congenital** and therefore identified when patients are young. Therefore, it is important to address **paediatric considerations,** including maintenance of blood glucose, and temperature regulation.

Often, patients with a PSS **present with neurological signs** due to hepatic encephalopathy from raised blood ammonia.

Medical stabilisation is therefore required (often for some weeks) before attempting sedation or anaesthesia. This **medical stabilisation includes antibiotics, lactulose, and dietary management;** with the aim of decreasing the bacterial population in the intestines and minimizing the production of toxins. Lactulose promotes the expulsion of faecal matter, as well as decreasing the bacterial load in the colon, whilst antibiotics help to eliminate bacteria that promote the formation of toxins.

These patients have **decreased liver function** (usually indicated by increased bile acids). This decreased function means less exothermic activity (predisposing to **hypothermia**) and **slower biotransformation (metabolism) of drugs.** Other haematological and biochemical abnormalities include low plasma proteins including albumin, microcytic normochromic anaemia, and decreased clotting factors.

If possible, **short acting drugs should be used,** those with an alternate route of metabolism, or those that can be antagonised. Benzodiazepines have historically been avoided because endogenous (produced in the body) benzodiazepines are implicated in the pathogenesis of hepatoencephalopathy.

Portosystemic shunts are usually attenuated via a laparotomy approach. There are both intrahepatic and extrahepatic shunts, and the risk of blood loss is greater with intrahepatic shunts as liver dissection is required.

Once the shunt is ligated, certain problems can occur, sometimes during surgery, but also during the recovery phase. When central venous pressure is measured, a significant decrease may be seen after shunt ligation because the same blood volume is now flowing through an additional new capillary network (i.e. the liver). Intestinal perfusion may become compromised at this time.

Complications after surgery include portal hypertension, which can lead to loss of proper blood circulation to abdominal organs and death. Animals may show signs of:
- ascites (fluid distension in the abdomen)
- vomiting
- diarrhoea
- depression
- respiratory distress.

A rare complication is **seizures which are refractory to treatment;** the cause of these seizures is unknown. Seizures may be managed with antiseizure medication e.g. levetiracetam.

Renal Dysfunction and Anaesthesia

The kidneys are one of the hardest working organs in the body with their functions including **urine production, blood pressure and osmolarity regulation, hormone secretion, and acid-base balance.** Therefore, if the kidneys are not functioning properly, the effects are wide ranging.

Preanaesthetic blood tests and urine specific gravity (USG) results help indicate whether azotaemia (an increase in urea +/- creatinine) is prerenal, renal, or postrenal.

Prerenal azotaemia is due to circulatory disturbances which decrease renal blood flow such as **dehydration or hypovolaemia.** Prerenal azotaemia is usually distinguished from renal azotaemia by clinical signs (evidence of dehydration or hypovolaemia) and urinalysis (urine is adequately concentrated, i.e. >1.030 in the dog, >1.035 in the cat), but there is usually no evidence of renal tubule dysfunction (such as excessive proteinuria).

Renal azotaemia is when more than 75% of the nephrons (functional unit of the kidney) **are non-functional.** Renal azotaemia may be due to primary intrinsic renal disease (glomerulonephritis, ethylene glycol toxicity) or renal injury which occurs secondary to renal ischaemia (such as from prerenal causes), or urinary tract obstruction (postrenal azotaemia). **Isosthenuria** (where the specific gravity is no different to that of plasma, USG 1.008–1.012) is common in renal azotaemia. Other evidence of renal tubular dysfunction in urinalysis includes excessive proteinuria, casts, and glucosuria without hyperglycaemia.

Postrenal azotaemia results from obstruction or rupture of urinary outflow tracts. Urine specific gravity results are quite variable, so it is best to diagnose these based on clinical signs.

These types of renal failure are not mutually exclusive, e.g. a dog with urethral obstruction has postrenal azotaemia as they are unable to void urine, however the back pressure onto the kidneys can cause renal failure, and the animal can develop prerenal failure if they become dehydrated through vomiting and poor oral intake. (Figure 9).

Acute Renal Failure

Ideally anaesthesia should not be performed on an animal with acute renal failure as anaesthesia may further negatively

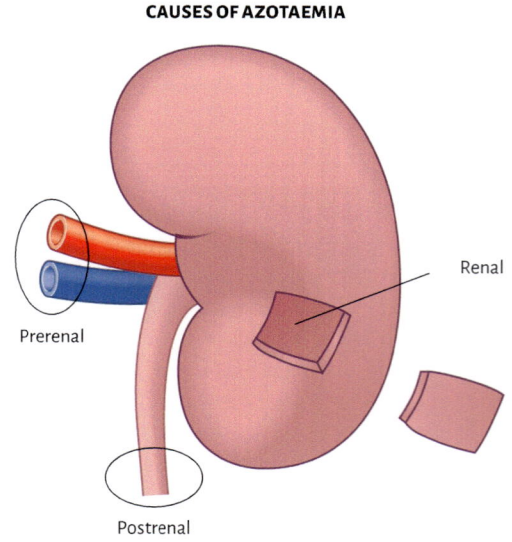

Figure 9. Prerenal, renal and postrenal failure.

impact the kidneys, but sometimes anaesthesia is needed to treat the cause of the acute renal failure. These are usually obstructive postrenal failure cases such as urethral obstruction or ruptured bladders.

Animals presenting with renal failure may exhibit signs of the following:
— **Dehydration** and potential hypovolaemia if dehydration is severe; from fluid shifts, third space losses (e.g. uroabdomen), decreased oral intake of water and food, gastrointestinal losses such as vomiting. Hydration and volume status should be assessed and corrected with fluid therapy before anaesthesia.
— **Electrolyte imbalances** and acid-base imbalances.
— **Uraemia** indicates that urea (a nitrogenous waste product usually excreted by the kidneys) is building up in the blood stream. This can cause nausea and vomiting, dullness and depression, seizures, hypothermia, and a decreased metabolic rate. Generally, **lower doses of sedatives and induction agents are required** because of central nervous system depression. The patient's body temperature should be monitored and warming undertaken if needed. Fluid therapy administration will decrease blood levels of urea.
— **Pain,** especially postrenal failure cases, where the bladder, or urethra are distended, as this produces visceral pain. Uroabdomen causes peritonitis which is also painful.

In acute renal failure, potassium ions and hydrogen ions which are usually excreted in the urine, are retained. Hydrogen ions are acidic and acidaemia develops if they cannot be excreted in the urine and accumulate in the blood stream. As it is of metabolic origin, it is termed **metabolic acidosis.** (See figure 10 to check the electrolyte secretion in the kidneys).

If there is a **primary acid-base derangement** (such as metabolic acidosis) the body tries to compensate using the other body system (in this case the respiratory system). Carbon dioxide is an acidic gas and therefore the patient breaths faster to increase elimination.

Potassium is mainly an intracellular ion, but once outside cells it can be problematic. **Hyperkalaemia is** where serum potassium levels increase above the normal range (3.5–5.5 mmol/l). Hyperkalaemia occurs because the only route of excretion of potassium from the body is via the urine, so **if urine cannot be voided potassium accumulates.** Hyperkalaemia causes muscle weakness, and neurological abnormalities, but of more concern to the anaesthetist is the possibility of **dysrhythmias.** Typical dysrhythmias include bradycardia, spiky T waves, flattened or lost P waves, and QRS complexes which look like they have been picked up at each end and pulled apart. (Figure 11).

Metabolic acidosis worsens hyperkalaemia because as hydrogen ions move into cells, potassium ions are pushed out. (Figure 12).

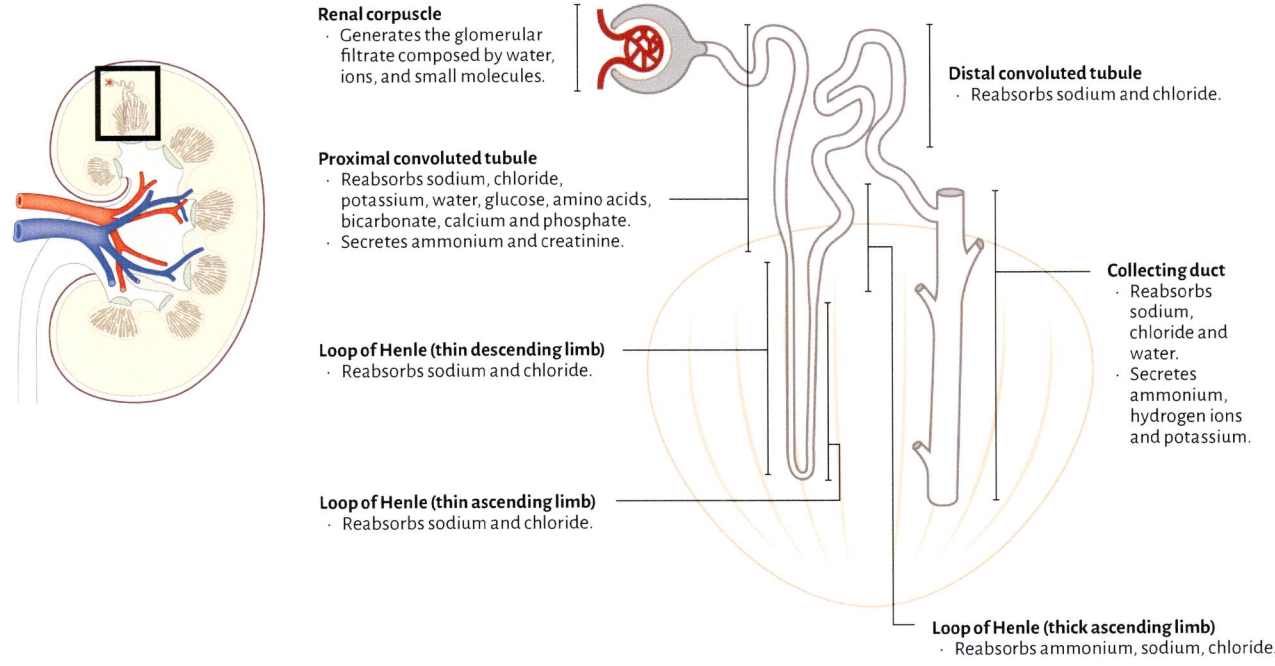

Figure 10. Electrolyte secretion in the kidney.

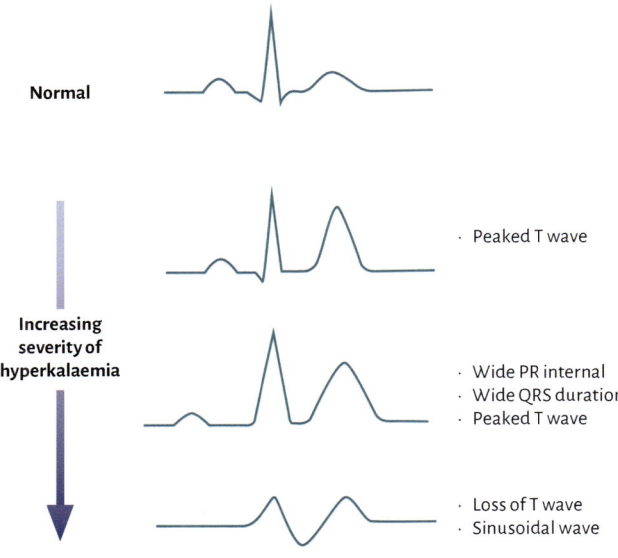

Figure 11. Bradyarhythmias commonly associated with hyperkalaemia.

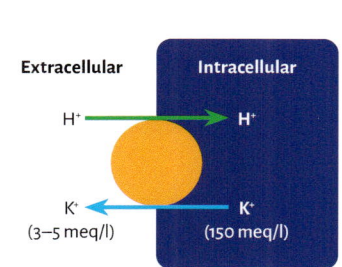

Figure 12. The effect of acidosis on serum potassium.

Stabilisation

Dehydration, hypovolaemia, uraemia, metabolic acidosis and hyperkalaemia are all improved with fluid therapy. Preanaesthesic boluses can be used until the patient is sufficiently stabilised for anaesthesia. Guidelines released by the American Animal Hospital Association (Grubb et al., 2020) suggest **animals should not be anaesthetised until pH has improved to at least >7.2, and potassium <6 mmol/l** (although ideally, they should be back to normal). During anaesthesia, fluid administration should be continued to support blood pressure, as well as postanaesthesia for at least 24 hours if any obstruction has been relieved as there is usually 24 hours' worth of postobstruction diuresis.

A good choice of isotonic crystalloids is either **0.9% NaCl or Hartmann's solution (Lactated Ringers).** Acetated Ringers, available in some countries, has a similar composition to Hartmann's solution but with acetate rather than lactate.

Many people are concerned about using Hartmann's in these cases because Hartmanns solution contains potassium, and the patients are already hyperkalaemic. However, the level of potassium in the fluid is low, and administering a crystalloid fluid dilutes the potassium. Also, as it is an alkalinising solution (because of the lactate), the pH is brought back up, which encourages the potassium to go back into the cells (where it is safely locked away) and actually reduces potassium serum concentrations.

Some vets feel concerned about giving fluid therapy to an animal with obstructive renal disease in case of bladder rupture. These animals are probably dehydrated and hypovolaemic so renal blood flow, and therefore glomerular filtration rate, is lower. In addition, back pressure from the obstruction reduces the impetus to produce urine, so **until the blockage is relieved little urine is produced.**

If fluid therapy boluses are insufficient to bring potassium down to safe levels for anaesthesia, then a further option aims to shift the potassium back into cells:
- **Glucose (+/- insulin)** can be used to shift potassium back into the cell via a cotransporter system as glucose is taken up. (Figure 13).
- If this is unsuccessful, the use of **calcium compounds** can cause a temporary stabilisation of the cardiac action potential, although this effect is only transient and does not affect serum potassium levels.

Intravenous fluid therapy, with Hartmann's solution can improve metabolic acidosis due to the lactate it contains. In severe situations, **sodium bicarbonate** can be infused slowly (ensuring it is not mixed with a calcium containing solution otherwise precipitation occurs which may potentially block the catheter), however it can produce multiple side effects including hypernatraemia, hypocalcemia, hypokalaemia, and carbon dioxide production, so it is usually reserved unless the base excess is more negative than -10 mmol/l.

In addition to stabilising the electrolyte and acid-base disorders, the patient should be provided with **adequate pain relief,** (usually opioid based) and their body temperature maintained.

Chronic Renal Failure and Anaesthesia

Animals with chronic renal disease often have clinical changes that affect anaesthesia. Many of these are **evident on haematological or biochemical blood panels** and therefore it

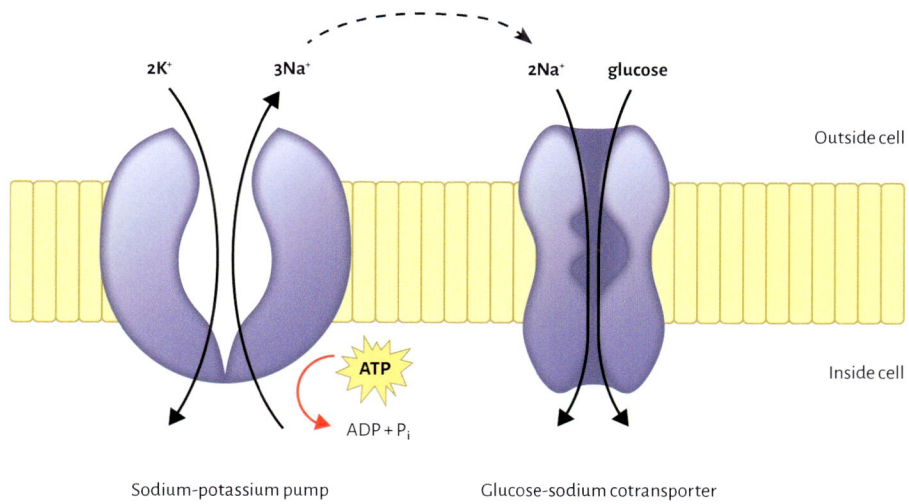

Figure 13. Glucose potassium cotransporter.

is easy to check the test results to see which clinical sequelae are relevant in each case.

- **Anaemia:** when kidneys are diseased or damaged, they do not make enough erythropoietin (a hormone that stimulates bone marrow to make red blood cells) and as a result the patient may be anaemic (Figure 14). In addition, high levels of urea suppress bone marrow production of red blood cells, and increase the fragility of red bloods cells, limiting their life span. Uraemia can also cause blood loss anaemia through gastrointestinal ulceration. This alters the animal's oxygen carrying capacity.
- **Hypoalbuminaemia** (where a protein losing nephropathy is present). Hypoalbuminaemia means more drug is free and active and therefore animals are at a higher risk of overdose.
- **Calcium phosphorus derangements** may predispose to arrhythmias.
- **Hypertension:** renal disease, especially chronic kidney disease (CKD), is the most common cause of hypertension in dogs and cats. The renin angiotensin aldosterone system (RAAS) (a hormone system within the body that is essential for the regulation of blood pressure and fluid balance) is regulated by the rate of renal blood flow and is therefore stimulated in CKD, producing hypertension. Chronic hypertension may lead to cardiomegaly and ventricular hypertrophy.
- **Bleeding tendencies** may occur due to intrinsic platelet defects, decreased platelet aggregation and impaired platelet adhesiveness; therefore, if from the history there is suspicion of coagulopathies, clotting times should be checked before large bore vessels are cannulated or surgery performed.

CKD: ERYTHROPOIESIS DISRUPTED FEEDBACK LOOP

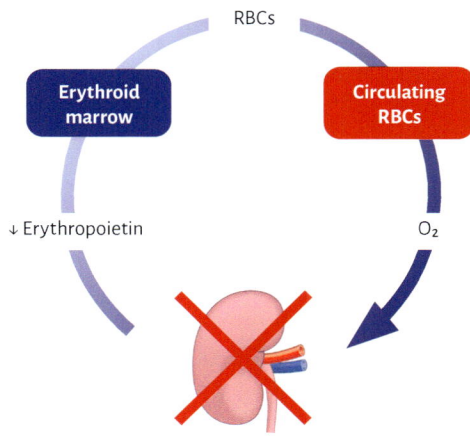

Figure 14. Regulation of erythropoiesis. Adapted from Erslev and Beutler. In: Williams' Hematology, 5th ed. 1995:425–441.

- **Acid-base abnormalities:** uraemia may cause nausea and vomiting which predisposes to acid-base abnormalities and dehydration.
- **Immunosuppression:** high levels of urea suppress bone marrow function and therefore immunosuppression; care should therefore be taken with skin preparation for catheters and surgeries.
- **Decreased drug clearance:** there is decreased renal clearance of some drugs, especially those with active metabolites. In anaesthesia, examples of these drugs include some opioids and some neuromuscular blockers.

Deleterious Effects of Anaesthesia on the Kidneys

Anaesthesia and certain drugs can be detrimental to kidney function, and in a patient with compromised renal function it is important to minimise or prevent further damage. Therefore, the main aims during anaesthesia (whether the patient has acute or chronic renal failure) are to **maintain renal blood flow and oxygenation of the renal tissue.**

There are several different mechanisms by which anaesthesia can alter renal perfusion, which matters because decreasing perfusion of an already dysfunctional organ is likely to make matters worse.

Renal blood flow is autoregulated across a bandwidth (usually 60–160 mmHg) of mean arterial pressure, it does not matter where within that range the blood pressure lies, the renal blood flow stays the same (Figure 15). Ideally an animal's arterial blood pressure should be kept within this bandwidth during anaesthesia. However, if an animal suffers from chronic hypertension, in this circumstance the aim must be to maintain blood pressure within the higher end of the bandwidth range.

Getting the depth of anaesthesia correct is very important. If the patient is too deeply anaesthetised, blood pressure may fall below the autoregulation bandwidth which reduces renal blood flow. However, if the patient it too light and they respond to nociception, the stimulation of the sympathetic nervous system causes vasoconstriction of the renal blood vessels, again affecting blood flow.

The kidneys rely on certain **prostaglandins such as PGI2 and PGE2** (amongst other substances) to maintain renal blood flow at times of low blood pressure. These prostaglandins are blocked by non-steroidal anti-inflammatory drugs (NSAIDs) and therefore during anaesthesia normotension cannot be guaranteed and **NSAIDs should not be used.**

There is evidence in cats with stable IRIS stage 2 and stage 3 renal failure (http://www.iris-kidney.com/pdf/IRIS_Staging_of_CKD_modified_2019.pdf), that low dose meloxicam or robenocoxib can be used long term for osteoarthritis pain without worsening renal disease, although a more recent prospective study suggested that cats receiving meloxicam had increased proteinuria six months into treatment (KuKanich et al., 2021). Even if these cats are on long term NSAIDs, these should be withheld around the time of anaesthesia.

Other than NSAIDs, the other class of drugs with the **potential for nephrotoxicity are volatile agents.** Two older agents, **methoxyflurane and enflurane** have been shown to be nephrotoxic because of a fluoride ion they yield. Metabolism of sevoflurane also yields fluoride, however, studies in animals and humans have not shown evidence of fluoride-induced nephrotoxicity, despite serum fluoride concentrations in this range that cause nephrotoxicity from other drugs. Sevoflurane does also however, produce a vinyl ether called Compound A which is produced when it is used in rebreathing systems during low flow anaesthesia. Compound A has been implicated in causing renal dysfunction in rats. In all other veterinary species, Compound A should cause few problems, however sevoflurane manufacturers suggest the volatile agents should not be used at low flows in circle systems for long periods of time.

Anaesthesia for Endocrinopathies

The endocrine system plays a major role in the maintenance of the body's internal environment. Alterations in function of the endocrine system can alter the response of the patient to anaesthesia. The **endocrine system consists of different glands which secrete hormones into the blood stream, which affect the activity of cells at another site in the body.** Therefore, this system is integral to homeostasis (i.e. regulation of a range of body system functions). Different pathophysiological changes are produced depending on what endocrine organ is affected.

Diabetes Mellitus

Diabetes mellitus is a chronic disorder of carbohydrate metabolism resulting from absolute or relative deficiency of insulin. Insulin is responsible for inhibition of gluconeogenesis

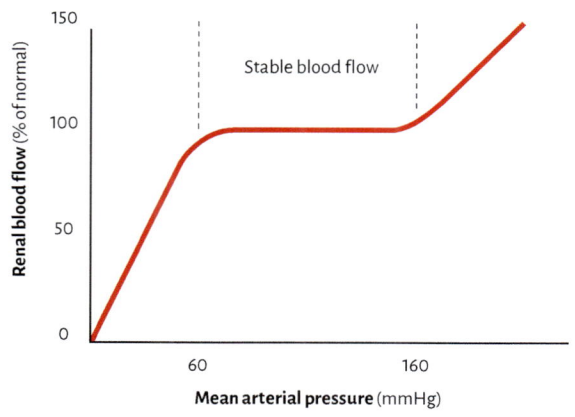

Figure 15. Renal blood flow is autoregulated over a range of blood pressures.

(production of glucose) and stimulation of glucose uptake into cells. Animals with unstable diabetes are usually polyphagic, polyuric, polydipsic, and lose weight.

Many diabetic patients are sedated or anaesthetised for reasons unrelated to their condition (e.g. cruciate rupture). However, there are a few situations when anaesthesia is required to treat or investigate conditions associated with diabetes, for example:
- **Ovariohysterectomy:** entire female dogs with diabetes mellitus tend to destabilise during oestrus or pregnancy due to the production of progesterone, therefore, ovariohysterectomy is often performed in diabetic bitches to aid stabilisation.
- **Phaecoemulsion:** animals with diabetes can develop diabetic cataracts due to sorbitol deposition in the lens. Phaecoemulsification for the treatment of cataracts (where the lens is emulsified and then aspirated from the eye) requires general anaesthesia.
- **Abdominal ultrasound:** may be required to investigate why a patient's diabetes is poorly controlled and sedation may be required to facilitate this.

Normal blood glucose is approximately 3–7 mmol/l. Both hyperglycaemia and hypoglycaemia can occur in a diabetic patient, which is dangerous if this occurs under anaesthesia. Hyperglycaemia causes glucosuria (if the blood glucose goes over the renal threshold) causing osmotic diuresis and dehydration. Severe hyperglycaemia can lead to coma, through dehydration, lactic acidosis, and hyperosmolality. Hypoglycaemia produces neurological damage (blood glucose <2.7 mmol/l).

Diabetic patients may also have chronic organ dysfunction. The renal system can suffer from diabetic nephropathy, prerenal azotaemia, and urinary tract infections; the liver can be affected by lipidosis, impaired function, or hepatomegaly. There are also electrolyte imbalances where total body stores of potassium and sodium become depleted.

Diabetic patients may be **immunosuppressed** because of the negative effects of elevated blood sugars on the immune system. Their loss of body and muscle mass can influence drug distribution and an increased potential for heat loss.

> The aims of anaesthesia for a diabetic patient are:
> - Maintain glucose within an appropriate range to prevent ketoacidosis (a possibility with hyperglycaemia) and neurological damage (a possibility with hypoglycaemia).
> - Maintain pH and electrolytes.
> - Rapid return to eating and drinking postoperatively.
> - Prevent sepsis.

Preoperatively, the patient should ideally be stabilised with insulin, and their electrolyte and acid-base status checked and corrected where necessary. It is important to know the patient's normal insulin and feeding regime. Unfortunately, there is some disruption to this routine due to the need for starvation for anaesthesia.

The American Animal Hospital Guidelines (Grubb et al., 2020) suggests the following **starvation and insulin protocol for a diabetic patient:**
- The procedure should be performed first on the day's list.
- The patient should be given a half-portion of their normal food 2–4 hours before anaesthesia and then starved.
- Water should be offered until the time of preanaesthetic medication.
- A half-dose of insulin should be given 2–4 hours before anaesthesia.

This is a generic protocol and does not take into account individual animal's blood glucose levels.

An alternative more individualised approach would be to starve from midnight, feed no breakfast, and then the morning of anaesthesia check blood glucose levels and administer the appropriate dose of insulin:
- blood glucose <6 mmol/l: no insulin given
- blood glucose 6–15 mmol/l: half-dose of insulin given
- blood glucose >15 mmol/l: full-dose of insulin given.

Again, the aim should be to undertake the anaesthetic first on the list, so the animal can feed before the nadir (the lowest point of the blood glucose curve). (Figure 16).

Blood glucose should be checked prior to induction and then every 15–30 minutes throughout the anaesthetic; this can be via blood draw, indwelling catheter, or pinprick samples.

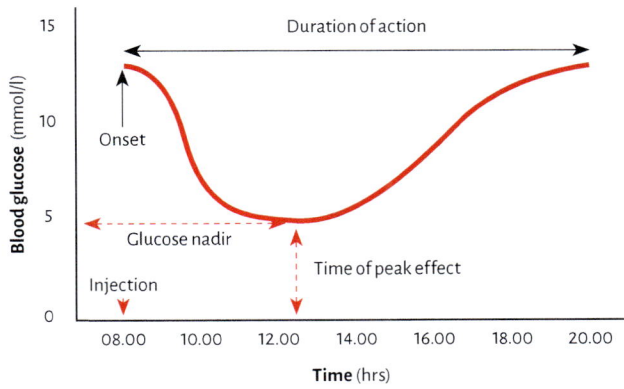

Figure 16. The nadir is the lowest point on the blood glucose curve after insulin administration.

If blood glucose levels are fluctuating or low normal, then sampling should be more frequent. When sampling via a catheter, it should be ensured that it is not used to give glucose containing fluids.

If the blood glucose decreases below 3 mmol/l, 0.25–0.5 g/kg glucose slow IV should be administered. **Glucose stock solution is hypertonic and therefore must be diluted with a crystalloid to avoid thrombophlebitis.** If blood glucose becomes excessively high, soluble insulin (0.1 IU/kg/hr) **intramuscularly** should be administered, to decrease the blood glucose concentration.

Postoperative nausea may delay a return to feeding, so administering **an antiemetic such as maropitant** should be considered. Likewise, over sedating with premedication should be avoided as the patient needs to recover from anaesthesia quickly to eat; **an opioid +/- low dose acepromazine** is an appropriate choice of premedication. α-2 adrenergic agonists block insulin and can disrupt glucose control and should be taken into account if these drugs are used in the anaesthetic protocol. The benefit of an α-2 adrenergic agonist is that they can be antagonised, which hastens recovery from anaesthesia.

Short acting drugs for anaesthetic induction should be used along with low solubility volatile agents for maintenance so that the patient can recover from anaesthesia quickly.

Multimodal analgesia is appropriate, especially as an animal in pain is unlikely to eat. Before administering a non-steroidal anti-inflammatory drug, the veterinary surgeon should ensure the patient is not suffering from diabetic nephropathy or prerenal azotaemia. **Fluid therapy should be administered** at 5 ml/kg/hr (dogs) and 3 ml/kg/hr (cats), which is reduced by 25% every hour of anaesthesia until the patient's maintenance rate is reached.

If using an individualised recovery protocol, as soon as animal can sit up and swallow a small test feed should be offered. If the patient eats and does not vomit, then the animal's usual breakfast should be offered. If the breakfast is eaten, the remainder of the insulin (which had not been given that morning) should be administered. Ideally, a return to the animal's normal insulin and feeding routine should be implemented as soon as possible. Sometimes, animals will not eat their breakfast and, in this situation, blood glucose should be monitored over the remainder of the day and further insulin given if blood glucose concentrations start to increase significantly.

Insulinomas

Insulinomas are malignant functional pancreatic tumours of the beta (β) cells, which retain the ability to produce and secrete insulin. Insulinomas are the most common pancreatic neuroendocrine tumour in **dogs**, which induce a variety of clinical signs that result from **hypoglycaemia and secondary neurological effects** (including collapse and seizures) to adrenergic effects from catecholamine release including anxiety. They are rarely reported in cats.

Anaesthesia for insulinoma resection is of increased risk for the patient, primarily due to the **risks of developing hypoglycaemia** under anaesthesia when CNS signs are less noticeable, in addition to the high sympathetic tone and possibility of arrhythmias (as catecholamines are counter regulatory to insulin).

These cases require thorough preoperative assessment, including blood biochemistry and electrolyte evaluation, particularly potassium. Prolonged preanaesthetic starvation should not be undertaken in these patients due to the risk of development of hypoglycaemia. Removing food at midnight with a small calorie dense meal at 4 am is one option, as is administering a glucose containing solution intravenously during the starvation time. Blood glucose should be checked before preanaesthetic medication, and if levels are low then it should be corrected with intravenous glucose before inducing anaesthesia. It is recommended that blood samples are taken every **fifteen minutes during anaesthesia,** and more regularly when the pancreas is handled, as this may cause additional release of insulin into the blood stream. The aim should be to maintain blood glucose within the range of 3–7 mmol/l. It is recommended that multiparameter monitoring (including electrocardiogram (ECG), and blood pressure) is performed in addition to regular blood glucose assessment.

Laparotomy is required to resect the tumour, with **multimodal analgesia** as part of the anaesthesia plan. **Preanaesthetic medication should include opioid analgesia plus a low dose of either an α-2 adrenergic agonist or acepromazine.** The choice between these agents depends on the animal's temperament and medical history. Guedes & Rude (2013) compared acepromazine and morphine with medetomidine and morphine preanaesthetic medication in dogs undergoing surgery to remove insulinomas. They found that medetomidine preanaesthetic medication significantly decreased plasma insulin concentrations and increased plasma glucose concentrations and the intraoperative glucose administration rate was significantly less in the animals that received medetomidine compared to those that did not. This stems from α-2 adrenergic agonists action of blocking insulin. The authors concluded these findings support the judicious use of medetomidine at low doses (the dose used in this study was 5 µg/kg intramuscularly) as an adjunct to the anaesthetic management of dogs with insulinoma. Additional analgesic techniques could include epidural analgesia, and lidocaine continuous rate infusions.

Alfaxalone or propofol can be used to induce anaesthesia. There have been occasional reports of pancreatitis following propofol administration in people due to the high lipid content of the drug, and this could be a potential reason to choose alfaxalone over propofol in these cases. The risk of pancreatitis following surgery is fairly high due to handling of the pancreas and should be monitored for (in addition to signs of diabetes mellitus) postoperatively.

Hypoadrenocorticism (Addison's disease)

Hypoadrenocorticism is characterised by glucocorticoid and/or mineralocorticoid deficiency due to a failure of the adrenal glands. The paired adrenal glands have an outer cortex and inner medulla. The cortex is composed of a further three layers, each responsible for secreting different substances:
- **outer zona glomerulosa:** production of mineralocorticoids (e.g. aldosterone)
- **middle zona fasciculata:** production of glucocorticoids (e.g. cortisol)
- **inner zona reticularis:** production of sex hormones (e.g. androgens and oestrogens).

Of these, glucocorticoids and mineralocorticoids in abnormal amounts have the potential to have an impact on anaesthesia.

Glucocorticoids such as cortisol are vital for:
- gluconeogenesis
- fat and protein metabolism
- immunity
- blood pressure regulation
- counteracting the effects of stress.

When planning an anaesthetic for a patient with hypoadrenocorticism, it is important to understand the pathophysiology of the disease to be able to adapt the plan accordingly.

Dogs deficient in mineralocorticoids may exhibit the following clinical signs:
- hyperkalaemia
- hyponatraemia
- azotaemia
- hypovolaemia/dehydration
- bradycardia, due to the hyperkalaemia (despite being hypovolaemic).

Dogs deficient in glucocorticoids usually have vague clinical signs such as:
- lethargy/weakness
- polyuria/polydipsia
- vomiting/diarrhoea
- abdominal pain
- weight loss.

Depending on the severity of the gastrointestinal signs, anaemia, hypoalbuminaemia, or metabolic acidosis may also be present.

The clinical presentation of a case of hypoadrenocorticism is often **waxing and waning,** with worsening illness in times of stress. However, a dog may be presented in an **Addisonian crisis where there is a life threatening episode** due to the combined hormone deficiencies. In these situations, treatment with aggressive intravenous fluid therapy with either normal saline or Hartmann's solution is used to restore fluid volume, improve renal perfusion, and decrease potassium concentrations.

Replacement of glucocorticoids (e.g. IV dexamethasone) and potentially **mineralocorticoids** in the acute setting can improve clinical signs and also any abnormalities in the clinical pathology results. Long term management of Addisonian patients requires daily replacement of either/and mineralocorticoids or glucocorticoids.

Addison's is a disease that rarely requires anaesthesia for treatment but it may be necessary to perform diagnostic tests to investigate the endocrinopathy. More commonly Addisonian patients are anaesthetised for a reason completely unrelated to their endocrinopathy.

Patients with hypoadrenocorticism should not be anaesthetised whilst experiencing an Addisonian crisis, as this places the patient at high risk of cardiovascular collapse due to the decreased venous return, peripheral vasoconstriction, and decreased cardiac output and contractility. Instead, they should be stabilised and well controlled with medication before attempting anaesthesia.

Clinical signs associated with hypoadrenocorticism worsen during times of stress as glucocorticoids are vital in counteracting the effects of stress. When planning an anaesthetic, care should be taken to **identify stressors and minimise them.** Surgical stress is not an all or nothing phenomenon, and the level of stress experienced is patient specific, combined with surgical, and anaesthetic factors.

Any abnormalities in potassium or sodium serum concentrations or acid-base abnormalities should be corrected before anaesthesia. In the first instance, fluid therapy should be administered with a balanced electrolyte solution. Abnormal sodium serum concentrations should not be corrected any faster than 0.5 mmol/hr to avoid demyelinating parts of the brain. Hartmann's solution or normal saline can be used to aid in stabilisation.

Usual morning doses of glucocorticoid and/or mineralocorticoid medication should be administered and sufficient time allowed for absorption if given orally.

Anaesthesia +/- surgery procedures are stressors in themselves and the latter can increase cortisol levels by 5–10 times (Sinclair, 2012). For this reason, in addition to the long term glucocorticoid supplementation, **additional steroid should be given in the perianaesthetic period.**

Therapeutic glucocorticoids for supplementation include hydrocortisone (structurally identical to cortisol) and related synthetics, dexamethasone and prednisolone. There are a variety of protocols for supplementation of steroids in the perianaesthetic period for dogs. The veterinary surgeon's decision should be based on the anticipated level of stress and whether mineralocorticoid activity is required.

Steroid supplementation may need to continue for several days after more stressful procedures. In all cases, long term mineralocorticoid and glucocorticoid medication should be continued as per the usual dosing schedule.

Anaesthetic Protocol

When the patient is fully stabilised, the choice of general anaesthetic is based on the procedure and preanaesthetic assessment of the patient (including their signalment).

High doses of vasodilatory drugs such as acepromazine should be avoided due to the long duration of vasodilation produced, which may exacerbate hypotension during an adrenal crisis.

Propofol or alfaxalone should be administered intravenously to effect, as appropriate choices for anaesthetic induction. Etomidate is an induction agent known for preserving cardiovascular stability. However, after injection it rapidly suppresses cortisol production by inhibiting 11-β-hydroxylase, a final step catalyst in cortisol biosynthesis. Although steroids are exogenously supplemented in Addisonian patients, any residual endogenous cortisol production is suppressed and therefore the author does not recommend this drug in these patients.

Addisonian patients are predisposed to hypoventilation and therefore it is appropriate to **choose a breathing system which is appropriate for positive pressure ventilation.**

A pre-emptive, multimodal analgesic approach, incorporating a local anaesthetic technique, if at all possible, is recommended. The only class of analgesics which **are contraindicated in these patients are non-steroidal anti-inflammatory drugs (NSAIDs).** This is because of the concurrent administration of steroids, and the potential for hypotensive episodes under anaesthesia.

If the patient's serum electrolyte concentrations are within normal limits, fluid therapy during anaesthesia with a balanced polyelectrolyte solution such as Hartmann's is warranted.

Capnography is valuable to identify hypoventilation and as an early indicator of cardiac insufficiency. Also, an ECG is appropriate to monitor for bradydysrrythmias which may occur due to changing electrolyte serum concentrations during anaesthesia. **Monitoring blood pressure,** directly or indirectly, identifies hypotension which is potentially suggestive of an adrenal crisis. These monitors should be used **in addition to pulse oximetry and routine manual monitoring.**

When there is an insufficient cortisol response to surgical or anaesthetic stress, there is a progressive loss of vasomotor tone and impaired α-adrenergic responses to noradrenaline. If the stressors continue, this **may lead to hypotension and eventually shock.** Often this hypotension is not responsive to fluid therapy boluses. In such a case, intervention with 2–4 mg/kg hydrocortisone IV or 5–10 mg/kg prednisolone IV has been suggested (Sinclair, 2012).

Hyperadrenocorticism (Cushing's disease)

This disease involves the overproduction of cortisol; either by an adrenal gland or pituitary gland tumour (the latter being a gland in the brain that produces ACTH, which in turn makes the adrenal glands produce cortisol). (Figure 17).

Cortisol is a steroid hormone that regulates a wide range of processes throughout the body, including metabolism and the immune response. It also has **an important role in helping the body respond to stress.** The clinical signs associated with too much cortisol in the blood stream are polyuria/polydipsia, polyphagia, pendulous abdomen, hepatomegaly, muscle weakness, and thinned skin.

Cushing's disease mainly affects dogs, is uncommon in cats, and is often associated with older age. Whilst hypoadrenocorticism (Addison's) is associated with hypovolaemia, hyperadrenocorticism tends to produce **hypervolaemia and fluid retention.**

Patients with Cushing's disease can have heart conditions due to the hypertension secondary to hypervolemia. This causes an increase in the workload of the myocardium and results in **myocardial hypertrophy.** This may be complicated by older animals having chronic valvular disease.

The **muscle weakness** that is of most concern to the anaesthetist is that associated with the **ventilatory muscles.** In addition to **hepatomegaly** limiting thoracic excursion, positive pressure ventilation may be required. Dogs with Cushing's may have **an increased risk of catheter infections** because of the effects of high levels of cortisol suppressing the immune system.

– steroids need supplementing during anaesthesia and for several days post operatively to **avoid an Addisonian crisis.** The opposite adrenal gland has suppressed cortisol production and it takes time for it to become fully functional again.

If a pituitary gland tumour is the reason for the hyperadrenocorticism, it may be resected via a hypophysectomy (Figure 18), which is a surgical approach through the soft palate. Anaesthetic considerations include:
- sharing an airway with the surgeon
- airway protection
- a potential for major blood loss
- cardiovascular and respiratory responses to tumour manipulation.

Following hypophysectomy, hormone replacement therapy consists of lifelong administration of cortisone acetate and thyroxine and temporary administration of desmopressin, a synthetic vasopressin analogue.

Hypothyroidism

Hypothyroidism is a reduced function of the thyroid gland. This endocrinopathy is very rare in cats, and most patients that present with hypothyroidism are dogs.

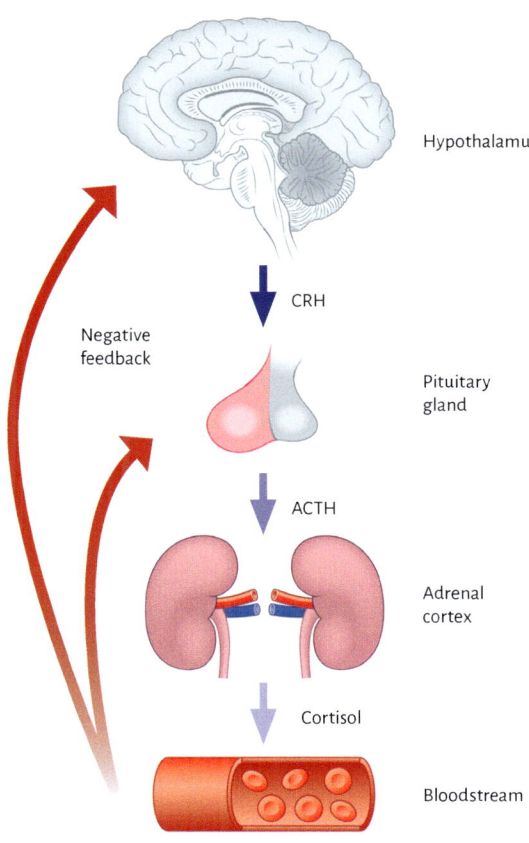

Figure 17. Hypothalamic pituitary adrenal axis.

Therefore, strict asepsis must be used when obtaining intravenous access. Placement of catheters may be more difficult as skin thickness is abnormal and veins fragile.

As with any disease of the endocrine system, unnecessary stressors should be avoided. Sedation or anaesthesia of a Cushing's patient is often for an unrelated reason, but sometimes sedation is required for an abdominal ultrasound as part of the diagnostic tests to investigate the disease. There are also surgical options to remove the tumours that produce the excessive cortisol which require carefully planned anaesthesia, and excellent surgical and intensive care facilities.

When an adrenal mass is identified as the cause, adrenalectomy may be required. Considerations for this anaesthetic are:
- excellent **muscle relaxation** as the adrenal glands are located deep within the abdomen;
- there is a potential of **major blood loss** as adrenal masses tend to invade the vena cava. The patient should be blood typed before anaesthesia and blood products should be available. Arterial blood pressure is the most accurate method of monitoring blood pressure, especially if there is major blood loss (which should also be monitored); and

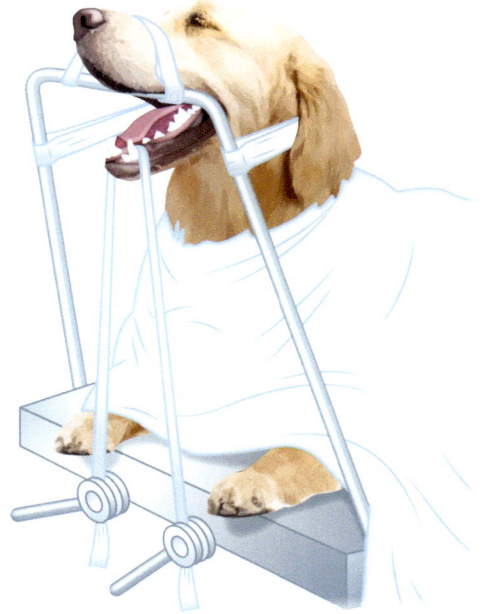

Figure 18. Surgical set up for hypophysectomy.

The hypothalamus regulates the secretion of thyroid hormone (Figure 19). The hypothalamus secretes thyrotropin releasing hormone (TRH), which acts on the pituitary gland by stimulating it to secrete thyroid stimulating hormone (TSH), which in turn, acts on the thyroid gland by stimulating it to secrete T3 and T4. Thyroid hormones predominantly affect the animal's metabolic rate.

Ideally, **hypothyroidism is identified before anaesthesia** and the patient made euthyroid by thyroid hormone supplementation. If supplementation has not taken place or the clinical signs associated with hypothyroidism are still apparent, the following anaesthetic considerations should be taken into account.

Affected dogs are often middle aged to older, and therefore geriatric considerations should be kept in mind. They have a **slower metabolic rate,** which makes them predisposed to **mild hypothermia** and **slower metabolism of anaesthetic drugs.** Dogs are often also obese, lethargic, and with mental obtundation; which means **lower sedative doses are required.** Dogs may be **anaemic** because of the effects of thyroid hormones on bone marrow function. Hypothyroid patients often have **peripheral neuropathies** (e.g. laryngeal paralysis), megaoesophagus, and a slow gastrointestinal transit time.

Hypothyroid dogs are **prone to bradyarrhythmias and have a slower circulation time.** Anaesthetic induction drugs must be given slowly and to effect. Their cardiac output may also be reduced, increasing the chances of intraoperative hypotension. Additional concerns are coagulopathies and skin changes.

Feline Hyperthyroidism

The vast majority of patients that present with hyperthyroidism are cats, due to **adenomas or carcinoma tumours of the thyroid gland producing excessive levels of thyroid** hormone. Thyroid carcinomas are reported in the dog; however these tumours are generally not productive (e.g. they do not affect the concentration of thyroid hormones in the blood stream).

Feline hyperthyroidism is often a disease associated with advancing age and therefore geriatric considerations are relevant. The most common clinical sign of hyperthyroidism is **weight loss** due to the increased rate of metabolism despite an increased appetite. Affected cats can be **restless and aggressive,** which often makes the cats difficult to handle.

When a normal healthy cat is difficult to handle, intramuscular injections of drugs that would cause profound sedation

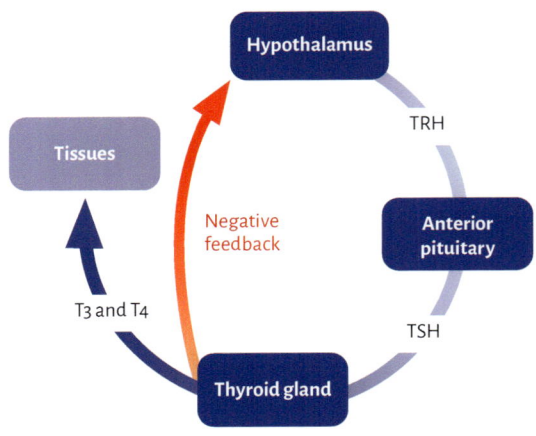

Figure 19. Synthesis of thyroid hormones.

or anaesthesia may be considered, however thyroid hormones affect many body systems causing multiorgan dysfunction and therefore extra care is required. The multi organ dysfunctions can include:
- **Liver:** elevated thyroid hormones can be hepatotoxic.
- **Kidneys:** hyperthyroidism causes damage to the feline kidney by several mechanisms including:
    - glomerular hypertension, which results in an accelerated decline in functional nephron mass;
    - hyperphosphatemia that could result in mineralization of soft tissues and worsening of renal function; and
    - whether the hyperthyroidism is causing damage to the kidneys, or the cat has chronic kidney disease, hyperthyroidism can mask declining renal function. Excess thyroid hormones artificially increase renal blood flow and glomerular filtration rate which decreases the serum concentrations of urea and creatinine. Treatment of hyperthyroidism decreases glomerular filtration, and the true urea and creatinine concentrations become apparent. Approximately 30% of patients develop overt chronic renal failure after treatment of hyperthyroidism.
- **Heart:** excessive thyroid hormones influence the heart, initially causing the heart to pump faster and with greater force. Eventually the heart becomes enlarged with a thicker wall to meet this increased demand. This disease is called **hypertrophic cardiomyopathy (HCM).** Hypertrophic cardiomyopathy is termed a high output cardiac failure because whilst the heart is pumping hard and often producing a high arterial blood pressure, the perfusion of the heart muscle itself is limited due to raised wall tension and increased volume of muscle. Sometimes the thickness of the heart muscle creates a subaortic occlusion during systole, momentarily causing outflow obstruction from the left ventricle.

Tumour Effects on Anaesthesia

The bulk of the tumour can influence anaesthesia; large tumours can press on the trachea and compromise airways and potentially cause problems for endotracheal intubation. The tumour may also press on the oesophagus and cause dysphagia. It can also cause laryngeal nerve dysfunction, potentially resulting in Horner's syndrome.

It may be necessary to anaesthetise the hyperthyroid patient for an unrelated reason, but more commonly for surgical resection of the affected thyroid gland. In this situation, how the surgery itself produces considerations for anaesthesia should be taken into account:
- tumours are highly vascular and can bleed during surgery, and the surgical site is near to large vessels and nerves in the neck; and
- the head area is shared with the surgeon, impacting on the breathing system and monitoring choices.

Postoperative complications include **laryngeal paralysis** (if the recurrent laryngeal nerve is damaged during surgery), this is seen as airway obstruction on recovery from anaesthesia. **Hypocalcemia** may also occur up to a week after surgery if the parathyroid glands (which lie next to the thyroid glands) are damaged.

Approach to Anaesthesia

These cats should be stabilised with antithyroid drugs before anaesthesia. Drugs that produce tachycardia such as ketamine should be avoided; the sympathomimetic effect that allows ketamine to increase cardiovascular parameters (cardiac output, heart rate, and arterial blood pressure) increases myocardial work and oxygen consumption and is detrimental to cats with HCM, potentially causing ventricular arrhythmias.

The major vasodilatory effects of drugs such as acepromazine should also be avoided. This is because reducing afterload exacerbates the pressure gradient across the left ventricular outflow tract. In addition, hypotension resulting from α-1 blockade may decrease coronary perfusion pressure.

In these cases, **mild bradycardia and mild vasoconstriction is often beneficial.** In one study, when administered intramuscularly, medetomidine had beneficial effects of reducing heart rate and eliminating left ventricular outflow tract obstruction (Lamont et al., 2002).

In addition, adequate oxygenation should be ensured and preload maintained with intravenous fluid therapy. As the cat may not be easy to handle, **intramuscular preanaesthetic medication** usually helps facilitate intravenous access, and as always **multimodal analgesia** should be considered. For premedication, opioids (+/- a low dose of an α-2 adrenergic agonist) should be considered, followed by intravenous anaesthetic induction. If, even after preanaesthetic medication, intravenous access cannot be achieved, a volatile agent chamber induction is a possibility (preferably with **sevoflurane** rather than isoflurane). Anaesthesia should be maintained with isoflurane or sevoflurane.

REFERENCES

- Doebeli, A., Michel, E., Bettschart, R., Hartnack, S. and Reichler, I.M., (2013) Apgar score after induction of anaesthesia for canine caesarian section with alfaxalone versus propofol. *Theriogenology*. 80, 850–4.
- Guedes, A.G., Rude, E.P. (2013) *Vet Anaesth Analg*. 40, 472–81.
- KuKanich, K., George, C., Roush, J.K., Sharp, S., Farace, G., Yerramilli, M., Peterson, S. and Grauer, G.F., (2021) Effects of low-dose meloxicam in cats with chronic kidney disease. *J Feline Med Surg*. 23, 138–148.
- Lamont, L.A., Bulmer, B.J., Sisson, D.D., Grimm, K.A. and Tranquilli, W.J., (2002) Doppler echocardiographic effects of medetomidine on dynamic left ventricular outflow tract obstruction in cats. *JAVMA*. 221, 1276–1281.
- Romagnoli, N., Barbarossa, A., Cunto, M., Ballotta, G., Zambelli, D., Armorini, S., Zaghini, A. and Lambertini, C., (2019) Evaluation of methadone concentrations in bitches and in umbilical cords after epidural or systemic administration for caesarean section: A randomized trial. *Veterinary Anaesthesia & Analgesia*. 46, 375–383.
- Sinclair (2012) Proceedings of the NAVC 2012 conference.
- Subramaniam, R. (2019) Anaesthetic concerns in preterm and term neonates. *Indian J Anaesth*. 63(9), 771–779.
- Vilar, J.M., Batista, M., Pérez, R., Zagorskaia, A., Jouanisson, E., Díaz-Bertrana, L. and Rosales, S., (2018) Comparison of three anaesthetic protocols for the elective caesarian-section in the dog: Effects on the bitch and the newborn puppies. *Anim Reprod Sci*. 190, 53–62.

Self-assessment

Test

1. Which of the following increases during pregnancy?
   a. Functional residual capacity.
   b. Systemic vascular resistance.
   c. Serum creatinine.
   d. Cardiac output.

2. Which of these parameters is included in the modified APGAR score?
   a. Temperature.
   b. Capillary refill time.
   c. Mucous membrane colour.
   d. Palpebral reflex.

3. Which of the following statements about aortocaval compression is correct?
   a. The vena cava is most easy to compress it lies to the right.
   b. The aorta is most easy to compress, and it lies to the right.
   c. The vena cava is most easy to compress, and it lies to the left.
   d. The aorta is most easy to compress, and it lies to the left.

4. Which of these is a shunt between the right and left side of the heart in the foetal circulation?
   a. Ductus venosus.
   b. Right aortic arch.
   c. Foramen ovale.
   d. Sphincter of Oddi.

5. The minimum alveolar concentration in geriatric animals is reduced by what percentage compared to a younger adult animal?
   a. 20%.
   b. 30%.
   c. 40%.
   d. 50%.

6. Which of these respiratory parameters is increased in the geriatric animal?
   a. Functional residual capacity.
   b. Vital capacity.
   c. Chest wall compliance.
   d. Ventilation/perfusion mismatch.

7. Hepatoencephalopathy is due to an increased blood concentration of:
   a. Albumin.
   b. Bilirubin.
   c. Ammonia.
   d. Lactulose.

Answers on page 240

8. Which of the following treatment modalities has no effect on serum potassium?
   a. Hartmann's solution.
   b. Glucose.
   c. Insulin.
   d. Calcium salts.

9. The bandwidth of renal blood flow autoregulation is normally between which approximate mean arterial blood pressures?
   a. 20–120 mmHg.
   b. 40–140 mmHg.
   c. 60–160 mmHg.
   d. 80–180 mmHg.

10. Which of the following clinical conditions involve the adrenal glands?
    a. Insulinoma.
    b. Diabetes mellitus.
    c. Addison's disease.
    d. Pancreatitis.

Clinical Case

A 12-year-old Italian Spinone presents for upper gastrointestinal endoscopy to investigate chronic diarrhoea. He has a PCV of 22% and total protein of 55 g/dl. His albumin level is 18 g/dl. Recently he has been diagnosed as hypothyroid and is yet to be stabilised.

1. If the maximum life expectancy of an Italian Spinone is 14 years, is this dog considered geriatric?

2. On clinical exam, what deviations from the normal might you expect in this dog because of its hypothyroidism?

3. What influence do the anaemia and low albumin levels have on the patient's anaesthetic?

4. How should anaesthetic induction be approached in this patient?

5. What volatile agent requirements will this patient have?

6. During the gastroscopy, the medic inflates the stomach with air to improve visualisation. What impact could this have on the anaesthetic?

Notes

Self-assessment

CORRECT ANSWERS:

TEST

1. d
2. c
3. a
4. c
5. b
6. d
7. c
8. d
9. c
10. c

CLINICAL CASE

1. **Is this dog considered geriatric?**
   Yes, as 12/14 x 100 is 86%, which is over the 80% cut off value.

2. **What deviations from the normal might you expect in this dog because of its hypothyroidism?**
   The dog is likely to be overweight. His heart rate and body temperature may be lower than usual.

3. **What influence do the anaemia and low albumin levels have on the patient's anaesthetic?**
   If a patient is moderately to severely anaemic this will influence their oxygen carrying capacity, and their anaesthetic requirements (e.g. a lower MAC value of volatile agents). The ability of the human eye to detect cyanosis can also be influenced by moderate to severe anaemia. Cyanosis (blue discoloration) can be seen by the human eye when the deoxygenated haemoglobin level is above 5 g/dl. However, if the patient is anaemic, their haemoglobin concentration in total (i.e. oxygenated and deoxygenated) may not even reach 5 g/dl, so it does not matter how hypoxic the patient is, the person responsible may not be able to see the blue discoloration. Decreased albumin will mean less drug is bound, and more drug is free (active). Induction agents must be given slowly to effect to avoid overdose.

4. **How should anaesthetic induction be approached in this patient?**
   Hypothyroid dogs may have laryngeal paralysis and megaoesophagus, therefore preoxygenation by mask would be indicated. This is due to the possibility of aspiration pneumonia if the dog has a megaoesophagus and regurgitates. Upper respiratory tract obstruction is also possible if the dog has a paralysed larynx. A head up induction is indicated to prevent regurgitation (a possibility with the megaoesophagus and slower gut emptying). Circulation time may be slower, and in addition to the lower albumin levels, both should prompt a slow intravenous anaesthetic induction "to effect".

5. **What volatile agent requirements will this patient have?**
   In general, geriatric patients have a 30% reduction in MAC, therefore their volatile agent requirement should be lower.

6. **What impact could this have on the anaesthetic?**
   Gastric dilation can limit tidal volume (which may lead to hypercapnia), reduce functional residual capacity, which may influence oxygenation, and be noxious/stimulating under anaesthesia.

Nursing Anaesthesia

Notes

Notes

Notes